热带医学特色高等教育系列教材

英汉对照

热带社区医学实验指导
Practical for Tropical Community Medicine

张帆 主编

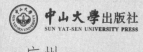

·广州·

版权所有　翻印必究

图书在版编目（CIP）数据

热带社区医学实验指导：英汉对照/张帆主编．—广州：中山大学出版社，2022.6
（热带医学特色高等教育系列教材）
ISBN 978-7-306-07499-7

Ⅰ.①热…　Ⅱ.①张…　Ⅲ.①热带医学—社区医学—医学院校—教材—汉、英　Ⅳ.①R197.1

中国版本图书馆 CIP 数据核字（2022）第 065316 号

出 版 人：	王天琪
项目策划：	徐　劲
策划编辑：	吕肖剑
责任编辑：	周明恩
封面设计：	林绵华
责任校对：	李昭莹
责任技编：	靳晓虹
出版发行：	中山大学出版社
电　　话：	编辑部 020-84111996，84110283，84111997，84110771
	发行部 020-84111998，84111981，84111160
地　　址：	广州市新港西路 135 号
邮　　编：	510275　传　真：020-84036565
网　　址：	http://www.zsup.com.cn　E-mail: zdcbs@mail.sysu.edu.cn
印 刷 者：	佛山市浩文彩色印刷有限公司
规　　格：	787mm×1092mm　1/16　18 印张　440 千字
版次印次：	2022 年 6 月第 1 版　2022 年 6 月第 1 次印刷
定　　价：	58.00 元

如发现本书因印装质量影响阅读，请与出版社发行部联系调换

《热带社区医学实验指导》编委会

主　编：张　帆
副主编：肖　莎　赵婵娟
编　委：（以姓氏笔画为序）
　　　　于德娥　苏　晶　李彦川　肖　莎
　　　　张　帆　周永江　赵婵娟　曹文婷

前言

社区医学（Community Medicine）是临床医学学士学位［Bachelor of Medicine & Bachelor of Surgery（MBBS）］来华留学生的必修课，与我国临床医学教育体系中的预防医学相对应，但其覆盖范围更为宽泛。该课程实践性强，理论与实践相辅相成，但目前国内尚无面向 MBBS 来华留学生的社区医学实验教材。《热带社区医学实验指导》在编写团队 5 年全英文教学实践的基础上修订完成，在编写中尽可能体现社区医学的学科内涵，确保教材的思想性、系统性、科学性、先进性和可扩展性。

本教材为英汉对照版专业课实践教材，在英语语言的应用上吸收国外同类教材的语言特点，同时考虑国内学术研究现状，尽量采用简单英语语法和标准词汇，做到言简意赅、深入浅出。本教材英文版可作为高等医学院校 MBBS 来华留学生甚至硕士研究生的实践教材；中文版除便于 MBBS 来华留学生学习和掌握对应的中文规范表达外，也适用于临床医学或其他专业的预防医学实验课、PBL 课程教学。此外，本教材还可作为从事公共卫生与预防医学、人群健康教育等专业技术人员及其他有关专业师生的学习参考书。本教材在使用时可根据本专业的教学要求、教学时数酌情增删。

本教材依托学科特点，参考培养要求，共分 6 章，每章编写了 2～7 个案例，按照"生物统计—流行病学和疾病控制—环境卫生—职业卫生—营养和食物—健康教育"的顺序进行编排，其中第一章生物统计学、第二章流行病学、第六章健康教育学还配备了习题。本教材从社区医学研究的方法学到实践应用案例，内容合理、循序渐进，涵盖了必要的基础知识和重点内容，重在梳理关键知识点，强化培养医学生的问题解决能力和团队合作能力，培养临床医学生的公共卫生理念和技能。

《热带社区医学实验指导》深度结合热带地区特色，其素材来源于热带地区常见的疾病案例、食物和环境样品，结合热带地区的自然环境特点和人群特征对热带社区医学进行实践探索，是根据中国国情和海南地方特色编写的具备科学性、实用性、趣味性、可操作性的社区医学实验指导教材。本教材在编写中参考和吸收了国内外有关教材和文献中新的观点和方法，在此谨向有关作者表示敬意和感谢。本教材的编写得到编者所在单位的领导和同事们的关心和支持，得到中山大学出版社的帮助，在此我谨代表全体编委一并表示衷心感谢。

在编写过程中，全体编委尽心尽力、通力合作，力图使本教材有所创新和突破。但由于编写时间短，加之编者水平有限，难免有疏漏之处，恳请使用本教材的广大师生和读者不吝指正，以便教材修订完善。

张　帆
2021 年 2 月 10 日

Contents 目 录

Chapter One Practical for Medical Statistics
第一章 生物统计学案例及习题 ·· 1

Experiment 1 Descriptive Statistics of Data ·· 3
实验一 数据的统计描述 ··· 6

Experiment 2 Normal Distribution ·· 8
实验二 正态分布 ··· 12

Experiment 3 Confidence Interval ·· 17
实验三 置信区间 ··· 19

Experiment 4 t-test ·· 21
实验四 t 检验 ·· 26

Experiment 5 Analysis of Variance ·· 30
实验五 方差分析 ··· 36

Experiment 6 Chi-square Test ··· 41
实验六 χ^2 检验 ··· 49

Chapter Two Practical for Epidemiology
第二章 流行病学案例及习题 ··· 57

Experiment 7 Disease Frequency Measurements ···································· 59
实验七 疾病频率测量 ··· 64

Experiment 8 Disease Distribution ··· 67
实验八 疾病的分布 ·· 72

Experiment 9 Cross-sectional Study ··· 77
实验九 现况研究 ··· 80

Experiment 10　Case-control Study ……………………………………………………… 83
实验十　病例对照研究 ……………………………………………………………… 87

Experiment 11　Cohort Study …………………………………………………………… 90
实验十一　队列研究 ………………………………………………………………… 94

Experiment 12　Experimental Epidemiological Study ………………………………… 97
实验十二　实验流行病学研究 …………………………………………………… 103

Experiment 13　Screening Evaluation ………………………………………………… 108
实验十三　筛检评价 ……………………………………………………………… 113

Chapter Three　Practical for Environmental Health
第三章　环境卫生学实验及案例 …………………………………………………… 117

Experiment 14　Determination of Particulate Matter in the Air …………………… 119
实验十四　大气中颗粒物的测定 ………………………………………………… 124

Experiment 15　Monitoring and Evaluation of Negative Ions in Air ……………… 128
实验十五　大气中负氧离子的监测与评价 ……………………………………… 132

Experiment 16　Determination of Biochemical Oxygen Demand in Water ………… 135
实验十六　水中生化需氧量的测定 ……………………………………………… 140

Experiment 17　Determination of Available Chlorine in Bleaching Powder and the
　　　　　　　　Amount of Residual Chlorine in Water ……………………………… 143
实验十七　漂白粉中有效氯含量、水中余氯量的测定 ………………………… 147

Experiment 18　Cases Study of the Relationship Between Environmental Pollution and
　　　　　　　　Human Health ……………………………………………………… 151
实验十八　环境污染与人群健康的案例分析 …………………………………… 154

Experiment 19　Investigation on the Effects of Environmental Arsenic Pollution on the
　　　　　　　　Health of Population ………………………………………………… 157
实验十九　环境砷污染对居民健康影响的调查研究 …………………………… 163

Chapter Four　Practice for Occupational Hygiene
第四章　职业卫生学实验及案例 …………………………………………………… 169

Experiment 20　Determination of δ-amino-γ-ketovalic Acid（δ-ALA）in Urine ……… 171
实验二十　尿中δ–氨基–γ–酮戊酸（δ-ALA）的测定 ………………………… 173

Experiment 21　Determination of Cholinesterase Activity in Whole Blood by
　　　　　　　　Spectrophotometry—by Ferric Trichloride Method ………………… 176
实验二十一　全血胆碱酯酶的测定——三氯化铁比色法 ……………………… 178

Experiment 22　Determination of Total Dust Concentration and Dispersion ……………… 181
实验二十二　总粉尘浓度及分散度的测定 ……………………………………………… 186

Experiment 23　Case Study of Occupational Diseases and Occupational Health ……… 190
实验二十三　职业病与职业卫生案例分析 ……………………………………………… 195

Experiment 24　The Measurement and Evaluation of Productive Noise ……………… 199
实验二十四　生产性噪声的测定与评价 ………………………………………………… 200

Experiment 25　Determination of Meteorological Conditions ………………………… 202
实验二十五　气象条件的测定 …………………………………………………………… 204

Chapter Five　Experiments and Cases of Nutrition and Food Hygiene
第五章　营养与食品卫生学实验及案例 ……………………………………………… 207

Experiment 26　Determination of Reducing Sugar Content in Food …………………… 209
实验二十六　食品中还原糖含量的测定 ………………………………………………… 211

Experiment 27　Determination of Vitamin C Content in Foods ………………………… 213
实验二十七　食品中维生素 C 含量的测定 ……………………………………………… 216

Experiment 28　Determination of Methanol Content in Liquor ………………………… 218
实验二十八　白酒中甲醇含量的测定 …………………………………………………… 220

Experiment 29　Anthropometric Measuring …………………………………………… 222
实验二十九　人体测量 …………………………………………………………………… 225

Experiment 30　Dietary Survey ………………………………………………………… 226
实验三十　膳食调查 ……………………………………………………………………… 230

Experiment 31　Case Analysis of Nutrition Intervention ……………………………… 233
实验三十一　营养干预案例分析 ………………………………………………………… 235

Experiment 32　Case Analysis of Food Poisoning Investigation and Treatment ……… 237
实验三十二　食物中毒调查处理案例分析 ……………………………………………… 241

Chapter Six　Cases and Practices of Health Education
第六章　健康教育案例与实践 …………………………………………………………… 245

Experiment 33　Design and Evaluation of Audience-centered Health Communication Materials …………………………………………………………… 247
实验三十三　以受众为中心的健康传播材料设计与评价 ……………………………… 252

Experiment 34　Assessment of Community Health Education ………………………… 256
实验三十四　社区健康教育诊断 ………………………………………………………… 263

Answers for Exercises ………………………………………………………… 270

习题参考答案 …………………………………………………………………… 272

参考文献 ………………………………………………………………………… 274

Chapter One | Practical for Medical Statistics

第一章 | 生物统计学案例及习题

Chapter One Practical for Medical Statistics

Experiment 1 Descriptive Statistics of Data

Ⅰ. Objectives

(1) To describe the important role of descriptive statistics in data analysis.

(2) To compare different measures of central tendency and dispersion of quantitative variables.

(3) To illustrate the difference and use of ratio, frequency and intensity of qualitative variables.

Ⅱ. Principles

(1) Statistical tables are usually used to summarize a set of observations, usually for different types of numerical data.

(2) Statistical graphs are usually used to visualize the data as a geometric chart, and express the quantitative relationship between the observations or variables by using different notations, such as the location of a dot, the elevation of a line, the length of a bar, or the size of an area.

(3) Descriptive statistics is a simple method to describe the main features of a collection of data quantitatively.

(4) Measures of location/central tendency are the center of a set of data, i.e., the point around which the observations tend to cluster, such as arithmetic mean, geometric mean and median.

(5) Another characteristic of a data set due to the spread of the observations, which is called variation, such as range, inter-quartile range, variance and standard deviation, coefficient of variation.

(6) Ratio is the proportion of any quantity to another.

(7) Relative frequency is a special type of ratio that both the numerator and denominator are frequencies, with the numerator as a part of the denominator.

(8) Intensity is another special type of ratio that the denominator is the total observed person-years during a certain period, and the numerator is the frequency of a certain event occurred during that period.

Ⅲ. Materials

Pompholyx often occurs among the patients with hyperhidrosis in spring and summer, even autumn in tropical or subtropical area. A research is aimed to observe the effect of some herbal lotion on pompholyx. 100 cases of pompholyx patients were divided into treatment and control groups, each group had 50 cases. Herbal lotion was used in the soaking treatment of treatment group, control group was treated with glycerol salicylic acid liniment. Both groups were given the necessary oral vitamin supplementation and the same dressing materials. 10 days for a course of treatment. 3 indexes including the itching/burning sensation disappearing time (d), the blisters drying time (d), desquamation recovering time (d) were observed. After a course of treatment, 48 of 50 cases in treatment group were cured (96.0%), 2 patients turned to be better (4.0%). 41 of 50 cases in the control group were cured (82.0%), 9 patients turned to be better (8.0%). The difference in itching/burning sensation disappearing time, the blisters drying time, desquamation recovering time and cure rate in two groups had statistical significance ($P < 0.05$). Then the researcher concluded that the herbal lotion had a significant clinical effect on pompholyx. Symptom improvement and treatment effect were compared between the two groups as follows.

Table 1-1 Symptom improvement comparison ($\bar{x} \pm s, d$)

Group	n	Itching/burning sensation disappearing time	Blisters drying time	Desquamation recovering time
treatment	50	3.0 ± 1.0	5.0 ± 1.0	8.0 ± 1.0
control	50	5.0 ± 1.0	8.0 ± 1.0	10.0 ± 2.0

Table 1-2 Treatment effect comparison [n, %]

Group	n	Cured	Better	Ineffective	Effective
treatment	50	48 (96.0)	2 (4.0)	0	50 (100.0)
control	50	41 (82.0)	9 (8.0)	0	50 (100.0)

Ⅳ. Procedures

(1) Identify which values represent the sample statistics and which values represent the population parameters.

Sample means, the average itching/burning sensation disappearing time of treatment group = 3.0, the average itching/burning sensation disappearing time of control group = 5.0. The average blisters drying time of treatment group = 5.0, the average blisters drying time of control group = 8.0. The average desquamation recovering time of treatment group = 8.0, the average desquamation recovering time of control group = 10.0.

Sample standard deviations, the itching/burning sensation disappearing time standard deviations of treatment group = 1.0, the itching/burning sensation disappearing time standard deviations of control group = 1.0. The blisters drying time standard deviations of treatment group = 1.0, the blisters drying time standard deviations of control group = 1.0. The desquamation recovering time standard deviations of treatment group = 1.0, the desquamation recovering time standard deviations of control group = 2.0.

Sample relative frequency (proportion), the effective rate of treatment group = 100.0%, the effective rate of control group = 100.0%.

Population parameters were not provided in the materials.

(2) Determine the shape of the distribution of numerical variables according to the descriptive statistics.

The distributions of itching/burning sensation disappearing time, blisters drying time, desquamation recovering time for each group are likely symmetric as their standard deviations are around 1/3 of their means.

(3) Specify whether the mean or median would be the best representative as a typical observation in the data, and whether the variability of observations would be the best representative using the standard deviation or inter-quartile range.

The distributions of itching/burning sensation disappearing time, blisters drying time, desquamation recovering time from each group are likely symmetric. Therefore the center would be described by the mean best, and variability would be described by the standard deviation best.

V. Exercises

(1) The following show how old each of eight kids were when they started kindergarten: 4, 4, 5, 4, 5, 4, 3, 4. Using this data, we'd better create (   )

A. a frequency table   B. a graph   C. both   D. none

(2) Frequency table could be created for which data set variables? (   )

A. categorical variables   B. continuous variable   C. both   D. none

(3) Which variable is a poor candidate for mean calculation? (   )

A. ID number   B. age   C. height   D. weight

(4) The distance of an observation and its mean is (   )

A. distribution   B. deviation   C. histogram   D. individuals

(5) Using the data along with appropriate computations, which of the following charts could not be constructed? (   )

Marital status	Frequency
Single	3
Married	5
Divorced	2
Separated	4
Total	14

A. a relative frequency table   B. a pie chart for percentages
C. a side-by-side bar chart   D. a Pareto chart

实验一　数据的统计描述

一、实验目的

（1）理解统计描述在数据分析中的重要性。

（2）掌握并比较用于描述定量变量集中、离散趋势的统计指标。

（3）了解定性变量的率、频率和强度指标的区别和应用。

二、实验原理

（1）统计表是将统计调查或实验所得来的原始数据，经过整理、汇总，使之呈现不同数值变量观测值的一种简单形式。

（2）统计图指将数据形象化为几何图，并通过使用不同的符号，如点的位置、线的高度、线的长度或面积的大小，来表达观察值或变量之间的数量关系的一种形式。

（3）统计描述是量化地描述一组数据的主要特征。

（4）数据位置或集中趋势的度量是指对一组数据中心位置的度量，即观察结果倾向于聚集的点，如算术平均值、几何平均值和中位数。

（5）数据变异的度量是数据集由于观测值的分散而产生的另一个特征，如极差、四分位数间距、方差、标准差和变异系数。

（6）比率是任何数量与另一数量的比值，用来表示两个观测值数量上的倍数或分数关系。

（7）相对频率在统计学中也称为频率，即分子和分母都是频率的一种特殊比值，分子是分母的一部分。

（8）强度是另一种特殊类型的比值，其分母为某一时期所观察到的人年总数，分子为某一事件在该时期发生的频数，即单位时间内某现象发生的频率。

三、实验材料

在热带或亚热带地区，手部汗疱疹常发病于多汗症患者身上，多见于春季和夏季，甚至秋季。某研究欲观察某中药洗液治疗手部汗疱疹的效果。将 100 例手部汗疱疹患者分为治疗组和对照组各 50 例，治疗组用某中药洗液稀释涂搽，对照组用水杨酸甘油搽剂涂搽，两组均给予必要的口服维生素补充和相同包扎材料，10 天为 1 个疗程，通过瘙痒/烧灼感消失时间（天）、水疱干涸时间（天）、脱屑/皲裂愈合时间（天）3 项指标观察治疗效果。1 个疗程后，治疗组治愈 48 例（96.0%），好转 2 例（4.0%）；对照组治愈 41 例（82.0%），好转 9 例（18.0%）；两组瘙痒/烧灼感消失时间、水疱干涸时间、脱屑/皲裂愈合时间及治愈率比较，差异均有统计学意义（$P<0.05$）。研究者认为，该中药洗液治疗手部汗疱疹效果显著。两组患者的症状改善情况及治疗效果比较详见表 1-1 和表 1-2。

表1-1　两组患者症状改善情况比较（$\bar{x} \pm s$, d）

组别	例数	瘙痒/烧灼消失	水疱消失	脱屑/皲裂愈合
治疗组	50	3.0±1.0	5.0±1.0	8.0±1.0
对照组	50	5.0±1.0	8.0±1.0	10.0±2.0

表1-2　两组患者临床疗效比较 [n,%]

组别	例数	治愈	好转	无效	总有效
治疗组	50	48（96.0）	2（4.0）	0	50（100.0）
对照组	50	41（82.0）	9（18.0）	0	50（100.0）

四、实验步骤

（1）确定哪些值表示样本统计量，哪些值表示总体参数。

样本均值：治疗组瘙痒/灼烧感消失平均时间=3.0天，对照组瘙痒/灼烧感消失平均时间=5.0天。治疗组水疱干燥平均时间=5.0天，对照组水疱干燥平均时间=8.0天。治疗组脱屑/皲裂愈合平均时间为8.0天，对照组脱屑/皲裂愈合平均时间为10.0天。

样本标准差：治疗组瘙痒/灼烧感消失时间标准差=1.0天，对照组瘙痒/灼烧感消失时间标准差=1.0天。治疗组水疱干燥时间标准差=1.0天，对照组水疱干燥时间标准差=1.0天。治疗组脱屑/皲裂愈合时间标准差=1.0天，对照组脱屑/皲裂愈合时间标准差=2.0天。

样本相对频率：治疗组有效率=100.0%，对照组有效率=100.0%。

资料中没有提供总体参数信息。

（2）根据统计描述结果判断研究中定量变量的大致分布形态。

由于瘙痒/灼烧感消失时间、水疱干燥时间和脱屑/皲裂愈合时间在两组中的样本标准差均在样本平均数的1/3内，据此大致判断这些变量在不同组别中的分布形态为对称分布。

（3）指出平均数或中位数是否能最好地代表研究中的定量数据，以及观察值的变异性是否能用标准差或四分位数间距表示。

由于各组瘙痒/烧灼感消失时间、水疱干燥时间、脱屑/皲裂愈合时间在各组间的分布大致是对称的，因此，中心位置/集中趋势最好用平均数来描述，而变异性最好用标准差来描述。

五、课后练习

（1）下面是8位儿童的幼儿园入学年龄（岁）：4，4，5，4，5，4，3，4。针对这些数据，用何种数据呈现工具较合适？（　　）

A. 频数表　　　　　B. 统计图　　　　　C. 两者均可　　　　　D. 两者都不行

(2) 频数表通常被用于哪类变量的描述?（   ）

A. 分类变量　　　　B. 连续变量　　　　C. 两者均可　　　　D. 两者都不行

(3) 下列哪个变量不适合计算平均数?（   ）

A. 身份编号　　　　B. 年龄　　　　　　C. 身高　　　　　　D. 体重

(4) 每个观测值与平均数之间的差距被称为(   )

A. 分布　　　　　　B. 离均差　　　　　C. 直方图　　　　　D. 个体

(5) 根据下表数据，哪一数据呈现形式是不恰当的?（   ）

婚姻状态	频数
未婚	3
已婚	5
离异	2
分居	4
合计	14

A. 频数表　　　　　B. 饼图　　　　　　C. 复合条图　　　　D. 帕累托图

Experiment 2　Normal Distribution

Ⅰ. Objectives

(1) To compare the differences between normal and skewed distributions.

(2) To show when a regular normal distribution can be transformed into a standard normal distribution.

(3) To introduce medical issues that arise in normal distribution application.

Ⅱ. Principles

(1) Normal distribution is often used as an initial approximation to describe continuous random variables that tend to cluster around a single mean value.

(2) Standard normal distribution is the special normal curve with $\mu = 0$ and $\sigma = 1$.

(3) Reference range is a range of values expected for a relative healthy individual.

Ⅲ. Materials

A study is to explore the reference range of the thickness of nuchal translucency (NT) of normal single fetal in early gestation in a coastal city. 1067 singleton pregnant women in the 11 to 13 weeks^{+6} of pregnancy were examined during January 2010 to December 2014 in local hospital. The NT thickness of fetal was measured by ultrasound, and pregnancy outcome was followed up.

The NT thickness of 1000 normal fetus in the first trimester were between 0.7～5.8 mm, following normal distribution and averagely 1.7 ± 0.6 mm. The 95% reference range of overall fetal NT thickness is 0.524 mm ～ 2.876 mm.

The fetal NT thickness among different maternal age, gestational week and fetal gender are shown as follows:

Table 2-1 Mean, median and 95% reference range of fetal NT thickness ($\bar{x} \pm s$, mm)

Variable	N	NT thickness/mm	M (P_{25}～P_{75})	Reference range
Maternal age				
<25	100	1.7 ± 0.5	1.7 (1.3～2.1)	0.72～2.68
25～	500	1.7 ± 0.5	1.7 (1.2～2.1)	0.72～2.68
30～	300	1.8 ± 0.6	1.7 (1.3～2.2)	0.62～2.98
35～	100	1.8 ± 0.6	1.8 (1.4～2.5)	0.62～2.98
Gestational week				
11^{+0}～11^{+6}	320	1.7 ± 0.5	1.7 (1.2～2.2)	0.72～2.68
12^{+0}～12^{+6}	340	1.7 ± 0.5	1.7 (1.4～2.3)	0.72～2.68
13^{+0}～13^{+6}	340	1.7 ± 0.6	1.8 (1.3～2.6)	0.52～2.88
Fetus gender				
male	520	1.8 ± 0.7	1.7 (1.1～2.6)	0.43～3.17
female	480	1.7 ± 0.6	1.6 (1.1～2.5)	0.52～2.88

Ⅳ. Procedures

1. Write down the shorthand for these normal distributions mentioned in the study

The NT thickness of 1000 normal fetus in the first trimester ～ $N(1.7, 0.6)$.

The NT thickness of normal fetus in the first trimester among maternal age <25 years old ～ $N(1.7, 0.5)$.

The NT thickness of normal fetus in the first trimester among maternal age between 25 and 30 years old ～ $N(1.7, 0.5)$.

The NT thickness of normal fetus in the first trimester among maternal age between 30 and 35 years old ～ $N(1.8, 0.6)$.

The NT thickness of normal fetus in the first trimester among maternal age >35 years old ～ $N(1.8, 0.6)$.

The NT thickness of normal fetus in gestational week 11 ～ $N(1.7, 0.5)$.

The NT thickness of normal fetus in gestational week 12 ～ $N(1.7, 0.5)$.

The NT thickness of normal fetus in gestational week 13 ～ $N(1.7, 0.6)$.

The NT thickness of normal male fetus in the first trimester ～ $N(1.8, 0.7)$.

The NT thickness of normal female fetus in the first trimester ～ $N(1.7, 0.6)$.

2. Draw a standard Normal distribution curve and mark $Z = -1.96$ and $Z = 1.96$

We need to put data onto a standardized scale. Using the standard deviation as a guide, Z-score can be calculated as

$$Z = \frac{x - \mu}{\sigma}$$

This commonly transformation may be employed for any normal distributions. We can visualize the 95% area as the shading shown in the following figure.

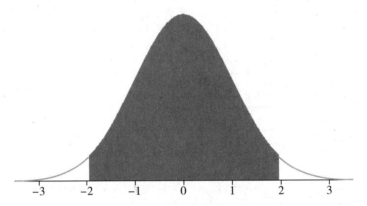

Figure 2-1 The shading area represents the majority (95%) observations

(Drawing tool: http://onlinestatbook.com/2/calculators/normal_dist.html)

As $P_{(-1.96 < Z < 1.96)} = 0.95$, the NT thickness of 1000 normal fetus in the first trimester:

$$Z_1 = \frac{x_1 - \mu}{\sigma} = \frac{x_1 - 1.7}{0.6} = -1.96, \quad x_1 = 0.524$$

$$Z_2 = \frac{x_2 - \mu}{\sigma} = \frac{x_1 - 1.7}{0.6} = 1.96, \quad x_1 = 2.876$$

Thus the 95% reference range of overall fetal NT thickness is 0.524 ~ 2.876 mm. Similar calculation can be conducted for 95% reference range of NT thickness among different groups.

3. Further application

(1) Find any individual's percentile of NT thickness for the population observed.

For example, for a pregnant woman younger than 25 years, her tested NT thickness result is 1.0 mm. She scored 1.4 standard deviations below the mean on the NT thickness of normal fetus in the first trimester among maternal age < 25 years old [(1.0 - 1.7)/0.5 = -1.4]. According to the probability table, $P_{(Z < -1.4)} = 0.0808$, thus her percentile of NT thickness is 8.08%.

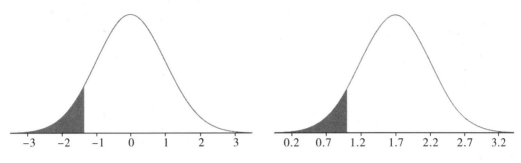

a. Area under standard normal distribution   b. Area under $N(1.7, 0.5)$

Figure 2 –2 Area under the normal curve ($Z < X$)

(2) Find the probability of any specified outcome.

For any randomly selected woman at 12 weeks pregnant from this population, what is the probability of NT thickness result higher than 1.2mm?

As

$$Z = \frac{x - \mu}{\sigma} = \frac{1.2 - 1.7}{0.5} = -1$$

According to the probability table, $P_{(Z > -1)} = 1 - P_{(Z < -1)} = 0.8413$, thus the probability of NT thickness result higher than 1.2mm is 84.13%.

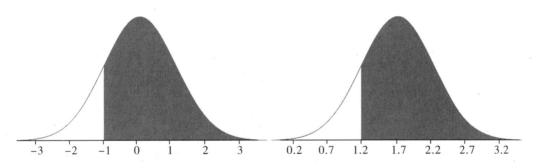

a. Area under standard normal distribution   b. Area under $N(1.7, 0.5)$

Figure 2 –3 Area under the normal curve ($Z > X$)

(3) Find the alarm for the relevant disease.

Suppose the risk of Down syndrome is about 1 in 1000, according to the probability table, $P_{(Z > 3.09)} = 0.001$, as

$$Z = \frac{x - \mu}{\sigma} = \frac{x - 1.7}{0.6} = 3.09, x = 3.554$$

Thus, it should be alarmed when NT thickness outcome is higher than 3.554 mm.

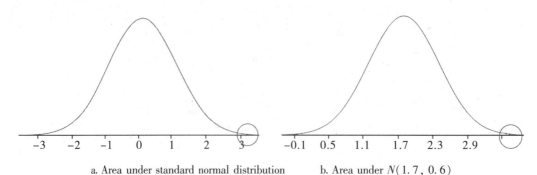

a. Area under standard normal distribution   b. Area under $N(1.7, 0.6)$

Figure 2-4 Area under the normal curve ($Z > X$)

V. Exercises

(1) According to the 68-95-99.7 rule, almost 95% of all observations in normal distribution are contained within a distance of how many standard deviations around the mean? (   )

A. 1　　　　　　　B. 2　　　　　　　C. 3　　　　　　　D. 4

(2) Use the standard normal distribution table to find $P_{(0<Z\leq1)}$ = (   ). ($P_{Z<-1}$ = 0.1587)

A. 0.0398　　　　B. 0.1666　　　　C. 0.3159　　　　D. 0.3413

(3) What percent of a standard normal distribution $N(\mu=0, \sigma=1)$ is found in $Z > -1.13$? (   ) ($P_{Z<-1.13}$ = 0.1292)

A. 0.1292　　　　B. 0.8708　　　　C. 0.68　　　　　D. 0.95

(4) Heights of 10 years old, regardless of gender, closely follow a normal distribution with mean 143 cm and standard deviation 5.6 cm. What is the probability that a randomly chosen 10 years old is shorter than 132 cm? (   ) ($P_{Z<-1.96}$ = 0.025)

A. 0.1292　　　　B. 0.975　　　　C. 0.025　　　　D. 0.95

(5) Heights of 10 years old, regardless of gender, closely follow a normal distribution with mean 143 cm and standard deviation 5.6 cm. What is the probability that a randomly chosen 10 years old is between 152 and 155 cm? (   ) ($P_{Z<-1.61}$ = 0.0537, $P_{Z<-2.14}$ = 0.0162)

A. 0.0537　　　　B. 0.0162　　　　C. 0.0375　　　　D. 0.0699

实验二　正态分布

一、实验目的

(1) 比较正态分布和偏态分布的差异。

(2) 掌握标准正态分布的概念，了解正态分布何时可转换为标准正态分布。

(3) 了解正态分布在解决医学问题中的应用。

二、实验原理

(1) 正态分布又名高斯分布,用来描述连续性随机变量的分布形式,通常呈单峰对称的钟形曲线。

(2) 标准正态分布是均数为 0(即对称轴为 Y 轴)、标准差为 1 的正态分布,记为 $N(0,1)$。

(3) 医学参考值范围亦称正常值范围,指大多数正常人的解剖、生理、生化等各种指标观测值的波动范围,用于划分正常与异常的界限。

三、实验材料

某研究欲探讨某沿海城市及周边地区妊娠早期正常单胎胎儿颈项透明层厚度(nuchal translucency,NT)的参考值范围。连续型选择 2010 年 1 月至 2014 年 12 月期间在当地三甲医院行产前超声检查的孕 11~13 周$^{+6}$的单胎孕妇 1067 例。对胎儿进行超声 NT 厚度测量,并随访妊娠结局。

最终纳入 1000 例正常妊娠结局者,妊娠早期正常胎儿的 NT 厚度在 0.7~5.8 mm 之间,经正态性检验,数据正态分布,平均 1.7 ± 0.6 mm。正常单胎胎儿 NT 厚度的 95% 参考值范围为 0.524~2.876 mm。

不同孕龄、孕周及胎儿性别的胎儿 NT 厚度见表 2-1。

表 2-1 胎儿 NT 厚度平均数、中位数及参考值范围($\bar{x} \pm s$, mm)

变量	N	NT 厚度/mm	M (P_{25}~P_{75})	参考值范围
孕妇年龄/岁				
<25	100	1.7 ± 0.5	1.7(1.3~2.1)	0.72~2.68
25~	500	1.7 ± 0.5	1.7(1.2~2.1)	0.72~2.68
30~	300	1.8 ± 0.6	1.7(1.3~2.2)	0.62~2.98
35~	100	1.8 ± 0.6	1.8(1.4~2.5)	0.62~2.98
孕周				
11^{+0}~11^{+6}	320	1.7 ± 0.5	1.7(1.2~2.2)	0.72~2.68
12^{+0}~12^{+6}	340	1.7 ± 0.5	1.7(1.4~2.3)	0.72~2.68
13^{+0}~13^{+6}	340	1.7 ± 0.6	1.8(1.3~2.6)	0.52~2.88
胎儿性别				
男性	520	1.8 ± 0.7	1.7(1.1~2.6)	0.43~3.17
女性	480	1.7 ± 0.6	1.6(1.1~2.5)	0.52~2.88

四、实验步骤

1. 写出研究中所有提到的正态分布的简写

1000 例正常产前胎儿妊娠早期 NT 厚度～$N(1.7,0.6)$。
年龄 <25 岁孕妇的正常胎儿妊娠早期 NT 厚度～$N(1.7,0.5)$。
25～30 岁孕妇的正常胎儿妊娠早期 NT 厚度～$N(1.7,0.5)$。
30～35 岁孕妇的正常胎儿妊娠早期 NT 厚度～$N(1.8,0.6)$。
年龄 >35 岁孕妇的正常胎儿妊娠早期 NT 厚度～$N(1.8,0.6)$。
正常胎儿妊娠 11 周 NT 厚度～$N(1.7,0.5)$。
正常胎儿妊娠 12 周 NT 厚度～$N(1.7,0.5)$。
正常胎儿妊娠 13 周 NT 厚度～$N(1.7,0.6)$。
正常男性胎儿妊娠早期 NT 厚度～$N(1.8,0.7)$。
正常女性胎儿妊娠早期 NT 厚度～$N(1.7,0.6)$。

2. 将正态分布转换为标准正态分布并找出 $Z=-1.96$ 和 $Z=1.96$ 的临界值

根据正态分布转换原理,可以将任意服从正态分布的随机变量观测值一一对应转换为 Z 分值:

$$Z = \frac{x - \mu}{\sigma}$$

结合标准正态分布曲线下分布面积规律,我们可以将中间 95% 的观测值对应标注为曲线下阴影部分,对应的 Z 分值分别为 -1.96 和 1.96。

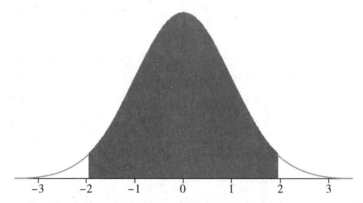

图 2-1　标准正态分布下 95% 的观测值对应曲线下阴影部分面积
(绘图工具:http://onlinestatbook.com/2/calculators/normal_dist.html)

1000 例正常产前胎儿妊娠早期 NT 厚度分布对应观测值:

$$Z_1 = \frac{x_1 - \mu}{\sigma} = \frac{x_1 - 1.7}{0.6} = -1.96, \ x_1 = 0.524$$

$$Z_2 = \frac{x_2 - \mu}{\sigma} = \frac{x_1 - 1.7}{0.6} = 1.96, \ x_1 = 2.876$$

因此，1000 例正常产前胎儿妊娠早期 NT 厚度的 95% 参考值范围为 0.524 ～ 2.876 mm。同理可依次计算出不同分组正常产前胎儿妊娠早期 NT 厚度的 95% 参考值范围。

3. 推广应用

（1）给定某一观测值推算其所在百分位数。

如一位年龄小于 25 岁的孕妇经 B 超测量其胎儿 NT 厚度为 1.0 mm。经标准正态变化，此观测值距离其均值有 1.4 个标准差［因为 (1.0 - 1.7)/0.5 = -1.4］。根据标准正态分布曲线下面积分布规律，$P_{(Z<-1.4)} = 0.0808$，因此这样的观测结果在总体中的百分位数为 8.08%。

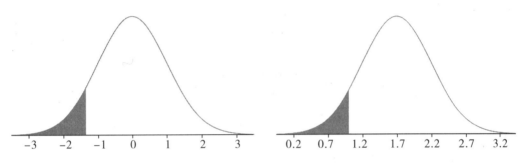

图 2 - 2　正态分布曲线下阴影面积（$Z < X$）

（2）推算某一观测范围的概率。

预知某一妊娠 $12^{+0} \sim 12^{+6}$ 周的孕妇观测得到 NT 厚度大于 1.2 mm 的可能性，可先经标准正态变化得

$$Z = \frac{x - \mu}{\sigma} = \frac{1.2 - 1.7}{0.5} = -1$$

根据标准正态曲线下面积分布规律，$P(Z > -1) = 1 - P(Z < -1) = 0.8413$，因此 NT 厚度大于 1.2 mm 的概率为 84.13%。

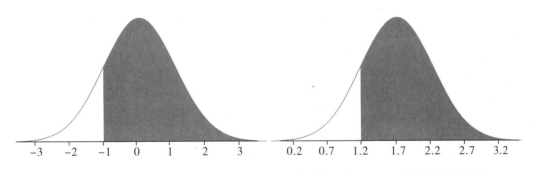

图 2 - 3　正态分布曲线下阴影面积（$Z > X$）

（3）根据相关疾病的患病风险推算警戒线。

假定新生儿患唐氏综合征的风险为1‰，根据标准正态曲线面积下分布规律，$P_{(Z>3.09)}=0.001$，反推当$Z=3.09$时对应的观测值为：

$$Z=\frac{x-\mu}{\sigma}=\frac{x-1.7}{0.6}=3.09, \quad x=3.554$$

因此当该人群中胎儿的NT厚度观测结果大于3.554 mm时，应当引起警惕。

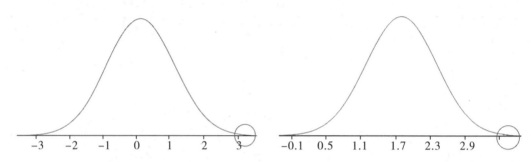

a. 标准正态分布曲线下阴影面积　　　b. 正态分布$N(1.7, 0.6)$曲线下阴影面积

图2-4　正态分布曲线下阴影面积（$Z>X$）

五、课后练习

（1）根据68-95-99.7法则，正态分布数据的95%观测值大约距离其均值（　　）个标准差。

A. 1　　　　　　B. 2　　　　　　C. 3　　　　　　D. 4

（2）查询标准正态分布概率表，$P(0<Z\leqslant 1)=$（　　）。（$P_{Z<-1}=0.1587$）

A. 0.0398　　　　B. 0.1666　　　　C. 0.3159　　　　D. 0.3413

（3）在标准正态分布中，Z取值大于-1.13的概率是（　　）。（$P_{Z<-1.13}=0.1292$）

A. 0.1292　　　　B. 0.8708　　　　C. 0.68　　　　　D. 0.95

（4）10岁孩童的身高无论性别，都遵循正态分布，假定其平均身高为143 cm，标准差为5.6 cm，那么随机抽取的一名10岁孩童小于132 cm的概率是（　　）。（$P_{Z<-1.96}=0.025$）

A. 0.1292　　　　B. 0.975　　　　C. 0.025　　　　D. 0.95

（5）10岁孩童的身高无论性别，都遵循正态分布，假定其平均身高为143 cm，标准差为5.6 cm，那么随机抽取的一名10岁孩童介于152 cm和155 cm的概率是（　　）。（$P_{Z<-1.61}=0.0537, P_{Z<-2.14}=0.0162$）

A. 0.0537　　　　B. 0.0162　　　　C. 0.0375　　　　D. 0.0699

Experiment 3 Confidence Interval

Ⅰ. Objectives

(1) To define point estimate and interval estimate of parameter inference.

(2) To compare properties of normal distribution and t-distribution.

(3) To illustrate the use of Central Limit Theorem in confidence interval.

Ⅱ. Principles

(1) Sampling Error occurs when different samples drawn from the same population could have different values of the sample statistics, which due to the nature of sampling.

(2) Sampling n-subjects from a normal distribution, the ratio between the difference of sample means to population mean and sampling error follows t-distribution centered at 0.

(3) The sample statistics are considered to be the point estimate of the corresponding population parameter.

(4) Instead of a point estimate, the interval around population parameter (such that there is with assumed probability that the true population parameter falls into this interval) is the estimate of interest.

Ⅲ. Materials

A study is to investigate the actual capacity of suspended red blood cells from a tropical blood center. One hundred bags of 1U suspended red blood cells and 100 bags of 2U suspended red blood cells were collected in the center. The capacity was assessed by microcomputer liquid withdrawal weighing controller, and actual capacity of suspended red blood cells was calculated. The measurements were tested following normal distributions and the results are shown as below:

Table 3 – 1 Capacity of suspended red blood cells (mL)

Units	n	Mean	Standard Deviation	Standard Error	95% Confidence Interval
1U	100	188.4	11.2	1.12	(186.2, 190.6)
2U	100	327.9	1.7	0.17	(327.6, 328.2)

Ⅳ. Procedures

(1) State the population and sample under consideration and whether the parameter of

interest is mean or proportion.

The sample is 100 bags of 1U suspended red blood cells and 100 bags of 2U suspended red blood cells collected in a tropical blood center. We might be tempted to generalize the population to represent all blood bags of suspended red blood cells collected in this region.

The parameter of interest is mean. Each measurement report a numerical value: capacity of suspended red blood cells.

(2) Identify the point estimate for the parameter and the statistic we can use to measure the uncertainty of the point estimate.

Estimate the parameter using the sample means: $\bar{X}_{1U}$ = 188.4 mL, $\bar{X}_{2U}$ = 327.9 mL

We can use standard error (SE) to measure the uncertainty of the point estimate:

$$SE_{1U} = \frac{S}{\sqrt{n}} = \frac{11.2}{\sqrt{100}} = 1.12,$$

$$SE_{2U} = \frac{S}{\sqrt{n}} = \frac{1.7}{\sqrt{100}} = 0.17$$

(3) Create a 95% confidence interval for the mean capacity of suspended red blood cells. Also interpret the confidence interval in the context of the study.

Recall that the general formula for 95% confidence interval in large sample is point estimate $\pm Z_{0.05/2} \times SE$.

1U: The point estimate is 188.4 mL, $Z_{0.05/2}$ = 1.96 for a 95% confidence level, and SE = 1.12. Then plug the values into the formula: 188.4 ± 1.96 × 1.12 = (186.2 mL, 190.6 mL). We are 95% confident that the mean capacity of 1U suspended red blood cell collected in this region is between 186.2 mL and 190.6 mL.

2U: The point estimate is 327.9 mL, $Z_{0.05/2}$ = 1.96 for a 95% confidence level, and SE = 0.17. Then plug the values into the formula: 327.9 ± 1.96 × 0.17 = (327.6 mL, 328.2 mL). We are 95% confident that the mean capacity of 2U suspended red blood cells collected in this region is between 327.6 mL and 328.2 mL.

V. Exercises

(1) The mean age of a sample individuals (n = 25) is 21.5, std = 3.26, what is the 95% confidence interval for this population mean? (　　) ($t_{0.05/2, 24}$ = 2.064)

　　A. (18.24, 24.76)　　　　　　　　B. (20.85, 22.15)
　　C. (20.15, 22.85)　　　　　　　　D. (19.44, 23.56)

(2) The mean age of a sample individuals (n = 25) is 21.5, std = 3.26, what is the 90% confidence interval for this population mean? (　　) ($t_{0.10/2, 24}$ = 1.711)

　　A. (18.24, 24.76)　　　　　　　　B. (20.85, 22.15)
　　C. (20.15, 22.85)　　　　　　　　D. (20.38, 22.62)

(3) The 95% CI for the μ is (　　)

A. contains the sample mean with 95% certainty

B. is less likely to contain the μ than 99% CI
C. contains 95% of the observations
D. is approximately equal to the $\overline{X} \pm 2S$

（4）Consider an sample of size 16 from a normally distributed population with $\sigma = 16$, if *sample mean* is 12, and *standard deviation* = 12, what is the appropriate formula for a 95% confidence interval for μ? （   ）

A. $\overline{X} \pm Z_{0.05/2} \times \dfrac{\sigma}{\sqrt{n}}$ 　　　　　　　B. $\overline{X} \pm Z_{0.05/2} \times \dfrac{S}{\sqrt{n}}$

C. $\overline{X} \pm t_{0.05/2, n-1} \times \dfrac{\sigma}{\sqrt{n}}$ 　　　　　D. $\overline{X} \pm t_{0.05/2, n-1} \times \dfrac{S}{\sqrt{n}}$

（5）Consider an sample of size 16 from a normally distributed population, if *sample mean* is 12, and *standard deviation* = 12, what is the appropriate formula for a 95% confidence interval for μ? （   ）

A. $\overline{X} \pm Z_{0.05/2} \times \dfrac{\sigma}{\sqrt{n}}$ 　　　　　　　B. $\overline{X} \pm Z_{0.05/2} \times \dfrac{S}{\sqrt{n}}$

C. $\overline{X} \pm t_{0.05/2, n-1} \times \dfrac{\sigma}{\sqrt{n}}$ 　　　　　D. $\overline{X} \pm t_{0.05/2, n-1} \times \dfrac{S}{\sqrt{n}}$

实验三　置信区间

一、实验目的

（1）掌握参数估计的两大基本方法：点估计和区间估计。
（2）学会比较正态分布与 t 分布的区别与联系。
（3）尝试理解抽样分布的中心极限定理及其在置信区间计算中的应用。

二、实验原理

（1）由抽样引起的样本统计量与总体参数不同，甚至样本之间的统计量也有所差异，称为抽样误差。
（2）在正态分布总体中进行抽样，样本平均数的离均差与标准误的比值服从自由度为 $n-1$ 的 t 分布，该分布是以 0 为中心的对称分布。
（3）样本统计量通常被认为是相应总体参数的点估计。
（4）不同于点估计，以既定的概率估计未知总体参数所在的范围，这个范围即置信区间。

三、实验材料

某研究欲调查热带地区人群悬浮红细胞实际容量情况。选取来自某血液中心的 1U 悬浮红细胞、2U 悬浮红细胞血液成分各 100 袋，用采液控制器称量其容量（mL），经正态性检验发现数据均服从正态分布，测量结果如下。

表 3-1 悬浮红细胞容量统计分析结果（mL）

项目	n	平均数	标准差	标准误	95% 置信区间
1U	100	188.4	11.2	1.12	(186.2, 190.6)
2U	100	327.9	1.7	0.17	(327.6, 328.2)

四、实验步骤

（1）先确定研究中的总体和样本，以及所求总体参数是均数还是比率。

本研究中的样本为来自某热带地区血液中心的 1U 悬浮红细胞、2U 悬浮红细胞血液成分各 100 袋，背后所代表的总体为该热带地区采集的所有 1U、2U 悬浮红细胞成分血袋中悬浮红细胞的容量。

本研究中的兴趣参数为均数。所以，每个观测结果读取的是每袋血成分的悬浮红细胞容量，单位为 mL，为定量变量。

（2）找出对总体参数的点估计值，并计算衡量点估计值不确定性的指标。

利用样本平均数作为总体平均数的点估计值：

$\bar{X}_{1U} = 188.4$ mL, $\bar{X}_{2U} = 327.9$ mL

用标准误来衡量点估计值的不确定性（样本统计量的变异）：

$$SE_{1U} = \frac{S}{\sqrt{n}} = \frac{11.2}{\sqrt{100}} = 1.12,$$

$$SE_{2U} = \frac{S}{\sqrt{n}} = \frac{1.7}{\sqrt{100}} = 0.17.$$

（3）计算该热带地区 1U、2U 悬浮红细胞成分容量的总体平均数的 95% 置信区间，并对其进行解释。

回顾大样本 95% 置信区间的计算公式：点估计值 $\pm Z_{0.05/2} \times SE$.

1U：点估计值为 188.4 mL，95% 置信水平的 Z 界值为 $Z_{0.05/2} = 1.96$，标准误 $SE = 1.12$。将数值代入公式计算得 $188.4 \pm 1.96 \times 1.12 =$ (186.2 mL, 190.6 mL)。我们有 95% 的把握认为此区间包含了该地区未知的 1U 悬浮红细胞成分平均容量。

2U：点估计值为 327.9 mL，95% 置信水平的 Z 界值为 $Z_{0.05/2} = 1.96$，标准误 $SE = 0.17$。将数值代入公式计算得 $327.9 \pm 1.96 \times 0.17 =$ (327.6 mL, 328.2 mL)。我们有 95% 的把握认为此区间包含了该地区未知的 2U 悬浮红细胞成分平均容量。

五、课后练习

（1）25 个研究对象的平均年龄是 21.5 岁，标准差为 3.26，总体平均年龄的 95% 置信区间是（   ）。（$t_{0.05/2, 24} = 2.064$）

A．（18.24，24.76） B．（20.85，22.15）
C．（20.15，22.85） D．（19.44，23.56）

（2）25个研究对象的平均年龄是21.5岁，标准差为3.26，总体平均年龄的90%置信区间是（   ）（$t_{0.10/2,24} = 1.711$）

A．（18.24，24.76） B．（20.85，22.15）
C．（20.15，22.85） D．（20.38，22.62）

（3）总体平均数的95%置信区间是（   ）

A．有95%的把握包含样本平均数
B．比99%置信区间包含未知总体平均数的可能性要小
C．包含95%的观测值
D．大约等于样本平均数 ± 2 × 标准差

（4）一个正态总体的标准差 $\sigma = 16$，如果从中抽取一个 $n = 16$ 的样本，得到样本平均数为12，样本标准差为12，则总体平均数的95%置信区间的计算公式为（   ）

A．$\bar{X} \pm Z_{0.05/2} \times \dfrac{\sigma}{\sqrt{n}}$ B．$\bar{X} \pm Z_{0.05/2} \times \dfrac{S}{\sqrt{n}}$

C．$\bar{X} \pm t_{0.05/2, n-1} \times \dfrac{\sigma}{\sqrt{n}}$ D．$\bar{X} \pm t_{0.05/2, n-1} \times \dfrac{S}{\sqrt{n}}$

（5）从一个正态总体中抽取一个 $n = 16$ 的样本，样本平均数为12，样本标准差为12，则总体平均数的95%置信区间的计算公式为（   ）

A．$\bar{X} \pm Z_{0.05/2} \times \dfrac{\sigma}{\sqrt{n}}$ B．$\bar{X} \pm Z_{0.05/2} \times \dfrac{S}{\sqrt{n}}$

C．$\bar{X} \pm t_{0.05/2, n-1} \times \dfrac{\sigma}{\sqrt{n}}$ D．$\bar{X} \pm t_{0.05/2, n-1} \times \dfrac{S}{\sqrt{n}}$

（赵婵娟）

Experiment 4　*t*-test

Ⅰ．Objectives

(1) To understand the meaning of hypothesis test.

(2) To familiarize with the basics of *t*-test and steps of hypothesis test.

(3) To be capable of using one sample *t*-test, paired samples *t*-test, two independent samples *t*-test in practice.

Ⅱ．Principles

(1) Hypothesis test is a major part of statistical inference, there has distinct and related to the confidence interval. The basic principles of hypothesis testing can be summarized as small

probability and reduction absurdum.

(2) Test hypotheses include null hypothesis and alternative hypothesis. Null hypothesis, also called original hypothesis, use symbol "H_0" to express, while alternative hypothesis using "H_1". They make assumptions about the population characteristics, according to the purpose of the study. Two hypotheses are a interrelated and contradictory pair.

(3) Significant level is denoted by α. Before hypothesis testing, the researcher may assume the size and one-sided/two-sided according to the purpose of test or professional knowledge. Commonly the used level of significant in practice is 0.05 and marked as $\alpha = 0.05$.

(4) P-value is the probability of obtaining current statistic and those test statistics which are even more extreme than the current statistic by random sampling if H_0 is correct. Compare P-value with significant level α, if $P \leq \alpha$, then reject the null hypothesis H_0 according to the small probability theory and accept the alternative hypothesis H_1. If $P > \alpha$, then not reject the null hypothesis H_0.

(5) One sample t-test is used to test whether there is a statistically significant difference between the mean of unknown population (μ) and the mean of a known population (μ_0). The assumption is that the sample is collected from a population with normal distribution. t statistic is calculated as

$$t = \frac{\bar{x} - \mu_0}{s_{\bar{x}}} \quad \nu = n - 1 \quad \text{(Formula 4-1)}$$

(6) Paired samples t-test is used to estimate whether the means of two related samples are significantly different. This test is used when two samples are in matched pair design. A paired samples t-test, which is similar to one sample t-test, is used to assess whether the mean of difference within each pair is significantly different from 0. Calculate t value by

$$t = \frac{\bar{d}}{s_{\bar{d}}} \quad \nu = \text{Number of pairs} - 1 \quad \text{(Formula 4-2)}$$

(7) Two independent samples t-test is a parametric test used to determine whether the difference between two sample means is significant. The two sample are randomly drawn from independent populations which follow normal distribution and have homogeneous variance. Calculate t value by

$$t = \frac{\bar{x}_1 - \bar{x}_2}{s_{\bar{x}_1 - \bar{x}_2}} \quad \nu = n_1 + n_2 - 2 \quad \text{(Formula 4-3)}$$

$$s_{\bar{x}_1 - \bar{x}_2} = \sqrt{s_c^2 \left(\frac{n_1 + n_2}{n_1 n_2}\right)} = \sqrt{\left[\frac{(n_1 - 1)s_1^2 + (n_2 - 1)s_2^2}{n_1 + n_2}\right]\left(\frac{n_1 + n_2}{n_1 n_2}\right)} \quad \text{(Formula 4-4)}$$

(8) Type I error is the error of rejecting a true null hypothesis. The probability of type I error is α.

(9) Type II error is the error of not rejecting a false null hypothesis. The probability of type II error is β.

(10) The power of test is the probability of making the correct decision of rejecting a false

null hypothesis, which is defined as $(1 - \beta)$.

III. Materials

Material I

Patient with advanced *schistosomiasis* may require pericardial devascularization due to the rupture of esophageal and gastric fundus veins. A study was conducted to investigate the effect of the surgery on the internal diameter of portal vein. The internal diameter of portal vein before and after pericardial devascularization was measured among 8 advanced *schistosomiasis* patients with esophageal and gastric fundus vein rupture, the data are shown as below (Table 4-1). Does the diameter of the portal vein get back to normal after pericardial devascularization?

Table 4-1 Internal diameter of portal vein before and after surgery in 8 patients (mm)

Case	1	2	3	4	5	6	7	8
Before surgery	16	15	15	18	16	17	14	14
After surgery	15	14	13	14	15	16	13	12

Material II

A research was conducted to evaluate the preventive effect of niclosamide in situ sustained-release injection against *Schistosoma japonicum* infection in mice. 10 mice were randomly divided into two groups. One group received a subcutaneous low-concentration niclosamide in situ sustained-release injection (71 mg/mL) at a single dose of 450 mg/kg (drug group, $n = 5$), while the other group did not receive any treatment (control group, $n = 5$). After 15 days, the mice were infected with 80 ± 4 *Schistosoma japonicum* cercariae. 35 days later, the mice were killed and the adult worms were seized. Does niclosamide in situ sustained-release injection have preventive effect in the infection of *Schistosoma japonicum* in mice?

Table 4-2 The worm burden at 35 days after the infection

Drug group	10	12	15	29	24
Control group	32	37	42	48	45

IV. Procedures

Material I

1. Identify the design of the study

For each patient, the internal diameter of portal vein is measured before and after surgery, so the study is a paired design.

2. Identify the data type of outcome

The index variable of the study is the internal diameter of portal vein, and the measurement result is numerical value, so the data type is quantitative data.

3. Hypothesis testing

Paired design, quantitative data, paired design t-test should be performed.

(1) Set up the hypothesis and significant level.

$H_0: \mu_d = 0$, there is no change in portal vein diameter in patients after surgery.

$H_1: \mu_d > 0$, there is a change in portal vein diameter in patients after surgery.

one-sided $\alpha = 0.05$.

(2) Calculation.

Firstly, calculate the differences for each pair.

Table 4-3 The differences between before and after surgery in 8 patients (mm)

NO.	before	after	d = before - after
1	16	15	1
2	15	14	1
3	15	13	2
4	18	14	4
5	16	15	1
6	17	16	1
7	14	13	1
8	14	12	2

Secondly, calculate mean and standard deviation of the differences.

$$\bar{d} = \frac{\sum d}{n} = \frac{(1+1+2+4+1+1+1+2)}{8} = 1.6 \text{ (mm)}$$

$$s_d = \sqrt{\frac{\sum (d-\bar{d})^2}{n-1}} = \sqrt{\frac{(1-1.6)^2 + \cdots + (2-1.6)^2}{8-1}} = 1.1 \text{ (mm)}$$

Thirdly, calculate t value

$$t = \frac{\bar{d}}{s_{\bar{d}}} = \frac{1.6}{1.1/\sqrt{8}} = 4.333 \quad \nu = 8-1 = 7$$

(3) Determine the P value and make decision.

From student's t distribution critical value table, one-sided critical value of t distribution with $\nu = 7$ is $t_{0.05,7} = 1.895$. $t > t_{0.05,7}$, $P < \alpha$, according to the significant level, we can reject the null hypothesis H_0, accept the alternative hypothesis H_1, there is a significantly statistical difference. So we regard that the surgery can decrease the inner diameter of portal vein level.

Material Ⅱ

1. Identify the design of the study

In the experiment, the mice were randomly divided into two groups, so the study is a completely random design.

2. Identify the data type of outcome

At the end of the experiment, the number of adult worms in mice was examined, so it is quantitative data.

3. Hypothesis testing

Completely random design, two groups, quantitative data, two independent samples t-test should be used.

(1) Set up the hypothesis and significant level.

$H_0: \mu_1 = \mu_2$, the numbers of adult worms are same between drug group and control group.

$H_1: \mu_1 < \mu_2$, the number of adult worms in drug group is smaller than that in control group.

one-sided $\alpha = 0.05$.

(2) Calculation.

Firstly, calculate mean and standard deviation for two groups separately.

$x_1 = 18.0 \quad s_1 = 8.2$

$x_2 = 40.9 \quad s_2 = 6.5$

Secondly, calculate standard error of the differences between two sample means

$$s_{\bar{x}_1 - \bar{x}_2} = \sqrt{\left[\frac{4 \times 8.2^2 + 4 \times 6.5^2}{5 + 5}\right]\left(\frac{5 + 5}{5 \times 5}\right)} = 4.63$$

Thirdly, calculate t value

$$t = \frac{\bar{x}_1 - \bar{x}_2}{s_{\bar{x}_1 - \bar{x}_2}} = \frac{18.0 - 40.9}{4.63} = -4.924 \quad \nu = n_1 + n_2 - 2 = 8$$

(3) Determine the P value and make decision.

From student's t distribution critical value table, one-sided critical value of t distribution with $\nu = 8$ is $t_{0.05,8} = 1.860$. $|t| > t_{0.05,8}$, $P < \alpha$, according to the significant level, the null hypothesis H_0 should be rejected, and we can accept the alternative hypothesis H_1, which means there is a significantly statistical difference between the means of the two groups. So niclosamide in situ sustained-release injection can prevent the infection of *Schistosoma japonicum* in mice.

Ⅴ. Exercises

(1) Type Ⅰ error is (   )

A. reject a true null hypothesis H_0

B. not reject a true null hypothesis H_0

C. reject a false null hypothesis H_0

D. not reject a false null hypothesis H_0

(2) The aim for paired design is to (   )

A. improve the accuracy of the results

B. improve the precision of the results

C. improve comparability between groups

D. make the comparison more meaningful

(3) When the two samples are from the normal distribution population, and the variances are equal, then two samples t-test is applied, the difference has statistically significant, the smaller the P value is (   )

A. the greater the difference between the two sample means

B. the greater the difference between the two population means

C. the more reason to prove that the two populations means are different

D. the more reason to prove that the two samples means are different

(4) When the two samples are compared, the following test levels are used to determine, which has the largest type Ⅱ error? (   )

A. $\alpha = 0.05$ B. $\alpha = 0.01$ C. $\alpha = 0.10$ D. $\alpha = 0.20$

(5) Which of the following statements is true about hypothesis test? (   )

A. one-sided test is better than two-sided test

B. to apply paired t-test or two-sample t-test is determined by the method of experimental design

C. if the P value is greater than 0.05, the probability of accepting null hypothesis error is very little

D. paired t-test should be first concerned.

实验四 t 检验

一、实验目的

（1）熟悉假设检验的意义。

（2）掌握假设检验的基本思想和步骤。

（3）掌握单样本 t 检验、配对 t 检验和两个独立样本 t 检验的适用条件和实际应用。

二、实验原理

（1）假设检验是统计推断的一个方面，与置信区间既有区别又有联系。假设检验基本思想概括为小概率和反证法。

（2）检验假设是根据研究目的作出对总体特征的假设，包含无效假设和备择假设。无效假设，亦称为零假设、原假设，用 H_0 表示；备择假设用 H_1 表示。H_0 和 H_1 是相互联系且对立的一对假设。

（3）检验水准用 α 表示。假设检验前，研究者根据假设检验目的或专业知识可人为设定其大小和单/双侧。大小一般设定为 0.05，记为"$\alpha = 0.05$"。

（4）P 值是在 H_0 所规定的总体中随机抽样，获得等于及大于和（或）等于及小于本次抽样所得统计量的概率。通 P 值与检验水准 α 大小比较，作出统计推断结论；当 $P \leq \alpha$ 时，拒绝 H_0，接受 H_1；当 $P > \alpha$ 时，不拒绝 H_0。

（5）单样本 t 检验用于样本均数（$\bar{x}$）所代表的未知总体均数（μ）与已知总体均数（μ_0）比较。

应用条件：样本来自正态分布总体。

检验统计量计算公式：

$$t = \frac{\bar{x} - \mu_0}{s_{\bar{x}}} \quad \nu = n - 1 \qquad \text{（公式 4-1）}$$

（6）配对 t 检验用于配对设计，配对 t 检验的原理与单样本 t 检验相同，首先求一对数据的差值（d），比较样本差值（$\bar{d}$）与已知总体均数 0。

应用条件：样本差值服从正态分布。

检验统计量计算公式：

$$t = \frac{\bar{d}}{s_{\bar{d}}} \quad \nu = \text{对子数} - 1 \qquad \text{（公式 4-2）}$$

（7）两个独立样本 t 检验又称为成组 t 检验，应用于完全随机设计，比较两个样本均数（$\bar{x}_1, \bar{x}_2$）所代表的总体均数（μ_1, μ_2）。

应用条件：①两个样本均来自正态分布总体；②两个总体的方差齐。

检验统计量计算公式：

$$t = \frac{\bar{x}_1 - \bar{x}_2}{s_{\bar{x}_1 - \bar{x}_2}} \quad \nu = n_1 + n_2 - 2 \qquad \text{（公式 4-3）}$$

$$s_{\bar{x}_1 - \bar{x}_2} = \sqrt{s_c^2 \left(\frac{n_1 + n_2}{n_1 n_2}\right)} = \sqrt{\left[\frac{(n_1 - 1)s_1^2 + (n_2 - 1)s_2^2}{n_1 + n_2}\right]\left(\frac{n_1 + n_2}{n_1 n_2}\right)} \qquad \text{（公式 4-4）}$$

（8）Ⅰ型错误为拒绝了实际上成立的 H_0，称之为"弃真"，用 α 表示。检验水准本质是研究者制定的允许犯Ⅰ型错误最大概率。当检验结果拒绝 H_0，才有可能犯Ⅰ型错误，其实际概率为 P 值。

（9）Ⅱ型错误为不拒绝实际上不成立的 H_0，称为"存伪"，用 β 表示。当检验结果不拒绝 H_0，才有可能犯Ⅱ型错误，其大小比较难估计，但其与Ⅰ型错误 α 此消彼长。

（10）检验效能为总体间确实有差异，按检验水准 α，发现这个差异的能力，又称为把握度，用 $(1 - \beta)$ 表示。

三、实验材料

材料一

晚期血吸虫病患者因食管胃底静脉破裂出血，可能需要进行贲门周围血管离断术治疗，某研究拟探讨该手术对晚期血吸虫病门静脉内径的影响。收集 8 例食管胃底静脉破裂的晚期血吸虫患者，行贲门周围血管离断术前、术后静脉内径，数据如下。进行贲门周围血管离断术前后患者门静脉内径扩张是否有所改善？

表4-1 8例患者手术前后门静脉内径（mm）

病例号	1	2	3	4	5	6	7	8
术前	16	15	15	18	16	17	14	14
术后	15	14	13	14	15	16	13	12

材料二

某研究评价低浓度氯硝柳胺原位固化长效注射剂对小鼠抗感染日本血吸虫的预防效果。10只昆明小鼠随机成分2组。给药组5只，小鼠皮下注射低浓度氯硝柳胺原位固化长效注射剂（71 mg/mL）450 mg/kg 1次；对照组5只小鼠不做任何处理。15天后，采用腹部贴片法感染日本血吸虫尾蚴（80±4）条/鼠。感染35天后，处死小鼠，检获成虫，结果见表4-2。氯硝柳胺原位固化长效注射剂是否有预防小鼠感染日本血吸虫的效果？

表4-2 给药组和对照组小鼠感染日本血吸虫尾蚴35天后虫荷

给药组	10	12	15	29	24
对照组	32	37	42	48	45

四、实验步骤

材料一

1. **设计类型**

每例患者手术前后分别测量门静脉内径，属于自身前后对照，因此试验设计的类型为配对设计。

2. **数据类型**

门静脉内径为指标变量，测量结果是数值，因此数据类型为定量数据。

3. **假设检验方法**

配对设计，定量资料的比较，选用配对设计 t 检验。

（1）建立检验假设，确定检验水准。

$H_0: \mu_d = 0$，即手术后晚期血吸虫病患者门静脉内径无改变。

$H_1: \mu_d > 0$，即手术后晚期血吸虫病患者门静脉内径变窄。

单侧 $\alpha = 0.05$。

（2）计算检验统计量。

第一步：求差值，术前门静脉内径 - 术后门静脉内径。

表4-3 8例患者手术前后门静脉内径（mm）差值

病例号	术前	术后	差值 d = 术前 − 术后
1	16	15	1
2	15	14	1
3	15	13	2
4	18	14	4
5	16	15	1
6	17	16	1
7	14	13	1
8	14	12	2

第二步：计算差值的均数和标准差。

$$\bar{d} = \frac{\sum d}{n} = \frac{(1+1+2+4+1+1+1+2)}{8} = 1.6 \text{（mm）}$$

$$s_d = \sqrt{\frac{\sum(d-\bar{d})^2}{n-1}} = \sqrt{\frac{(1-1.6)^2 + \cdots + (2-1.6)^2}{8-1}} = 1.1 \text{（mm）}$$

第三步：计算检验统计量。

$$t = \frac{\bar{d}}{s_{\bar{d}}} = \frac{1.6}{1.1/\sqrt{8}} = 4.333 \quad \nu = 8 - 1 = 7$$

（3）确定P值大小，作出统计推断结论。

以自由度 $\nu = 7$，查 t 界值表，$t_{0.05,7} = 1.895$。检验统计量 $t > t_{0.05,7}$，$P < \alpha$，按检验水准 $\alpha = 0.05$，拒绝 H_0，接受 H_1，差异有统计学意义；可以认为进行贲门周围血管离断术后患者门静脉内径扩张有所改善。

材料二

1. 设计类型

实验中将小鼠随机分成两组，为完全随机设计。

2. 数据类型

实验结束时，检查小鼠体内成虫数，为定量数据。

3. 假设检验方法

完全随机设计，两组定量数据比较，应使用两个独立样本 t 检验。

（1）建立检验假设，确定检验水准。

$H_0: \mu_1 = \mu_2$，即氯硝柳胺原位固化长效注射剂无预防小鼠感染日本血吸虫的效果。

$H_1: \mu_1 < \mu_2$，即氯硝柳胺原位固化长效注射剂有预防小鼠感染日本血吸虫的效果。

单侧 $\alpha = 0.05$。

（2）计算检验统计量。

第一步：求均数和标准差。分别求出给药组和对照组虫荷的均数和标准差。

$\bar{x}_1 = 18.0 \quad s_1 = 8.2$

$\bar{x}_2 = 40.9$ $s_2 = 6.5$

第二步：计算两个样本均数之差的标准误

$$s_{\bar{x}_1-\bar{x}_2} = \sqrt{\left[\frac{4 \times 8.2^2 + 4 \times 6.5^2}{5+5}\right]\left(\frac{5+5}{5 \times 5}\right)} = 4.63$$

第三步：计算检验统计量

$$t = \frac{\bar{x}_1 - \bar{x}_2}{s_{\bar{x}_1-\bar{x}_2}} = \frac{18.0 - 40.9}{4.63} = -4.924 \quad \nu = n_1 + n_2 - 2 = 8。$$

（3）确定 P 值大小，作出统计推断结论。

以自由度 $\nu = 8$，查 t 界值表，$t_{0.05,8} = 1.860$。检验统计量 $|t| > t_{0.05,8}$，$P < \alpha$，按检验水准 $\alpha = 0.05$，拒绝 H_0，接受 H_1，差异有统计学意义；可以认为氯硝柳胺原位固化长效注射剂有预防小鼠感染日本血吸虫的效果。

五、课后练习

（1）假设检验中的 Ⅰ 型错误是（   ）
　A. 拒绝了实际上成立的 H_0　　　　　　B. 不拒绝实际上成立的 H_0
　C. 拒绝实际上不成立的 H_0　　　　　　D. 不拒绝实际上不成立的 H_0

（2）配对设计的目的是（   ）
　A. 提高结果精确性　　　　　　　　　　B. 提高结果准确性
　C. 提高组间可比性　　　　　　　　　　D. 使比较结果更有意义

（3）在资料呈正态、方差齐时，两样本比较作 t 检验，差别有统计学意义，P 值越小说明（   ）
　A. 两样本均数差别越大　　　　　　　　B. 两总体均数差别越大
　C. 越有理由认为两总体均数不同　　　　D. 越有理由认为两样本均数不同

（4）两样本比较时，分别取以下检验水准，哪一个的 Ⅱ 型错误最大？（   ）
　A. $\alpha = 0.05$　　　B. $\alpha = 0.01$　　　C. $\alpha = 0.10$　　　D. $\alpha = 0.20$

（5）关于假设检验，下列哪一项说法是正确的？（   ）
　A. 单侧检验优于双侧检验
　B. 采用配对 t 检验还是成组 t 检验是由实验设计方法决定
　C. 检验结果若 P 值大于 0.05，则接受 H_0 犯错误的可能性很小
　D. 首选配对 t 检验

Experiment 5　Analysis of Variance

Ⅰ. Objectives

（1）To familiarize with the basic idea of analysis of variance.

（2）To be able to apply analysis of variance in practical settings.

Ⅱ. Principles

(1) Analysis of variance is briefly marked ANOVA, also called as the F test, be used to compare means across many groups. The basic idea is to decompose the total variation (sum of mean difference squared) into its corresponding parts according to the cause of variation, and at the same time, the degree of freedom is also decomposed. The part of the mean square of the study factor is compared with the part of the mean square of the random error to construct the test statistic F.

(2) Analysis of variance for complete random design is referred to as one-way ANOVA, there is only one factor that has more than two levels. The total variation (SS_{total}) is divided into the variation due to differences between groups (SS_{group}) and the variation due to random error within groups (SS_{error}).

$$SS_{total} = SS_{group} + SS_{error} \quad \nu_{total} = \nu_{group} + \nu_{error} \quad \text{(Formula 5-1)}$$

$$MS_{group} = \frac{SS_{group}}{\nu_{group}} \quad MS_{error} = \frac{SS_{error}}{\nu_{error}} \quad \text{(Formula 5-2)}$$

$$F = \frac{MS_{group}}{MS_{error}} \quad \nu_1 = \nu_{group}, \nu_2 = \nu_{error} \quad \text{(Formula 5-3)}$$

(3) Analysis of variance for random block design evaluates the difference across several groups which are matched samples. There are two factor effects (i.e., the group factor and the block factor), therefore the method is referred to as two-way ANOVA. The total variation (SS_{total}) is divided into the variation due to differences between groups (SS_{group}), the variation due to differences between blocks (SS_{block}) and the variation due to random error within groups (SS_{error}).

$$SS_{total} = SS_{group} + SS_{block} + SS_{error} \quad \nu_{total} = \nu_{group} + \nu_{block} + \nu_{error} \quad \text{(Formula 5-4)}$$

$$MS_{group} = \frac{SS_{group}}{\nu_{group}} \quad MS_{block} = \frac{SS_{block}}{\nu_{block}} \quad MS_{error} = \frac{SS_{error}}{\nu_{error}} \quad \text{(Formula 5-5)}$$

$$F_1 = \frac{MS_{group}}{MS_{error}} \quad \nu_1 = \nu_{group}, \nu_2 = \nu_{error} \quad \text{(Formula 5-6)}$$

$$F_2 = \frac{MS_{block}}{MS_{error}} \quad \nu_1 = \nu_{block}, \nu_2 = \nu_{error} \quad \text{(Formula 5-7)}$$

Ⅲ. Materials

Material Ⅰ

A study compared the immune protective efficacy of BCG vaccine (BCG), *Mycobacterium tuberculosis* H37Ra strain (H37Ra) and a new tuberculosis vaccine strain (B/R strain) that merged by protoplast fusion technique with BCG vaccine and *Mycobacterium tuberculosis* H37Ra strain. 22 C57BL/6 mice were randomly divided into four groups: Saline group (5 mice), BCG group (5 mice), H37Ra group (6 mice) and B/R group (6 mice), they were intradermal vaccinated with sterile saline 0.1 mL, BCG suspension 0.1 mL of, H37Ra suspension 0.1 mL and B/R suspension 0.1 mL (containing viable count of 1×10^6). After 3 weeks, measured IL-2 level in mouse plasma. Is there any difference in IL-2 level in four groups of mice?

Table 5-1 The level of IL-2 in mice plasma after immunization (pg/mL)

Saline group	6.9	7.8	7.6	7.5	5.9	—
BCG group	47.3	51.0	47.5	47.3	47.2	—
H37Ra group	62.5	55.4	56.7	52.6	53.4	61.3
B/R group	57.9	57.5	56.0	53.7	59.9	55.3

Material Ⅱ

A project investigated the function of a transmission-blocking vaccine candidate *Pb*280 in *Plasmodium berghei*. Selected 18 female KM mice from 6 litters while 3 mice each litter, 3 mice from same litter were randomly assigned to the *Pb*280KO-C1 group (C1 group), *Pb*280KO-C2 group (C2 group) and the control group. Each mouse, were injected 5×10^6 with *Pb*280KO-C1, *Pb*280KO-C2 and wild-type (WT) *P. Berghei* through tail vein. After 3 days, tail vein blood of mice was mixed with zygote culture medium, the number of zygotes was counted 24 hours later. The results are shown in Table 5-2, is there a difference in the zygotes counts in three *Plasmodium* strains?

Table 5-2 The numbers of zygotes of *Plasmodium* strains

Block	C1 group	C2 group	Control group
1	409	558	735
2	501	574	829
3	396	537	838
4	389	554	732
5	457	546	781
6	344	553	798

Ⅳ. Procedures

Material Ⅰ

1. Identify the design of the study

22 C57BL/6 mice were randomly divided into four groups, so the study is a complete random design.

2. Identify the data type of outcome

The index variable is the IL-2 level in mouse plasma, and the measurement result is numerical value, so the data type is quantitative data.

3. **Hypothesis testing**

Complete random design, four groups, quantitative data, perform one-way ANOVA.

(1) Set up the hypothesis and significant level.

$H_0: \mu_1 = \mu_2 = \mu_3 = \mu_4$, the levels of IL-2 in four groups of mice are the same.

$H_1: \mu_1, \mu_2, \mu_3, \mu_4$ are not all the same, at least the IL-2 level of one group is different.

$\alpha = 0.05$.

(2) Calculation.

Firstly, calculate the overall mean ($\bar{x}$), each group mean ($\bar{x}_1, \bar{x}_2, \bar{x}_3, \bar{x}_4$).

$$\bar{x} = \frac{6.9 + \cdots + 47.3 + \cdots + 62.5 + \cdots + 57.9 + \cdots + 55.3}{22} = 43.6 \text{ pg/mL}$$

$$\bar{x}_1 = \frac{6.9 + 7.8 + 7.6 + 7.5 + 5.9}{5} = 7.1 \text{ pg/mL}$$

$$\bar{x}_2 = \frac{47.3 + 51.0 + 47.5 + 47.3 + 47.2}{5} = 48.1 \text{ pg/mL}$$

$$\bar{x}_3 = \frac{62.5 + 55.4 + 56.7 + 52.6 + 53.4 + 61.3}{6} = 57.0 \text{ pg/mL}$$

$$\bar{x}_4 = \frac{57.9 + 57.5 + 56.0 + 53.7 + 59.9 + 55.3}{6} = 43.6 \text{ pg/mL}$$

Secondly, calculate the total sum of squares (SS_{total}) and the associated degree of freedom (ν_{total}), the between groups sum of squares (SS_{group}) and the associated degree of freedom (ν_{group}), the variation due to random error within groups sum of squares (SS_{error}) and the associated degree of freedom (ν_{error}).

$$SS_{total} = \sum (x - \bar{x})^2 = (6.9 - 43.6)^2 + \cdots + (55.3 - 43.6)^2 = 8975.62$$

$$\nu_{total} = n - 1 = 22 - 1 = 21$$

$$SS_{group} = \sum n_i (\bar{x}_i - \bar{x})^2 = 5 \times (7.1 - 43.6)^2 + \cdots + 6 \times (56.7 - 43.6)^2 = 8854.72$$

$$\nu_{group} = k - 1 = 4 - 1 = 3$$

$$SS_{error} = \sum (x_i - \bar{x}_i)^2 = (6.9 - 7.1)^2 + (7.8 - 7.1)^2 + \cdots + (55.3 - 56.7)^2 = 120.90$$

$$\nu_{error} = n - k = 22 - 4 = 18$$

Thirdly, calculate the mean squares between groups and within groups.

$$MS_{group} = \frac{SS_{group}}{\nu_{group}} = \frac{8854.72}{3} = 2951.57$$

$$MS_{error} = \frac{SS_{error}}{\nu_{error}} = \frac{120.90}{18} = 6.72$$

And finally, calculate F value

$$F = \frac{MS_{group}}{MS_{error}} = \frac{2951.57}{6.72} = 439.22.$$

(3) Determine the *P* value and make decision.

From *F* distribution critical value table, the critical value of *F* distribution with $\nu_1 = 3$, $\nu_2 = 18$ is $F_{0.05(3,18)} = 3.16$. $F > F_{0.05(3,18)}$, $P < \alpha$, according to the significant level, we can reject the null hypothesis H_0, accept alternative hypothesis H_1, there is a statistical difference. Therefore, we conclude that there are at least two groups in the IL−2 level are significantly different.

Material Ⅱ

1. Identify the design of the study

The female mice in research were from 6 litters, and every 3 mice from the same litter were randomly divided into 3 groups, so the study is a random block design.

2. Identify the data type of outcome

The index variable is the number of zygotes, and the measurement result is numerical value, so the data type is quantitative data.

3. Hypothesis testing

Random block design, three groups, quantitative data, perform two-way ANOVA.

(1) Set up the hypothesis and significant level.

$H_0: \mu_1 = \mu_2 = \mu_3$, there is no difference in the number of zygotes in *Plasmodium* strains.

$H_1: \mu_1, \mu_2, \mu_3$ are not all the same, there is a difference in the number of zygotes in *Plasmodium* strains.

$\alpha = 0.05$.

(2) Calculation.

Firstly, calculate the overall mean ($\bar{x}$), each group mean and each block mean ($\bar{x}_i, \bar{x}_j$).

Table 5−3 The means of zygotes of *Plasmodium* strains

Block	C1 group	C2 group	Control group	$\bar{x}_j$
1	409	558	735	567.3
2	501	574	829	634.7
3	396	537	838	590.3
4	389	554	732	558.3
5	457	546	781	594.7
6	344	553	798	565.0
$\bar{x}_i$	416.0	553.7	785.5	585.1 ($\bar{x}$)

Secondly, calculate the total sum of squares (SS_{total}) and the associated degree of freedom (ν_{total}), the between groups sum of squares (SS_{group}) and the associated degree of freedom

(ν_{group}), the between blocks sum of squares (SS_{block}) and the associated degree of freedom (ν_{block}), the variation due to random error within groups sum of squares (SS_{error}) and the associated degree of freedom (ν_{error}).

$SS_{total} = \sum(x - \bar{x})^2 = (409 - 585.1)^2 + \cdots + (798 - 585.1)^2 = 444732.94$

$\nu_{total} = n - 1 = 18 - 1 = 17$

$SS_{group} = \sum n_i(\bar{x}_i - \bar{x})^2 = 6 \times (416.0 - 585.1)^2 + \cdots + 6 \times (785.5 - 585.1)^2 = 418458.11$

$\nu_{group} = k - 1 = 3 - 1 = 2$

$SS_{block} = \sum n_j(\bar{x}_j - \bar{x}_j)^2 = 3 \times (409 - 567.3)^2 + \cdots + 3 \times (798 - 565.0)^2 = 12035.61$

$\nu_{block} = b - 1 = 6 - 1 = 5$

$SS_{error} = SS_{total} - SS_{group} - SS_{block} = 444732.94 - 418458.11 - 12035.61 = 14239.22$

$\nu_{error} = \nu_{total} - \nu_{group} - \nu_{block} = 17 - 2 - 5 = 10$

Thirdly, calculate the mean squares between groups and the error.

$MS_{group} = \dfrac{SS_{group}}{\nu_{group}} = \dfrac{418458.11}{2} = 209229.06$

$MS_{error} = \dfrac{SS_{error}}{\nu_{error}} = \dfrac{14239.22}{10} = 1423.92$

And finally, calculate F value

$F = \dfrac{MS_{group}}{MS_{error}} = \dfrac{209229.06}{1423.92} = 146.94$

(3) Determine the P value and make decision.

From F distribution critical value table, the critical value of F distribution with $\nu_1 = 2$, $\nu_2 = 10$ is $F_{0.05(2,10)} = 4.10$. $F > F_{0.05(2,10)}$, $P < \alpha$, according to the significant level, we can reject the null hypothesis H_0, accept alternative hypothesis H_1, there is a significant difference. Therefore, we could say there is a difference in the number of zygotes in *Plasmodium* strains.

V. Exercises

(1) Which of the following statements is false? (   )

A. the variance divided by its degree of freedom is the mean square

B. ANOVA requires that the data within each group are nearly normal

C. ANOVA requires that the variability across the groups is about equal

D. in one-way ANOVA, the mean square within groups is the mean square of the error

(2) For two groups, for the same data, the result of ANOVA and the result of t-test (   )

A. completely equivalent, and $t = F$

B. the ANOVA is more accurate

C. the t-test is more accurate

D. completely equivalent, and $t = \sqrt{F}$

(3) Comparing a complete random design and random block design, which of the following

is true?(   )

A. two designs have a same efficiency

B. the error of random block design is certainly less than that of complete random design

C. the sources of variation in the random block design are more finely divided than those in the complete random design

D. none of them

(4) Which one can replace paired *t*-test?(   )

A. ANOVA for complete random design

B. ANOVA for random block design

C. both of them

D. none of them

(5) Comparing two means, which method can be used?(   )

A. ANOVA　　　　　　　　　　B. *t*-test

C. ANOVA or *t*-test　　　　　　D. homogeneity of variance test

实验五　方差分析

一、实验目的

(1) 熟悉方差分析的基本思想。

(2) 掌握完全随机设计和随机区组设计方差分析中变异和自由度的分解及假设检验过程。

二、实验原理

(1) 方差分析又称为 F 检验,可用于3组及以上定量数据的比较。其基本思想是根据引起变异的原因,将总变异(离均差平方和,SS)分解为相应的部分,同时总自由度(ν)也进行分解;各部分离均差平方和除以自由度得到均方(MS),即方差;研究因素的那部分均方与随机误差部分均方相比,构建检验统计量 F。

(2) 完全随机设计方差分析又称成组设计方差分析,将受试对象随机分配到多个处理组去,给予不同干预,比较各处理组间实验效应是否有差别。只分析处理因素,因此亦被称为单因素方差分析。

$$SS_{total} = SS_{group} + SS_{error} \quad \nu_{total} = \nu_{group} + \nu_{error} \quad \text{(公式 5-1)}$$

$$MS_{group} = \frac{SS_{group}}{\nu_{group}} \quad MS_{error} = \frac{SS_{error}}{\nu_{error}} \quad \text{(公式 5-2)}$$

$$F = \frac{MS_{group}}{MS_{error}} \quad \nu_1 = \nu_{group}, \quad \nu_2 = \nu_{error} \quad \text{(公式 5-3)}$$

(3) 随机区组设计方差分析又称配伍设计方差分析,将受试对象按某种属性或特征配成区组，区组内受试对象相同或最为相似，将同一区组内受试对象随机分配 k 个处理组接受不同的干预，可以比较不同处理组、不同区组之间两个因素的效应，因此亦被称为两因素方差分析。

$$SS_{total} = SS_{group} + SS_{block} + SS_{error} \quad \nu_{total} = \nu_{group} + \nu_{block} + \nu_{error} \quad （公式5-4）$$

$$MS_{group} = \frac{SS_{group}}{\nu_{group}} \quad MS_{block} = \frac{SS_{block}}{\nu_{block}} \quad MS_{error} = \frac{SS_{error}}{\nu_{error}} \quad （公式5-5）$$

$$F_1 = \frac{MS_{group}}{MS_{error}} \quad \nu_1 = \nu_{group}, \nu_2 = \nu_{error} \quad （公式5-6）$$

$$F_2 = \frac{MS_{block}}{MS_{error}} \quad \nu_1 = \nu_{block}, \nu_2 = \nu_{error} \quad （公式5-7）$$

三、实验材料

材料一

某研究拟比较卡介苗（BCG）、结核分枝杆菌国际标准无毒株（H37Ra）及利用原生质体融合技术以卡介苗和结核分枝杆菌国际标准无毒株为亲本菌株所构建的新型结核病疫苗株（B/R 菌株）的免疫保护效力。将 C57BL/6 小鼠 22 只随机分为 4 组：生理盐水组（5 只）、BCG 组（5 只）、H37Ra 组（6 只）、B/R 组（6 只），分别皮内接种无菌生理盐水 0.1 mL、BCG 菌悬液 0.1 mL、H37Ra 菌株悬液 0.1 mL、B/R 菌株悬液 0.1 mL（含活菌数为 $1×10^6$ 个），3 周后检测小鼠外周血中 IL-2 含量，结果见表 5-1。四组小鼠外周血 IL-2 水平是否有差别？

表 5-1 4 组小鼠接种 3 周后外周血 IL-2 含量（pg/mL）

生理盐水组	6.9	7.8	7.6	7.5	5.9	—
BCG 组	47.3	51.0	47.5	47.3	47.2	—
H37Ra 组	62.5	55.4	56.7	52.6	53.4	61.3
B/R 组	57.9	57.5	56.0	53.7	59.9	55.3

材料二

某课题研究传播阻断疫苗候选抗原 $Pb280$ 在伯氏疟原虫中的基因功能，从 6 窝昆明小鼠中每窝取 3 只雌鼠，同窝 3 只小鼠随机分配到基因敲除 C1 组、基因敲除 C2 组和对照组，每组小鼠分别经尾静脉注射 $5×10^6$ 个将 $Pb280$ 基因敲除疟原虫株 $Pb280$KO-C1 型、$Pb280$KO-C2 型和野生型伯氏疟原虫。感染 3 天后取小鼠尾静脉血与动合子培养基混合培养，24 小时后计算动合子数，结果见表 5-2。三型疟原虫株的动合子数是否不同？

表 5-2　三型疟原虫株的动合子数

窝别	C1 组	C2 组	对照组
1	409	558	735
2	501	574	829
3	396	537	838
4	389	554	732
5	457	546	781
6	344	553	798

四、实验步骤

材料一

1. 设计类型

22 只 C57BL/6 小鼠被随机分成 4 组，为完全随机设计类型。

2. 数据类型

结局指标是小鼠外周血中 IL-2 含量，为定量数据。

3. 假设检验方法

完全随机设计，多组定量数据比较，采用单因素方差分析。

（1）建立检验假设，确定检验水准。

$H_0: \mu_1 = \mu_2 = \mu_3 = \mu_4$，即 4 组小鼠外周血 IL-2 水平相同。

$H_1: \mu_1, \mu_2, \mu_3, \mu_4$ 不全相同，即 4 组小鼠外周血 IL-2 水平不全相同。

$\alpha = 0.05$。

（2）计算检验统计量。

第一步：计算总的样本均数 $\bar{x}$，各组样本数均数 $\bar{x}_1, \bar{x}_2, \bar{x}_3, \bar{x}_4$。

$$\bar{x} = \frac{6.9 + \cdots + 47.3 + \cdots + 62.5 + \cdots + 57.9 + \cdots + 55.3}{22} = 43.6 \,(\text{pg/mL})$$

$$\bar{x}_1 = \frac{6.9 + 7.8 + 7.6 + 7.5 + 5.9}{5} = 7.1 \,(\text{pg/mL})$$

$$\bar{x}_2 = \frac{47.3 + 51.0 + 47.5 + 47.3 + 47.2}{5} = 48.1 \,(\text{pg/mL})$$

$$\bar{x}_3 = \frac{62.5 + 55.4 + 56.7 + 52.6 + 53.4 + 61.3}{6} = 57.0 \,(\text{pg/mL})$$

$$\bar{x}_4 = \frac{57.9 + 57.5 + 56.0 + 53.7 + 59.9 + 55.3}{6} = 43.6 \,(\text{pg/mL})$$

第二步：计算总的离均差平方和 SS_{total} 和自由度 ν_{total}；处理因素离均差平方和 SS_{group} 和自由度 ν_{group}；误差离均差平方和 SS_{error} 和自由度 ν_{error}。

$$SS_{total} = \sum (x - \bar{x})^2 = (6.9 - 43.6)^2 + \cdots + (55.3 - 43.6)^2 = 8975.62$$

$\nu_{total} = n - 1 = 22 - 1 = 21$

$SS_{group} = \sum n_i(\bar{x}_i - \bar{x})^2 = 5 \times (7.1 - 43.6)^2 + \cdots + 6 \times (56.7 - 43.6)^2 = 8854.72$

$\nu_{group} = k - 1 = 4 - 1 = 3$

$SS_{error} = \sum (x_i - \bar{x}_i)^2 = (6.9 - 7.1)^2 + (7.8 - 7.1)^2 + \cdots + (55.3 - 56.7)^2 = 120.90$

$\nu_{error} = n - k = 22 - 4 = 18$

第三步：计算处理因素均方 MS_{group}，误差均方 MS_{error}。

$MS_{group} = \dfrac{SS_{group}}{\nu_{group}} = \dfrac{8854.72}{3} = 2951.57$

$MS_{error} = \dfrac{SS_{error}}{\nu_{error}} = \dfrac{120.90}{18} = 6.72$

第四步：计算 F 值。

$F = \dfrac{MS_{group}}{MS_{error}} = \dfrac{2951.57}{6.72} = 439.22$

（3）确定 P 值大小，作出统计推断结论。

以自由度 $\nu_1 = 3$，$\nu_2 = 18$，查 F 界值表，$F_{0.05(3,18)} = 3.16$。检验统计量 $F > F_{0.05(3,18)}$，$P < \alpha$，按检验水准 $\alpha = 0.05$，拒绝 H_0，接受 H_1，差异有统计学意义；可以认为 4 组小鼠外周血 IL-2 水平不全相同。

材料二

1. 设计类型

6 窝小鼠每窝取 3 只雌鼠，同窝 3 只小鼠随机分到基因敲除 C1 组、基因敲除 C2 组和对照组，为随机区组设计。

2. 数据类型

结局指标是小鼠尾静脉血与动合子培养基混合培养 24 小时后动合子数，为定量数据。

3. 假设检验方法

随机区组设计定量数据比较，采用两因素方差分析。

（1）建立检验假设，确定检验水准。

$H_0: \mu_1 = \mu_2 = \mu_3$，即三型疟原虫株的动合子数相同。

$H_0: \mu_1, \mu_2, \mu_3$ 不全相同，即三型疟原虫株的动合子数不全相同。

$\alpha = 0.05$。

（2）计算检验统计量。

第一步：计算总的样本均数，各组、各窝样本均数。

表 5-3 三型疟原虫株的动合子数均值

窝别	C1 组	C2 组	对照组	$\bar{x}_j$
1	409	558	735	567.3
2	501	574	829	634.7

续表 5-3

窝别	C1 组	C2 组	对照组	$\bar{x}_j$
3	396	537	838	590.3
4	389	554	732	558.3
5	457	546	781	594.7
6	344	553	798	565.0
$\bar{x}_i$	416.0	553.7	785.5	585.1（$\bar{x}$）

第二步：计算总的离均差平方和 SS_{total} 和自由度 ν_{total}；处理因素离均差平方 SS_{group} 和自由度 ν_{group}；区组因素离均差平方 SS_{block} 和自由度 ν_{block}；误差离均差平方和 SS_{error} 和自由度 ν_{error}。

$$SS_{total} = \sum (x - \bar{x})^2 = (409 - 585.1)^2 + \cdots + (798 - 585.1)^2 = 444732.94$$

$$\nu_{total} = n - 1 = 18 - 1 = 17$$

$$SS_{group} = \sum n_i(\bar{x}_i - \bar{x})^2 = 6 \times (416.0 - 585.1)^2 + \cdots + 6 \times (785.5 - 585.1)^2 = 418458.11$$

$$\nu_{group} = k - 1 = 3 - 1 = 2$$

$$SS_{block} = \sum n_j(x_j - \bar{x}_j)^2 = 3 \times (409 - 567.3)^2 + \cdots + 3 \times (798 - 565.0)^2 = 12035.61$$

$$\nu_{block} = b - 1 = 6 - 1 = 5$$

$$SS_{error} = SS_{total} - SS_{group} - SS_{block} = 444732.94 - 418458.11 - 12035.61 = 14239.22$$

$$\nu_{error} = \nu_{total} - \nu_{group} - \nu_{block} = 17 - 2 - 5 = 10$$

第三步：计算处理因素均方 MS_{group}，误差均方 MS_{error}。

$$MS_{group} = \frac{SS_{group}}{\nu_{group}} = \frac{418458.11}{2} = 209229.06$$

$$MS_{error} = \frac{SS_{error}}{\nu_{error}} = \frac{14239.22}{10} = 1423.92$$

第四步：计算 F 值。

$$F = \frac{MS_{group}}{MS_{error}} = \frac{209229.06}{1423.92} = 146.94$$

（3）确定 P 值大小，作出统计推断结论。

以自由度 $\nu_1 = 2$，$\nu_2 = 10$，查 F 界值表，$F_{0.05(2,10)} = 4.10$。检验统计量 $F > F_{0.05(2,10)}$，$P < \alpha$，按检验水准 $\alpha = 0.05$，拒绝 H_0，接受 H_1，差异有统计学意义；可以认为三型疟原虫株的动合子数有差异。整体比较有差异后若想进一步说明组间差异，需要进行两两比较，本书不做详细介绍。

五、课后练习

（1）以下说法不正确的是（　　）

A. 方差除以其自由度就是均方

B. 方差分析时要求各样本来自相互独立的正态总体

C. 方差分析时要求各样本所在总体的方差相等

D. 完全随机设计的方差分析，组内均方就是误差均方

（2）当组数等于 2 时，对于同一资料，方差分析结果与 t 检验结果（　　）

　　A. 完全等价且 $t = F$ 　　　　　　　　B. 方差分析结果更准确

　　C. t 检验结果更准确 　　　　　　　　D. 完全等价且 $t = \sqrt{F}$

（3）比较完全随机设计与随机区组设计，下列说法正确的是（　　）

　　A. 两种设计试验效率一样

　　B. 随机区组设计的误差一定小于完全随机设计

　　C. 随机区组设计的变异来源比完全随机设计分得更细

　　D. 以上说法都不对

（4）配对 t 检验可以用哪种设计类型的方差分析来替代？（　　）

　　A. 完全随机设计 　　　　　　　　　　B. 随机区组设计

　　C. 两种设计都可以 　　　　　　　　　D. 两种设计都不行

（5）两样本均数的比较，可用（　　）

　　A. 方差分析 　　　　　　　　　　　　B. t 检验

　　C. 方差分析与 t 检验均可 　　　　　　D. 方差齐性检验

Experiment 6　Chi-square Test

Ⅰ. Objectives

(1) To familiarize with chi-square test requirements.

(2) To master the application of chi-square test in practical settings.

Ⅱ. Principles

(1) χ^2 Distribution is positive skewness and tends to normal distribution while increasing the degree of freedom. The square sum of the k random variables, which are independent normal distributions, follows the χ^2 distribution with the degree of freedom of k.

(2) The basic of χ^2 test can be explained by the formula of χ^2. The value of χ^2 reflects the overall difference between the actual frequency and theoretical frequency.

$$\chi^2 = \sum \frac{(A - T)^2}{T}, \quad \nu = (R - 1) \times (C - 1) \qquad (\text{Formula } 6 - 1)$$

In which, A is the actual frequency, T is the theoretical frequency which is calculated on the basis of the null hypothesis H_0.

$$T = \frac{n_R n_C}{n} \qquad (\text{Formula } 6 - 2)$$

(3) χ^2 Test for four-fold table is used to compare two rates (proportions). Tables in the form of Table 6-1 are called four-fold tables as the four cells contain all information.

Table 6-1　The form of four-fold table

group	positive	negtive
treat	a	b
control	c	d

Calculate the χ^2 value besides by the basic formula, also through the specific formula.

When $n \geqslant 40$ and $T \geqslant 5$ in all cells, no need for correction:

$$\chi^2 = \frac{(ad-bc)^2 n}{(a+b)(c+d)(a+c)(b+d)} \quad \text{(Formula 6-3)}$$

When $n \geqslant 40$ and at least one cell $1 \leqslant T < 5$, use the corrected formula:

$$\chi_c^2 = \frac{(|ad-bc|-n/2)^2 n}{(a+b)(c+d)(a+c)(b+d)} \quad \text{(Formula 6-4)}$$

(4) McNemar χ^2 test for paired-sample four-fold table is to test whether the results of two methods are different. Paired-sample four-fold table is the table form of paired-sample design for binary data.

Table 6-2　the form of paired-sample four-fold table

| One method | Another method | | total |
	positive	negative	
positive	a	b	a+b
negative	c	d	c+d
total	a+c	b+d	a+b+c+d

When $b+c \geqslant 40$:

$$\chi^2 = \frac{(b-c)^2}{(b+c)}, \quad \nu = 1 \quad \text{(Formula 6-5)}$$

When $b+c < 40$:

$$\chi_c^2 = \frac{(|b-c|-1)^2}{(b+c)}, \quad \nu = 1 \quad \text{(Formula 6-6)}$$

(5) χ^2 test for the contingency table is used to compare multiple rates or two (or more) proportions. Contingency table or R × C table refers to the table with more than 2 rows or columns. Avoid the following situations that more than 20 percent of cells have theoretical frequency less than 5, or one cell theoretical frequency is less than 1. Besides the basic formula, the following formula can be used to compute the χ^2 value.

$$\chi^2 = n\left(\sum \frac{A^2}{n_R n_C} - 1\right), \quad \nu = (R-1) \times (C-1) \tag{Formula 6-7}$$

III. Materials

Material I

A research focused on the impact of ambient temperature on the vector competence of *Anopheles stephensi* to malaria parasites. *Anopheles stephensi* was infected with *Plasmodium yoelii* at 24℃ and 28℃ respectively. The midgut of *Anopheles stephensi* was dissected 9 days after infection. The development of *Plasmodium oocysts* was observed and counted under fluorescence microscope. The results are shown in Table 6-3. Please compare the infection rates of *plasmodium* under different temperature.

Table 6-3 Infection of *Anopheles stephensi* by *Plasmodium yoelii* under different temperatures

Groups	Uninfected counts	Infected counts	Total counts	Infection rate/%
24℃	3	33	36	91.7
28℃	30	19	49	38.3

Material II

In order to establish a more time-saving and specific real time fluorescent quantitative PCR method for early diagnosis of Dengue virus type 1, the results of fluorescent quantitative PCR in 166 serum from patients suspected of dengue virus type 1 were identical with those of dengue virus specific primers, and were compared with those of conventional PCR. Is the positive rate of real time PCR higher than that of conventional PCR?

Table 6-4 Comparison of different diagnostic methods

Fluorescent quantitative PCR	Conventional PCR		Total
	positive	negative	
Positive	36	90	126
Negative	0	40	40
Total	36	130	166

Material III

A randomized, controlled, multi-center clinical study was conducted to investigate the efficacy of medical ozone versus Ganlixin capsule in the treatment of chronic hepatitis B. 175 patients with chronic hepatitis B were randomly divided into 3 groups: 58 cases in group A (domestic medical ozone generator group), 62 cases in group B (German Hermes medical ozone generator group), 55 cases in group C (Ganlixin capsule oral treatment group). After 12 weeks of treatment, three group rates of patients with viral response are shown as follows, whether is there any difference in the effectiveness of the three treatments?

Table 6-5 Effects of medical ozone therapy on patients with CHB

Groups	n	Virological response counts	Response rate /%
A group	58	13	22.4
B group	62	10	16.4
C group	55	6	10.9
Total	175	29	17.6

IV. Procedures

Material I

1. Identify the design of the study

In this experiment, *Anopheles Stephensi* was infected with *Plasmodium yoelii* at 24℃ and 28℃, so the study is a completely random design.

2. Identify the data type of outcome

The outcome of the experiment was whether each *Anopheles mosquito* was infected with *Plasmodium yoelii*, and was classified into two categories.

3. Hypothesis testing

Completely random design, two groups, qualitative data, χ^2 test for four-fold table should be used.

(1) Set up the hypothesis and significant level.

$H_0: \pi_1 = \pi_2$, there is no difference in the infection rate of *Plasmodium yoelii* between. two temperatures

$H_1: \pi_1 \neq \pi_2$, there is a difference in the infection rate of *Plasmodium yoelii* between. two temperatures.

$\alpha = 0.05$.

(2) Calculation.

Firstly, find out the actual frequencies of a, b, c, d.

Table 6-6 The four-fold table of infection of *Anopheles stephensi* by *Plasmodium yoelii* under different temperatures

Group	Uninfected counts	Infected counts	Total
24℃	3 (a)	33 (b)	36
28℃	30 (c)	19 (d)	49
Total	33	52	85

Secondly, check the condition.

$n = n_1 + n_2 = 36 + 49 = 85 > 40$

$T_a = \dfrac{36 \times 33}{85} = 14.0 \qquad T_b = \dfrac{36 \times 52}{85} = 22.0$

$T_c = \dfrac{49 \times 33}{85} = 19.0 \qquad T_d = \dfrac{49 \times 52}{85} = 30.0$

Every theoretical frequency is more than 5, no need for correction.

Thirdly, calculate χ^2 value.

$\chi^2 = \dfrac{(ad-bc)^2 n}{(a+b)(c+d)(a+c)(b+d)}$
$= \dfrac{(3 \times 19 - 33 \times 30)^2 \times 49}{(3+33)(30+19)(3+30)(33+19)} = 24.444.$

(3) Determine the P value and make decision.

From χ^2 distribution critical value table, the critical value of χ^2 distribution with $\nu = 1$ is $\chi^2_{0.05,1} = 3.84$. $\chi^2 > \chi^2_{0.05,1}$, $P < \alpha$, according to the significant level, we can reject the null hypothesis H_0, accept alternative hypothesis H_1, there is a significantly statistical difference. So we regard that there is a difference in the infection rate of *plasmodium* yoelii between two temperatures.

Material Ⅱ

1. Identify the design of the study

In this study, each patient's serum was detected by both fluorescent quantitative PCR and conventional PCR, so it is the type of matched design.

2. Identify the data type of outcome

Fluorescent quantitative PCR and conventional PCR gave positive or negative results, so the data were classified into two categories.

3. Hypothesis testing

Matched design, two methods, qualitative data, *McNemar* χ^2 test for paired-sample four-fold table should be used.

(1) Set the hypothesis and significant level.

$H_0: B = C$, the positive rate of fluorescent quantitative PCR is the same as that of conventional PCR.

$H_1: B \neq C$, the positive rate of fluorescent quantitative PCR is different from that of conventional PCR.

$\alpha = 0.05$.

(2) Calculation.

Firstly, find out the actual frequencies of b, c.

Table 6-7 The paired-sample four-fold table of two different diagnostic methods

Fluorescent quantitative PCR	Conventional PCR		Total
	Positive	Negative	
Positive	36	90 (b)	126
Negative	0 (c)	40	40
Total	36	130	166

Secondly, check the condition.

$b + c = 90 + 0 = 90 > 40$, no need for correction.

Thirdly, calculate χ^2 value.

$$\chi^2 = \frac{(b-c)^2}{(b+c)} = \frac{(90-0)^2}{90+0} = 90.$$

(3) Determine the P value and make decision.

From χ^2 distribution critical value table, the critical value of χ^2 distribution with $\nu = 1$ is $\chi^2_{0.05,1} = 3.84$. $\chi^2 > \chi^2_{0.05,1}$, $P < \alpha$, according to the significant level, we can reject the null hypothesis H_0, accept alternative hypothesis H_1, there is a significantly statistical difference. We can consider that the positive rate of fluorescent quantitative PCR is different from that of conventional PCR.

Material Ⅲ

1. Identify the design method of the study

In the clinical trial, patients with chronic hepatitis B were randomly divided into 3 groups, which were treated by domestic medical ozone generator, German Hermes medical ozone generator and Ganlixin capsule respectively. It's a completely random design.

2. Identify the data type of outcome

After 12 weeks of treatment, examine the patient's response for viral which is a binary classification.

3. Hypothesis testing

Completely random design for three groups, the outcome index is whether the virus response, the data can be collated into $R \times C$ table. To determine whether there is a difference in viral response rates among the three groups, χ^2 test for the contingency table should be used.

(1) Set the hypothesis and significant level.

$H_0: \pi_1 = \pi_2 = \pi_3$, there was no difference in the effects of the three treatments.

H_1: at least two of π_1, π_2, π_3 are not equal, the effects of the three treatments are not all the same.

$\alpha = 0.05$.

(2) Calculation.

Firstly, find out the actual frequencies for all cells.

Table 6-8 The contingency table of the effects of different diagnostic methods on patients with CHB

Group	n	Virological response	No response
A group	58 (n_1)	13	45
B group	62 (n_2)	10	52
C group	55 (n_3)	6	49
Total	175 (n)	29	146

Secondly, check the condition.

The smallest theoretical frequency $T = \dfrac{n_R n_C}{n} = \dfrac{55 \times 29}{175} = 9.1 > 5$, that means no cell's theoretical frequency is less than 5.

Thirdly, calculate χ^2 value.

$$\chi^2 = n\left(\sum \dfrac{A^2}{n_R n_C} - 1\right) = 175 \times \left(\dfrac{13^2}{58 \times 29} + L + \dfrac{49^2}{55 \times 136} - 1\right) = 2.716$$

(3) Determine the P value and make decision.

From χ^2 distribution critical value table, the critical value of χ^2 distribution with $v = 2$ is $\chi^2_{0.05,2} = 5.99$. $\chi^2 < \chi^2_{0.05,2}$, $P > \alpha$, according to the significant level, we can't reject the null hypothesis H_0, there is no significantly statistical difference. We can't consider that there is any difference among the effects of the three therapies for chronic hepatitis B.

Ⅴ. Exercises

(1) The analysis of the data in the four-fold table, which circumstance is a continuous correction usually required? (   )

    A. $1 < T < 5$ and $n > 40$ B. $T < 5$
    C. $T < 1$ or $n < 40$ D. $T < 1$ and $n \geqslant 40$

(2) χ^2 test for four-fold table does not need correction formula, the application condition is (   )

    A. $n > 40$ and $T > 5$ B. $n < 40$ and $T > 5$
    C. $n > 40$ and $1 < T < 5$ D. $n < 40$ and $1 < T < 5$

(3) A study was conducted to investigate the threat of tropical high temperature and high humidity to nosocomial infection, and to monitor the rate of nosocomial infection in patients at Grade Ⅲ, Class A hospital, is the incidence of nosocomial infection different in four quarters? (   )

Table 6-9 The rates of nosocomial infection in four quarters

Quarter	Monitoring cases	Infection counts	Infection rate/%
I	24604	436	1.77
II	28979	575	1.98
III	28433	518	1.82
IV	30624	497	1.62
Total	112640	2026	1.80

A. χ^2 test for four-fold table, no need corrected
B. χ^2 test for four-fold table, corrected
C. McNemar χ^2 test for paired-sample four-fold table
D. χ^2 test for the contingency table

(4) Test 96 samples of drinking water by lactose multi-tube fermentation and enzyme substrate methods, the detection rate is 83.3% by lactose multi-tube fermentation, the detection rate is 89.6% by enzyme substrate method, and 78.1% by both methods, the hypothesis test that should be used to determine whether there is a difference in the detection rates between the two methods is (   )

A. χ^2 test for four-fold table
B. McNemar χ^2 test for paired-sample four-fold table
C. χ^2 test for the contingency table
D. t-test

(5) To explore the curative effect of Hainan tropical Chinese herbal medicine on knee osteoarthritis/osteodystrophy, 90 patients were randomly divided into 2 groups, the treatment group used Hainan tropical Chinese herbal fumigation knee joint, in the control group, diclofenac diethy lamine cream was applied locally to the affected knee joint. After 3 weeks, the results of treatment are shown in Table 6-10. The method to compare the efficiency of the two groups should be (   )

Table 6-10 Effection on knee osteoarthritis/osteodystrophy of two groups

Group	n	Effect	No-effect	Effective rate/%
Treat	45	42	3	93.3
Control	45	34	11	75.5

A. χ^2 test for four-fold table, no need corrected
B. χ^2 test for four-fold table, corrected
C. McNemar χ^2 test for paired-sample four-fold table
D. χ^2 test for the contingency table

实验六 χ^2 检验

一、实验目的
（1）熟悉卡方检验的基本思想。
（2）掌握卡方检验的方法及各种公式的适用条件。

二、实验原理
（1）χ^2 分布呈正偏态，随着自由度 k 的增大，趋于正态分布。k 个互相独立并呈标准正态分布的随机变量的平方和服从自由度为 k 的 χ^2 分布。

（2）χ^2 检验的基本思想是假设无效假设 H_0 成立前提下，计算理论频数 T；检验统计量 χ^2 值反映实际频数 A 与理论频数 T 的吻合情况；如果实际支持 H_0，实际频数 A 与理论频数 T 应相差不大，χ^2 应不大；反之 χ^2 大，即实际频数 A 与理论频数 T 相差较大，当超过抽样误差允许范围，有理由拒绝 H_0。

$$\chi^2 = \sum \frac{(A-T)^2}{T}, \quad \nu = (R-1) \times (C-1) \qquad （公式6-1）$$

式中，A 为实际频数；T 为理论频数，假设 H_0 成立时计算。

$$T = \frac{n_R n_C}{n} \qquad （公式6-2）$$

（3）四格表资料的 χ^2 检验用于完全随机设计两个比率或构成比的比较，数据可以整理成四格表。其检验统计量除用基本公式计算外，可用四格表资料的专用公式计算。

表 6-1 四格表资料的一般形式

组别	有效	无效
试验组	a	b
对照组	c	d

$n \geq 40$，且每个格子 $T \geq 5$ 时，专用公式：

$$\chi^2 = \frac{(ad-bc)^2 n}{(a+b)(c+d)(a+c)(b+d)} \qquad （公式6-3）$$

$n \geq 40$，任一格子 $1 \leq T < 5$ 时，校正公式：

$$\chi_c^2 = \frac{(|ad-bc|-n/2)^2 n}{(a+b)(c+d)(a+c)(b+d)} \qquad （公式6-4）$$

（4）配对四格表资料的 χ^2 检验又称 McNemar 检验，用于配对设计两个比率的比较。数据可以整理成配对四格表。

表6-2 配对四格表资料的一般形式

甲法	乙法		合计
	+	-	
+	a	b	a+b
-	c	d	c+d
合计	a+c	b+d	a+b+c+d

$b+c>40$ 时，公式：

$$\chi^2 = \frac{(b-c)^2}{(b+c)}, \quad \nu = 1 \tag{公式6-5}$$

$b+c \leqslant 40$ 时，校正公式：

$$\chi_c^2 = \frac{(|b-c|-1)^2}{(b+c)}, \quad \nu = 1 \tag{公式6-6}$$

（5）行×列表资料的 χ^2 检验用于完全随机设计多个率或构成比的比较，数据可以整理成列联表。适用条件是不能超过1/5格子的理论频数小于5或不能有任一格子的理论频数小于1。检验统计量除用基本公式计算外，可用下面公式。

$$\chi^2 = n\left(\sum \frac{A^2}{n_R n_C} - 1\right), \quad \nu = (R-1) \times (C-1) \tag{公式6-7}$$

三、实验材料

材料一

某研究探讨环境温度对斯氏按蚊传疟能力的影响，分别在24℃和28℃温度下利用约氏疟原虫感染斯氏按蚊，9天后解剖蚊中肠，荧光显微镜下观察疟原虫卵囊发育情况并计数，结果见表6-3。比较不同温度条件下的疟原虫感染率。

表6-3 不同温度下斯氏按蚊感染约氏疟原虫情况

组别	未感染按蚊数	感染按蚊数	按蚊总数	感染率/%
24℃	3	33	36	91.7
28℃	30	19	49	38.3

材料二

某研究欲建立更省时、特异，可对登革1型病毒进行早期诊断的实时荧光定量PCR方法，荧光定量PCR对166份疑似登革1型病人血清的检测结果与登革病毒种特异引物探针检测结果完全一致，并与常规PCR检测结果进行比较，结果见表6-4。荧光定量PCR阳性率是否高于常规PCR？

表6-4 荧光定量PCR和常规PCR

荧光定量PCR	常规PCR		合计
	阳性	阴性	
阳性	36	90	126
阴性	0	40	40
合计	36	130	166

材料三

某课题采用随机、对照、多中心试验探讨医用臭氧与甘利欣胶囊对照治疗慢性乙型病毒肝炎的疗效。将175例慢性乙肝患者随机分成3组，分别是A组（国产医用臭氧发生仪治疗组）58例，B组（德国赫美斯医用臭氧发生仪治疗组）62例，C组（甘利欣胶囊口服治疗组）55例。12周疗程后，3组患者病毒应答率如下表。3种疗法效果是否有差异？

表6-5 三组患者治疗12周后病毒应答情况

组别	例数	应答例数	应答率/%
A组	58	13	22.4
B组	62	10	16.4
C组	55	6	10.9
合计	175	29	17.6

四、实验步骤

材料一

1. 设计类型

实验是在24℃和28℃两个温度下，用约氏疟原虫感染斯氏按蚊，属于完全随机设计类型。

2. 数据类型

实验结局是每只按蚊是否感染约氏疟原虫，是或者否，属于二分类数据。

3. 假设检验方法

2个处理组，结局为两种分类，实验数据可以整理成四格表形式，比较2个温度条件下疟原虫感染率是否有差异，可以用四格表资料χ^2检验。

（1）建立检验假设，确定检验水准。

$H_0: \pi_1 = \pi_2$，即2个温度条件下疟原虫感染率无差异。

$H_1: \pi_1 \neq \pi_2$，即2个温度条件下疟原虫感染率有差异。

$\alpha = 0.05$。

（2）计算检验统计量。

第一步：资料整理成四格表形式，确定a, b, c, d 4个实际频数。

表6-6 不同温度下斯氏按蚊感染约氏疟原虫四格表

组别	未感染按蚊数	感染按蚊数	合计
24℃	3（a）	33（b）	36
28℃	30（c）	19（d）	49
合计	33	52	85

第二步：条件判断。

$n = n_1 + n_2 = 36 + 49 = 85 > 40$

$T_a = \dfrac{36 \times 33}{85} = 14.0 \qquad T_b = \dfrac{36 \times 52}{85} = 22.0$

$T_c = \dfrac{49 \times 33}{85} = 19.0 \qquad T_d = \dfrac{49 \times 52}{85} = 30.0$

4个格子理论频数都大于5，不需要校正，可以选择基本公式或专用公式。

第三步：计算检验统计量，采用专用公式。

$$\chi^2 = \dfrac{(ad-bc)^2 n}{(a+b)(c+d)(a+c)(b+d)}$$

$$= \dfrac{(3 \times 19 - 33 \times 30)^2 \times 49}{(3+33)(30+19)(3+30)(33+19)} = 24.444$$

（3）确定 P 值大小，作出统计推断结论。

以自由度 $\nu = 1$，查 χ^2 界值表，$\chi^2_{0.05,1} = 3.84$。检验统计量 $\chi^2 > \chi^2_{0.05,1}$，$P < \alpha$，按检验水准 $\alpha = 0.05$，拒绝 H_0，接受 H_1，差异有统计学意义；可以认为两个温度条件下疟原虫感染率有差异。

材料二

1. 设计类型

本研究中，每份病人血清分别用荧光定量 PCR 和常规 PCR 两种方法检测，故为配对设计类型。

2. 数据类型

荧光定量 PCR、常规 PCR 两种方法检测给出阳性或阴性两种结果，所以为二分类数据。

3. 假设检验方法

配对设计，两种方法检测结果为互不相容的两种，整理成配对四格表资料。比较荧光定量 PCR 阳性率是否高于常规 PCR，使用配对四格表资料 χ^2 检验。

（1）建立检验假设，确定检验水准。

$H_0: B = C$，即荧光定量 PCR 阳性率与常规 PCR 阳性率相同。

$H_1: B \neq C$，即荧光定量 PCR 阳性率与常规 PCR 阳性率不同。

$\alpha = 0.05$。

(2) 计算检验统计量。

第一步：确定 b，c 两个实际频数。

表6-7 荧光定量 PCR 和常规 PCR 配对四格表

荧光定量 PCR	常规 PCR		合计
	阳性	阴性	
阳性	36	90（b）	126
阴性	0（c）	40	40
合计	36	130	166

第二步：条件判断。

$b + c = 90 + 0 = 90 > 40$，不需要校正。

第三步：计算检验统计量。

$$\chi^2 = \frac{(b-c)^2}{(b+c)} = \frac{(90-0)^2}{90+0} = 90$$

(3) 确定 P 值大小，作出统计推断结论。

以自由度 $\nu = 1$，查 χ^2 界值表，$\chi^2_{0.05,1} = 3.84$。检验统计量 $\chi^2 > \chi^2_{0.05,1}$，$P < \alpha$，按检验水准 $\alpha = 0.05$，拒绝 H_0，接受 H_1，差异有统计学意义；可以认为荧光定量 PCR 阳性率高于常规 PCR。

材料三

1. 设计类型

临床试验中，将慢性乙肝患者随机分成3组，分别接受国产医用臭氧发生仪治疗、德国赫美斯医用臭氧发生仪治疗和甘利欣胶囊口服治疗，属于完全随机设计类型。

2. 数据类型

治疗12周后，检测患者体内病毒是否应答，为二分类数据。

3. 假设检验方法

完全随机设计3个处理组，结局指标为病毒是否应答，数据可以整理成行×列表形式。推断3组患者病毒应答率是否有差异，使用行×列表 χ^2 检验。

(1) 建立检验假设，确定检验水准。

$H_0: \pi_1 = \pi_2 = \pi_3$，即3种疗法效果无差异。

$H_1: \pi_1$、π_2、π_3 不全相同，即3种疗法效果不全相同。

$\alpha = 0.05$。

(2) 计算检验统计量。

第一步：资料整理成行×列表，确定每个格子的实际频数。

表6-8 3组患者治疗12周后病毒应答行×列表

组别	例数	应答例数	未答应例数
A组	58（n_1）	13	45
B组	62（n_2）	10	52
C组	55（n_3）	6	49
合计	175（n）	29	146

第二步：条件判断。

最小的理论频数 $T = \dfrac{n_R n_C}{n} = \dfrac{55 \times 29}{175} = 9.1 > 5$，故没有格子的理论频数小于5。

第三步：计算检验统计量。

$$\chi^2 = n\left(\sum \dfrac{A^2}{n_R n_C} - 1\right) = 175 \times \left(\dfrac{13^2}{58 \times 29} + L + \dfrac{49^2}{55 \times 136} - 1\right) = 2.716$$

（3）确定 P 值大小，做出统计推断结论。

以自由度 $\nu = 2$，查 χ^2 界值表，$\chi^2_{0.05,2} = 5.99$。检验统计量 $\chi^2 < \chi^2_{0.05,2}$，$P > \alpha$，按检验水准 $\alpha = 0.05$，不拒绝 H_0，差异无统计学意义；尚不能认为三种疗法治疗慢性乙肝病毒肝炎效果有差异。

五、课后练习

（1）分析四格表资料时，通常在什么情况下需要进行连续性校正？（　　）
A. $1 < T < 5$ 且 $n > 40$　　　　　　　B. $T < 5$
C. $T < 1$ 或 $n < 40$　　　　　　　　　D. $T < 1$ 且 $n \geq 40$

（2）四格表 χ^2 检验不需要校正公式的应用条件为（　　）
A. $n > 40$ 且 $T > 5$　　　　　　　　　B. $n < 40$ 且 $T > 5$
C. $n > 40$ 且 $1 < T < 5$　　　　　　　D. $n < 40$ 且 $1 < T < 5$

（3）某研究欲探讨热带地区特有的高温、高湿气候对医院感染的威胁，监测某三级甲等医院一年住院患者，按季度分析感染率的情况，结果见表6-9。四个季度医院感染发病率是否不同？（　　）

表6-9 不同季度医院感染发病率

季度	监测例数	感染例数	感染率/%
第一季度	24604	436	1.77
第二季度	28979	575	1.98
第三季度	28433	518	1.82
第四季度	30624	497	1.62
合计	112640	2026	1.80

A. 四格表 χ^2 检验，不校正公式
B. 四格表 χ^2 检验，校正公式
C. 配对设计 χ^2 检验
D. 行×列表 χ^2 检验

（4）采用乳糖多管发酵法与酶底物法同时检测 96 份生活饮用水样中大肠埃希菌的情况，乳糖多管发酵法检出率为 83.3%，酶底物法检出率为 89.6%，两法同为阳性率为 78.1%，推断两种方法检出率是否有差别应使用的假设检验方法是（　　）

A. 四格表 χ^2 检验
B. 配对设计 χ^2 检验
C. 行×列表 χ^2 检验
D. t 检验

（5）拟探讨海南热带中草药治疗膝骨性关节炎的疗效，将 90 例膝骨性关节炎患者随机分成 2 组，治疗组使用海南热带中草药熏洗膝关节，对照组选用双氯芬酸二乙胺乳局部外用，涂布于患侧膝关节，治疗 3 周后结果见表 6-10。比较两组有效率是否有差别选用的方法是（　　）

表 6-10　治疗组和对照组临床疗效的比较

组别	例数	有效	无效	有效率/%
治疗组	45	42	3	93.3
对照组	45	34	11	75.5

A. 四格表 χ^2 检验，不校正公式
B. 四格表 χ^2 检验，校正公式
C. 配对设计 χ^2 检验
D. 行×列表 χ^2 检验

（苏　晶）

Chapter Two | Practical for Epidemiology
第二章 | 流行病学案例及习题

Experiment 7   Disease Frequency Measurements

Ⅰ. Objectives

To master the definition, application conditions and calculation methods of disease frequency measurement indicators which are commonly used in epidemiological studies.

Ⅱ. Principles

(1) The key indicators for the measurement of incidence frequency include incidence rate, attack rate, and secondary attack rate.

(2) Incidence rate (IR) is defined as the number of new cases of a disease that occur during a specified period of time in a population at risk for developing the disease. The calculation formula is as below (Formula 7 – 1).

$$IR = \frac{\text{The number of new cases of a disease}}{\text{The number of exposed people in the same period}} \times K \quad \text{(Formula 7 – 1)}$$

$K = 100\%, 1000‰, \cdots$

Notes: If a person has multiple illnesses during the observation period, the number of cases should be counted as multiple, such as influenza, diarrhea, and other diseases. The number of people exposed to the disease during the same period is the number of people who are likely to develop the disease during the same period, and those who had the disease or have the immunity of the disease need to be excluded. The observation period, usually 1 year, is required to calculate the incidence rate.

(3) The attack rate (AR) is usually used to measure a disease outbreak within a geographic location and within a short period of time. The calculation formula is same as the incidence rate calculation formula, but the observation period is relative shorter, it can be a day, a week, ten days, a month. The AR is often used to calculate the incidence of outbreaks of food, occupational poisoning, and infectious diseases.

$$AR = \frac{\text{New cases of a disease during the observation period}}{\text{The number of exposed people in the same period}} \times K \quad \text{(Formula 7 – 2)}$$

$K = 100\%, 1000‰, \cdots$

(4) Secondary attack rate (SAR), also known as the second-generation incidence rate. It measures the proportion of the number of infected persons in the total number of susceptible persons from the shortest to the longest incubation period of a certain infectious disease. In epidemiological studies, SAR is often used to reflect the infectivity of infectious diseases.

$$SAR = \frac{\text{The number of cases in susceptible contacts during incubation period}}{\text{Total number of susceptible contacts}} \times 100\%$$

(Formula 7 – 3)

(5) The key indicators for the measurement of prevalence frequency include prevalence rate and prevalence of infection.

(6) Prevalence, also known as present rate, is the proportion of new and old cases of a disease in the total population at a given time. The prevalence can be divided into time point prevalence and time period prevalence according to different observation time. The observation period for the time point prevalence is generally no more than one month, while the observation period for the time period prevalence is usually several months to one year. The calculation formulas are as below (Formula 7-4 and 7-5).

$$\text{Time point prevalence} = \frac{\text{The number of new and old cases of a certain disease}}{\text{The total number of this population at that point time}} \times K$$

(Formula 7-4)

$$\text{Time period prevalence} = \frac{\text{The number of new and old cases of a certain disease}}{\text{The average number of this population at that period time}} \times K$$

(Formula 7-5)

$K = 100\%, 1000\text{‰}, \cdots$

The prevalence rate is usually used to reflect the current condition of the disease, which can reflect the prevalence of chronic diseases with a longer course of disease.

(7) Prevalence of infection is the proportion of infected persons (with a pathogen) in a population examined within a certain period of time. It is indeed the prevalence rate in the field of infectious diseases. The calculation formula is as below (Formula 7-6).

$$\text{Prevalence of infection} = \frac{\text{The number of infected subjects}}{\text{Total number of people examined}} \times 100\% \quad (\text{Formula 7-6})$$

(8) The key indicators for the measurement of mortality frequency include mortality rate, case fatality rate, and survival rate.

(9) Mortality rate is the proportion deaths in a given population in a given period of time. It is the most commonly used indicator for measuring death in a population. The numerator is the number of deaths and the denominator is the average population size in the same period. The observation time is often measured in years. The calculation formula is as below (Formula 7-7).

$$\text{Mortality rate} = \frac{\text{The total number of deaths in a given population in a given year}}{\text{The average size of the population in the same year}} \times K$$

(Formula 7-7)

$K = 100\%, 1000\text{‰}, \cdots$

The mortality rate calculated according to the above formula is also known as crude mortality rate. Crude mortality rates in different regions cannot be directly compared and need to be standardized. Mortality rate can be calculated according to different demographic characteristics (such as age, sex, occupation, ethnicity, etc.), which is called as specific mortality rate. For example, the specific mortality rates for different genders and ages are calculated as below (Formula 7-8 and 7-9).

$$\text{The male specific mortality rate} = \frac{\text{Total male deaths in a given year}}{\text{The average number of male in the same year}} \times K$$

(Formula 7 – 8)

The specific mortality rate between 40 and 50 years old =

$$\frac{\text{The total number of deaths in a given year among people aged 40 to 50}}{\text{The average number of people aged 40 to 50 in the same year}} \times K$$

(Formula 7 – 9)

$K = 100\%, 1000, ‰\cdots$

(10) The case fatality rate refers to the proportion of people who die of a disease in a given period of time. It is the probability of death due to a disease among patients whom diagnosed with this disease. It can reflect the severity of a disease, the level of a medical care, and/or treatment. It can be used for measuring infectious diseases or chronic diseases. The formula for calculation case fatality rate is calculated as below (Formula 7 – 10).

$$\text{Case fatality rate} = \frac{\text{The number of deaths caused by a disease in a given period}}{\text{The number of cases of a disease in the same period}} \times 100\%$$

(Formula 7 – 10)

(11) Survival rate refers to the proportion of patients receiving a particular treatment or with a disease who are still alive after n years of follow-up. The calculation formula is calculated as below (Formula 7 – 11).

$$\text{Survival rate} = \frac{\text{The number of patients who survived after } n \text{ years of follow-up}}{\text{The total number of cases after followed-up for } n \text{ years}} \times 100\%$$

(Formula 7 – 11)

Ⅲ. Materials

Material I

COVID – 19 pandemic has affected our lives tremendously. A study analyzed the epidemic characteristics of COVID – 19 in Ningxia Province, China, to provide some basis information for COVID preventing and controlling among different stakeholders including government sectors. Based on the data collected regarding the three – dimension distribution of newly diagnosed COVID – 19 cases in Ningxia from January 22 to March 31, 2020, it shows a total of 75 individuals were newly diagnosed. The characteristics of study population including age, sex, and geographic location are shown in Table 7 – 1.

Table 7-1 Distribution of COVID-19 cases in Ningxia Province

	Reported cases	Population	Incidence rate
Total	75	6818182	
Sex			
Males	41	3388430	
Females	34	3429752	
Years of age			
0～19	6	1714286	
20～39	35	2215190	
40～59	21	2000000	
60～79	13	866667	
Geographic location			
Yinchuan city	37	2256098	
Wuzhong city	28	1414141	
Guyuan city	5	1250000	
Zhongwei city	4	1176471	

Question: Please calculate the total incidence rate of COVID - 19 of the whole study population and the incidence rates of the subgroup of population with different characteristics.

Material Ⅱ

On May 1, 2019, at 9:00 pm, a city Center for Disease Control and Prevention (CDCP) received a report from a hospital emergency department reporting that there were more than 30 patients were sick with symptoms of nausea, vomiting, abdominal pain and diarrhea. All of them were from one company, thus were suspected suffering from a mass food poisoning outbreak. The CDCP started a rapid epidemiological investigation and found that, 400 employees in this company had joined "team building activities", and after had a meal together, 55 of them developed these symptoms within 2 days.

Question 1: Which indicator should be used to measure the disease frequency in this case?
Question 2: How to calculate that indicator?

Material Ⅲ

In order to know the infection of Toxoplasma in different border areas of Yunnan Province, China, 561 human blood samples were collected from three border areas of Yunnan Province between November 2015 and May 2016. Of these samples, 222 were form the China-Vietnam boarder, 170 from the China - Laos border, and 169 from the China - Myanmar border. The anti - toxoplasma IgG antibody in serum was detected using enzyme-linked immunosorbent assay (ELISA). The number of samples with IgG positive were 19, 15, and 10 from China - Laos, China - Vietnam, and China - Myanmar borders area, respectively.

Question 1: Which indicator should be used to measure the disease frequency in this case?
Question 2: Please calculate that indicator of the total population, China-Laos, China-

Vietnam and China-Myanmar border population, respectively.

Material Ⅳ

On January 1st, 2019, a team of researchers conducted a health examination among 1000 elderly (aged 65~90 years old) from a community, of whom, 250 were diagnosed with diabetes. The same year, on December 30th, another 300 elderly people in the community were diagnosed with diabetes. Between these two examinations, 40 individuals died including 10 died from diabetes.

Question 1: Please calculate the prevalence and incidence rate of diabetes in the elderly population in this community in 2019.

Question 2: What are the differences between the prevalence and incidence rate?

Question 3: Please calculate the mortality rate and diabetes fatality rate for the elderly population in this community in 2019.

Question 4: What are the differences between the calculation of mortality rate and case fatality rate?

Ⅳ. Exercises

(1) The subjects of epidemiology are (   )

A. Special patients　　B. Ordinary patients　　C. Healthy subject　　D. Population

(2) Incidence rate indicators are derived from (   )

A. Survey of hospitalized patients　　　　B. Survey of outpatients

C. Survey of community population　　　D. Survey of all patients

(3) Which of the following factors can account for the change in incidence rate? (   )

A. Effectiveness of epidemic prevention measures

B. Increase or decrease in diseases treatment level

C. Improvement of disease diagnosis

D. Changes in diagnostic criteria

(4) Which of the following factors is associated with the change in prevalence rate? (   )

A. Increase or decrease in disease incidence

B. Increase or decrease of case fatality rate

C. Total number of people increases or decreases

D. Survival time

(5) What index should be used to evaluate the clinical rescue effect of acute myocardial infarction? (   )

A. Incidence rate　　　　　　　　　　B. Prevalence rate

C. Mortality rate　　　　　　　　　　D. Case fatality rate

实验七　疾病频率测量

一、实验目的
掌握流行病学研究中常用的疾病频率测量指标的含义、应用条件及计算方法。

二、实验原理
(1) 发病频率测量关键指标：发病率、罹患率、续发率。

(2) 发病率，是指一定期间内，一定范围内人群中某病新发病例出现的频率。计算公式为：

$$发病率 = \frac{一定时期内某人群中某病新病例数}{同期该人群暴露人口数} \times K \quad （公式7-1）$$

$K = 100\%, 1000‰, \cdots$

注意：若观察期内一个人多次发病时，应计算为多个发病病例数，如流感、腹泻等疾病。同期该人群暴露人口数是指同期可能患该病的人群，那些已经患病或者具有免疫力不会患病的人需要排除。计算发病率时一般需要规定观察时间，一般是1年。

(3) 罹患率，通常指在某一局限范围短时间内的发病率。其计算公式与发病率相同，但它的观察时间较短，可以日、周、旬、月为单位，使用比较灵活。常用于计算食物、职业中毒及传染病暴发的发病率。

$$罹患率 = \frac{观察期间某病新病例数}{同期暴露人口数} \times K \quad （公式7-2）$$

$K = 100\%, 1000‰, \cdots$

(4) 续发率：也称二代发病率，指某些传染病在最短潜伏期到最长潜伏期之间，易感接触者中发病人数占所有易感接触者总数的百分比。续发率常用于传染病流行病学调查，可用于比较传染病传染力强弱。

$$续发率 = \frac{潜伏期内易感接触者中发病人数}{易感接触者总人数} \times 100\% \quad （公式7-3）$$

(5) 患病频率测量关键指标：患病率、感染率。

(6) 患病率，也称现患率，是指某特定时间内总人口中某病新旧病例所占的比例。患病率可按照观察时间不同分为时点患病率和期间患病率。时点患病率的观察时间一般不超过一个月，而期间患病率的观察时间通常为几个月至1年。计算公式分别为：

$$时点患病率 = \frac{某一时点某人群中某病新旧病例数}{该时点人口数} \times K \quad （公式7-4）$$

$$期间患病率 = \frac{某观察期间某人群中某病的新旧病例数}{同期的平均人口数} \times K \quad （公式7-5）$$

$K = 100\%, 1000‰, \cdots$

患病率通常用来反映疾病的现患状况，可反映病程较长的慢性病的流行情况。

（7）感染率，是指在某时间内被检人群中某病原体现有感染者人数所占比例，是患病率在传染病领域的应用。计算公式为：

$$\text{感染率} = \frac{\text{受检者中感染人数}}{\text{受检人数}} \times 100\% \tag{公式 7-6}$$

（8）死亡频率测量关键指标：死亡率、病死率、生存率。

（9）死亡率，表示一定期间内，某人群中总死亡人数在该人群中所占的比例，是测量人群死亡危险最常用的指标。分子为死亡人数，分母为该人群同期平均人口数。观察时间常以年为单位。计算公式为：

$$\text{死亡率} = \frac{\text{某人群某年总死亡人数}}{\text{该人群同年平均人口数}} \times K \tag{公式 7-7}$$

$K = 100\%，1000‰，\cdots$

根据上述公式计算得出的死亡率也叫作粗死亡率。不同地区死亡率不能直接进行比较，需要做标化处理。死亡率可按照不同人口学特征（如年龄、性别、职业、民族等）分别计算，则为死亡专率。如性别、年龄死亡专率的计算公式为：

$$\text{男性死亡专率} = \frac{\text{男性某年总死亡人数}}{\text{男性同年平均人口数}} \times K \tag{公式 7-8}$$

$$40 \sim 50 \text{ 岁死亡专率} = \frac{40 \sim 50 \text{ 岁人群某年总死亡人数}}{40 \sim 50 \text{ 岁人群同年平均人口数}} \times K \tag{公式 7-9}$$

$K = 100\%，1000‰，\cdots$

（10）病死率，表示一定时期内因某病死亡者占该病病人的比例，表示某病病人因该病死亡的危险性。病死率表示确诊某病病人的死亡概率，它可以反映疾病的严重程度，也可以反映医疗水平和诊治能力，常用于传染病，也可用于慢性病。计算公式为：

$$\text{病死率} = \frac{\text{某时期内因某病死亡人数}}{\text{同期某病的病人数}} \times 100\% \tag{公式 7-10}$$

（11）生存率，是指接受某种治疗的病人或某病病人中，经 n 年随访仍然存活的病人数所占的比例。计算公式为：

$$\text{生存率} = \frac{\text{随访满 } n \text{ 年仍然存活的病例数}}{\text{随访满 } n \text{ 年的病例数}} \times 100\% \tag{公式 7-11}$$

三、实验材料

材料一

2020 年，全球新型冠状病毒感染的肺炎（新冠肺炎）疫情大流行，严重影响人类健康。某研究分析了中国宁夏回族自治区新冠肺炎疫情流行特征，为疫情防控和策略制定提供依据。通过现场流行病学调查收集相关数据，采用描述流行病学的方法，分析 2020 年 1 月 22 日至 3 月 31 日宁夏新冠肺炎确诊病例的三间分布特征。其间累计报告新冠肺炎确诊病例共 75 例，无症状感染者 1 例。病例的性别、年龄、地区分布特征及基本人口数如表 7-1 所示。

表 7-1 宁夏新冠肺炎病例人群特征分布情况

	报告发病数	人口数	发病率
总体	75	6818182	
性别			
男	41	3388430	
女	34	3429752	
年龄			
0～19	6	1714286	
20～39	35	2215190	
40～59	21	2000000	
60～79	13	866667	
地区			
银川市	37	2256098	
吴忠市	28	1414141	
固原市	5	1250000	
中卫市	4	1176471	

问题：请计算宁夏新冠肺炎总体报告发病率及各专项报告发病率。

材料二

2019 年 5 月 1 日 21 时，某市疾病预防控制中心接到辖区某医院急诊科报告接诊 30 余名有恶心、呕吐、腹痛、腹泻等症状的患者，均为某公司职员，疑似群体食物中毒事件。疾控人员迅速介入，通过相应流行病学调查，发现该公司 400 名员工于 5 月 1 日当天进行了团建活动，并在同一酒店集体用餐，其中 55 人在 2 天内陆续发病，经治疗均好转。

问题 1：该案例应该计算何指标来反应疾病频率？

问题 2：该指标应该如何计算？

材料三

为了解中国云南省边境地区不同民族、不同人群弓形虫感染情况，2015 年 11 月到 2016 年 5 月期间在云南省中老、中越、中缅 3 个边境地区采集人群血样 561 份（中越边境 222 份、中老边境 170 份、中缅边境 169 份），应用酶联免疫吸附测定法（Enzyme Linked Immuno Sorbent Assay，ELISA）检测血清中抗弓形虫 IgG 抗体，其中中老、中越、中缅边境阳性人数分别为 19、15、10 人。

问题 1：该案例应该计算何指标来反应疾病频率？

问题 2：请分别计算总人群、中老、中越、中缅边境人群该指标具体值。

材料四

研究者于 2019 年 1 月 1 日对某社区老年人群（65～90 岁）进行健康检查，该小区共有 1000 名该年龄段的老年人，其中 250 人被确诊为糖尿病。2019 年 12 月 30 日再次对该小区老年人进行检查,其中 300 人被确诊为糖尿病。该人群两次体检间隔期内死亡人数 40 人,其中 10 人死于糖尿病。

问题 1:请计算 2019 年该社区老年人群糖尿病患病率及发病率。
问题 2:患病率和发病率计算方法有何区别?
问题 3:请计算 2019 年该社区老年人群死亡率及糖尿病病死率。
问题 4:死亡率和病死率计算方法有何区别?

四、课后练习

(1) 流行病学的研究对象是(　　)
A. 特殊患者　　　　　B. 普通患者　　　　C. 健康者　　　　D. 人群
(2) 发病率指标来自(　　)
A. 对住院病人的调查　　　　　　　　B. 对门诊病人的调查
C. 对社区人群的调查　　　　　　　　D. 对所有病人的调查
(3) 下列哪项因素可以引起发病率的变化?(　　)
A. 防疫措施有效与否　　　　　　　　B. 治疗水平的升高或降低
C. 疾病诊断水平的提高　　　　　　　D. 诊断标准的变化
(4) 下列哪项因素与患病率的变化有关?(　　)
A. 发病率的升高或下降　　　　　　　B. 病死率的升高或下降
C. 人口总数增加或减少　　　　　　　D. 存活时间
(5) 对急性心梗评价临床抢救效果应采用何指标?(　　)
A. 发病率　　　　　B. 患病率　　　　C. 死亡率　　　　D. 病死率

Experiment 8　Disease Distribution

Ⅰ. Objectives

To describe the forms and characteristics of distribution of disease in a population, and to master the description methods of the three-dimension distribution.

Ⅱ. Principles

(1) Distribution of disease, also known as three-dimension distribution, is the existence of diseases in different populations, different times, and different regions, as well as the pattern of their occurrence and development. It describes the group of phenomenon of disease including disease onset, development/prognosis, and death, as well as its characteristics and patterns. It is one of the fundamental elements of epidemiological research.

(2) Characteristics of disease distribution in population perspective: The distribution of diseases or health states of population can be described from different age, gender, occupation, race and ethnic

group, marriage status, family structures, behavior and lifestyle, etc. To study these characteristics can help us to identify the demographic factors of disease or health status of a population.

(3) Characteristics of disease distribution in regional perspective: It can describe characteristics of a disease (health states) distribution in global, domestic, urban, rural, or local perspective.

(4) Endemic clustering means that the frequency of incidence, prevalence or mortality in an area is significantly higher than that in the surrounding area, that is, the frequency of disease in the area exceeds the random probability.

(5) Endemic diseases refer to the diseases that are relatively stable and frequently occur in some specific areas, also known as local diseases.

(6) The characteristics of disease temporal distributions include rapid fluctuation, seasonality (seasonal variation), periodicity (cyclic variation) and secular trend (secular change).

(7) Rapid fluctuation generally refers to the epidemic or outbreak of a disease lasting a few days, weeks or months, which is a special mode of existence of a disease. Rapid fluctuation is similar in meaning to outbreak. The difference between these two terms is that outbreak is often used to describe a small number of people, while rapid fluctuation is often used to describe a large number of people.

(8) Seasonality refers to the phenomenon that the incidence of diseases increases in a certain season. Seasonality has two forms, including strict seasonality and seasonal increase.

(9) Strict seasonality means that the incidence of a disease is concentrated in a few months of the year, and no cases occur in the other months. In some areas, the occurrence of insect-borne infectious diseases may be strictly seasonal.

(10) Seasonal increase means that the incidence is all the year round, but only increases in a certain month/s. For example, there are cases of intestinal and respiratory infectious diseases throughout the year, but the incidence of intestinal infectious diseases is increased in summer and autumn, while the incidence of respiratory infectious diseases is increased in winter and spring.

(11) The periodicity of disease refers to the phenomenon that the disease frequency fluctuates regularly in accordance with a certain time interval, and an epidemic peak appears every few years. The change of disease periodicity sees respiratory tract infectious disease more, be like influenza, epidemic cerebrospinal membrane inflammation, whooping cough, chicken pox, and so on.

(12) Secular trend, also known as secular change, is a change in the clinical characteristics, distribution, prevalence, etc. of a disease over a relatively long period of time, usually a few years or decades. For example, some diseases may show a trend of increasing or decreasing incidence over several years or decades.

(13) Migrant epidemiology is a typical example of a comprehensive description of the immigrant population in terms of time distribution of a disease and is a way of exploring its etiology. It is to explore the relationship between the occurrence of diseases and genetic factors or environmental factors by observing the differences in the incidence rate or mortality rate of diseases

among the immigrants, the local residents of the resettled places and the population of the original places. Migration epidemiology is often used to investigate the etiology and epidemic factors of tumors, chronic diseases and some genetic diseases.

(14) Epidemic intensity refers to the change in the incidence of a disease among the population in a given area, and the degree of association between the cases in a given period of time. It is commonly expressed as sporadic, outbreak, epidemic, and pandemic.

(15) Sporadic means that the incidence rate of a disease is the general level over the years, and there is no obvious temporal and spatial connection between cases, showing sporadic occurrence. Sporadic is generally described for a large area. Sporadic incidence is generally compared with local incidence in the last three years.

(16) An outbreak is the sudden occurrence of many patients with the same symptoms within a short period of time in a local area or collective unit. Most of these people share the same source of infection and transmission. Most patients often appear between the shortest and longest incubation periods of the disease.

(17) Epidemic means that the incidence rate of a disease in a certain region significantly exceeds the incidence rate level of the disease in the past years. Compared with the sporadic incidence of the disease, there is an obvious temporal and spatial connection between cases when the epidemic occurs. For example, the epidemic of COVID-19 presents a typical temporal and spatial association.

(18) Pandemic means that the incidence of a disease significantly exceeds the incidence level of the disease in previous years, the disease spreads rapidly, and in a short period of time crosses provincial boundaries, national boundaries, and even peripheral boundaries to form a worldwide epidemic, such as COVID-19, which rapidly develops into a global pandemic.

Ⅲ. Materials

Material Ⅰ

Malignant tumors (cancers) have become one of the major public health problems that seriously threaten the health of the Chinese population. According to the latest statistics in China, malignant tumors caused death account for 23.91% of all deaths. The incidence and deaths of malignant tumors in the past decade have been raised and it more likely will continually to rise. The annual medical expenses caused by malignant tumors exceed 220 billion, and the prevention and control situation is severe. In January 2019, the National Cancer Center released the latest national cancer statistics. Since the data of the National Cancer Registry generally lag behind the release of 3 years, the data shown in Figure 8-1, 8-2 and Table 8-1 is the 2015 National Cancer Registry data. The report showed that about 3.929 million malignant tumors occurred in 2015 and about 2.338 million people died. On average, more than 10000 people are diagnosed with cancer every day, and 7.5 people are diagnosed with cancer every minute. The detailed data are shown in Figure 8-1, 8-2 and Table 8-1.

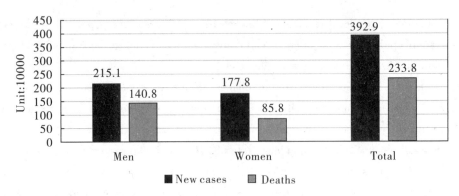

Figure 8-1　The new cancer cases and deaths in China, 2015

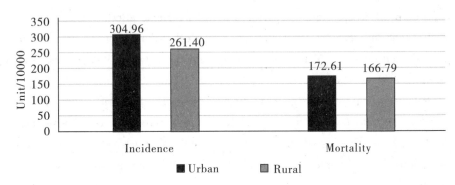

Figure 8-2　Distribution of cancer incidence rate and mortality rate in urban and rural in China, 2015

Table 8-1　Estimated cases and cancer incidences by geographic areas in China, 2015

Geographic areas	Gender	New cases (×1000)	Crude incidence (1/10^5)	ASIRC (1/10^5)[a]	ASIRW (1/10^5)[b]	Cumulative rate (0~74 years old)(%)
Eastern areas	Male	86.6	330.91	211.59	209.37	24.71
	Female	76.5	300.71	190.72	181.69	19.9
	Both	163.1	316.03	200	194.35	22.25
Middle areas	Male	72.2	303.71	212.67	211.79	25.23
	Female	58.6	261.67	174.58	168.48	18.72
	Both	130.8	283.33	192.51	189.03	21.94
Western areas	Male	56.3	274.98	197.58	196.34	22.92
	Female	42.7	222.43	154.9	149.42	16.63
	Both	99	249.51	175.5	172.15	19.75
All areas	Male	215.1	305.47	207.99	206.49	24.36
	Female	177.8	265.21	175.47	168.45	18.6
	Both	392.9	285.83	190.64	186.39	21.44

Notes: a: ASIRG: age-standardized incidence rate by Chinese standard population in 2000; b: ASIRW: age-standardized incidence rate by world standard population (Segi's population).

Question 1: Try to analyze the distribution characteristics of the number of new cases and deaths from cancer in 2015 in China as shown in Figure 8-1.

Question 2: Try to analyze the distribution characteristics of cancer incidence rate and mortality rate in China in 2015 as shown in Figure 8-2.

Question 3: Try to comprehensively analyze the characteristics of cancer incidence rate in China in 2015 as shown in Table 8-1.

Question 4: Based on the above information, what suggestions can be provided for tumor prevention?

Material Ⅱ

Malaria is an insect-borne infectious disease caused by the bite of anopheles mosquitoes or by the transmission of malaria parasites into the blood of people carrying malaria parasites through. It is also one of the most serious public health problems worldwide with high morbidity and mortality rates. Especially in tropical regions, malaria has severe impact on local populations. Sanya City, located in the southernmost tip of Hainan Province, is the only place in China with a typical tropical climate and used to be an area of high malaria prevalence. Try to analyze the characteristics of malaria prevalence and distribution in Sanya City during 1951-2018.

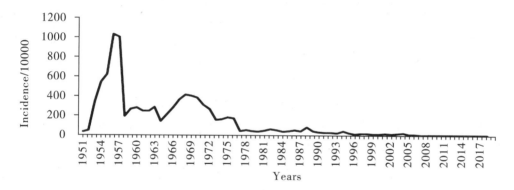

Figure 8-3 Trends of malaria incidence in Sanya City from 1951 to 2018

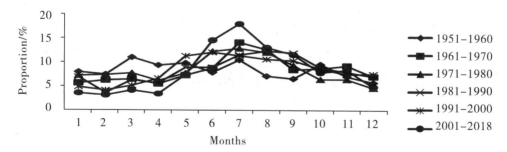

Figure 8-4 Seasonal distribution of malaria incidence in Sanya City, 1951-2018

Question 1: According to Figure 8-3, please analyze the characteristics of malaria distribution in Sanya City from 1951 to 2018.

Question 2: According to Figure 8-4, please analyze the seasonal distribution characteristics of malaria incidence in Sanya City from 1951 to 2018.

Question 3: What is seasonality in the temporal distribution of disease? What specific expression form does seasonality have?

Question 4: What characteristics are used to describe the temporal distribution of disease?

Ⅳ. Exercises

(1) The three-dimension distributions of diseases refer to ( )

A. Genetics, host, and environment

B. Human, space, and time

C. Age, gender, and occupation

D. Human, time, and heredity

(2) The fundamental principles of epidemiology do not include ( )

A. Describe the distribution characteristics of the disease

B. Explore the causes

C. Propose strategies for disease prevention

D. Provide individualized treatment to patients

(3) The time distribution of the disease does not include ( )

A. Epidemic   B. Outbreak   C. Periodicity   D. Seasonality

(4) Which epidemiological study can comprehensively describe the three-dimension distributions of the disease ( )

A. Birth cohort study   B. Cross-sectional study

C. Immigration Epidemiology study   D. Genetic epidemiology study

(5) The epidemic intensity of the disease includes ( )

A. Sporadic, outbreak, and epidemic

B. Epidemic, outbreak, and continuation

C. Outbreak, secondary, and epidemic

D. Renewed, secondary, and Sporadic

实验八 疾病的分布

一、实验目的

掌握流行病学研究中疾病在人群分布的形式及特点，掌握三间分布的描述方法。

二、实验原理

(1) 疾病的分布亦称三间分布，是指疾病在不同人群、不同时间、不同地区的存在状态及其发生、发展规律。疾病分布的主要内容是描述疾病的发病、患病和死亡的群体现象及其特点和规律。它是流行病学研究的基础。

（2）疾病的人群分布特征：可从不同年龄、性别、职业、种族和民族、婚姻与家庭、行为生活方式等角度描述疾病或健康状态的分布情况。研究这些相关特征，有助于探讨疾病或健康状态的影响因素或流行特征。

（3）疾病的地区分布特征：可以描述疾病或健康状态的全球分布特征、国内分布特征、城乡分布特征或地方性特征等。

（4）地区聚集性：某地区发病及患病等疾病频率高于周围地区的情况，该地区疾病频率超过了随机概率，称为疾病的地区聚集性。

（5）地方性疾病，是指局限于某些特定地区内相对稳定并经常发生的疾病，也称地方病。

（6）疾病的时间分布特征，包括短期波动、季节性、周期性、长期趋势。

（7）短期波动，一般是指持续几天、几周或几个月的疾病流行或疫情暴发，是疾病的特殊存在方式。其含义与暴发相近，区别在于暴发常用于少量人群，而短期波动常用于较大数量的人群。

（8）季节性，是指疾病在一定季节内呈现发病率增高的现象。季节性有两种表现形式，包括严格的季节性和季节性升高。

（9）严格的季节性，是指发病都集中在一年中的少数几个月，其余月份没有病例发生，某些地区以虫媒传播的传染病的发生可具有严格的季节性。

（10）季节性升高，是指一年四季均发病，但仅在一定月份发病率升高，如肠道传染病和呼吸道传染病，全年均有病例发生，但肠道传染病多见于夏秋季，而呼吸道传染病则在冬春季高发。

（11）疾病的周期性，是指疾病频率按照一定的时间间隔，有规律地起伏波动，每隔若干年出现一个流行高峰的现象。疾病周期性的变化多见于呼吸道传染病，如流行性感冒、流行性脑脊髓膜炎、百日咳、水痘等。

（12）长期趋势，也称长期变异或长期变动，是指在一个比较长的时间内、通常为几年或几十年，疾病的临床特征、分布状态、流行强度等方面所发生的变化。如某些疾病可表现出几年或几十年发病率持续上升或下降的趋势。

（13）移民流行病学是进行疾病人群、地区和时间分布综合描述的一个典型案例，是探讨疾病病因的一种方法。它是通过观察疾病在移民、移居地当地居民及原始地人群间的发病率或死亡率的差异，从而探讨疾病的发生与遗传因素或环境因素的关系。移民流行病学常用于肿瘤、慢性病及某些遗传病的病因和流行因素探讨。

（14）疾病流行强度是指一定时期内疾病在某地区人群中发病率的变化及其病例间的联系程度，常用散发、暴发、流行及大流行表示。

（15）散发，指发病率呈历年一般水平，各病例间在发病时间和地点上无明显联系，表现为散在发生。散发一般是对于范围较大的地区而言。散发一般与当地近 3 年的发病率进行比较。

（16）暴发，是指局部地区或集体单位，短时间内突然发生很多症状相同病人的现象。

这些人大多有相同的传染源和传播途径。大多数病人常同时出现在该病的最短和最长潜伏期之间。

（17）流行，是指在某地区某病的发病率显著超过该病历年发病率水平，相对于散发，流行出现时各病例之间呈现明显的时间和空间联系，如新冠肺炎的流行则呈现出典型的时间和空间关联。

（18）大流行，是指某病发病率显著超过该病历年发病率水平，疾病蔓延迅速，在短时间内跨越省界、国界甚至周界形成世界性流行，如新冠肺炎快速发展为大流行。

三、实验材料

材料一

恶性肿瘤（癌症）已经成为严重威胁中国人群健康的主要公共卫生问题之一。根据我国最新的统计数据，恶性肿瘤死亡占居民全部死因的23.91%，且近十几年来恶性肿瘤的发病率和死亡率均呈持续上升态势。每年恶性肿瘤所致的医疗花费超过2200亿元，防控形势严峻。2019年1月，国家癌症中心发布了最新一期全国癌症统计数据。由于全国肿瘤登记中心的数据一般滞后3年发布，图8-1和8-2以及表8-1展示数据为2015年全国肿瘤登记数据。该次报告主要发现2015年恶性肿瘤发病约392.9万人，死亡约233.8万人。平均每天超过1万人被确诊为癌症，每分钟有7.5个人被确诊为癌症。详细数据如图8-1和8-2以及表8-1所示。

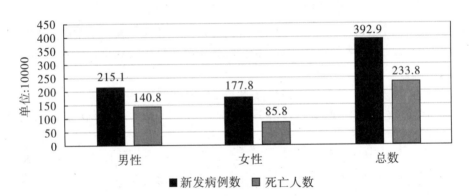

图8-1 我国2015年恶性肿瘤发病和死亡

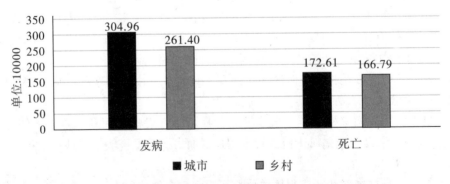

图8-2 我国2015年恶性肿瘤发病率和死亡率城乡分布情况

表 8-1 我国 2015 年不同地域恶性肿瘤新发病例数及发病率分布情况

地域	性别	新发病例数 (×1000)	粗发病率 (1/10^5)	中标发病率 (1/10^5)[a]	世标发病率 (1/10^5)[b]	0～74 岁累积发病率（%）
东部地区	男性	86.6	330.91	211.59	209.37	24.71
	女性	76.5	300.71	190.72	181.69	19.9
	总体	163.1	316.03	200	194.35	22.25
中部地区	男性	72.2	303.71	212.67	211.79	25.23
	女性	58.6	261.67	174.58	168.48	18.72
	总体	130.8	283.33	192.51	189.03	21.94
西部地区	男性	56.3	274.98	197.58	196.34	22.92
	女性	42.7	222.43	154.9	149.42	16.63
	总体	99	249.51	175.5	172.15	19.75
全国	男性	215.1	305.47	207.99	206.49	24.36
	女性	177.8	265.21	175.47	168.45	18.6
	总体	392.9	285.83	190.64	186.39	21.44

注：a. 中标发病率为按 2000 年中国标准人口计算的年龄标准化发病率；b. 世标发病率为按世界标准人口计算的年龄标准化发病率。

问题 1：试分析图 8-1 中 2015 年我国肿瘤新发病和死亡人数的分布特征。

问题 2：试分析图 8-2 中 2015 年我国肿瘤发病率和死亡率的分布特征。

问题 3：试综合分析表 8-1 中 2015 年我国肿瘤发病率的分布情况。

问题 4：根据以上信息，针对肿瘤的预防可以提供哪些意见和建议？

材料二

疟疾是经按蚊叮咬或输入带疟疾原虫者血液而感染疟原虫所引起的虫媒传染病，也是全球最严重的公共卫生问题之一，尤其在热带地区发病率和死亡率均高，对当地居民造成严重影响。海南省三亚市地处热带，是我国唯一一个具有典型热带气候的地区，曾是疟疾高流行地区。试分析 1951—2018 年三亚市疟疾流行与分布特征。

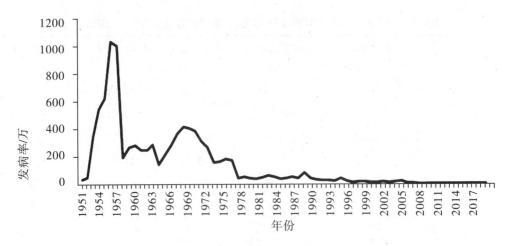

图8-3 三亚市1951—2018年疟疾发病率变化趋势

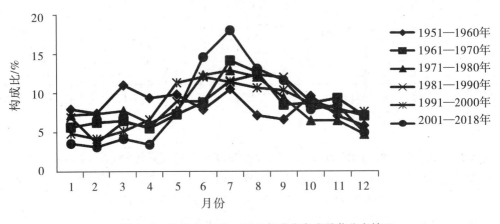

图8-4 三亚市1951—2018年疟疾发病季节分布情况

问题1：根据图8-3，试分析1951—2018年三亚市疟疾分布特征。

问题2：根据图8-4，试分析1951—2018年三亚市疟疾发病季节分布特征。

问题3：什么是疾病时间分布特征中的季节性？季节性有哪些具体的表现形式？

问题4：描述疾病时间分布特征总共有哪些？

四、课后练习

（1）疾病的三间分布是指（　　　）

A. 遗传、宿主、环境　　　　　　　　B. 人间、空间、时间

C. 年龄、性别、职业　　　　　　　　D. 人间、时间、遗传

（2）流行病学的基本任务不包括（　　　）

A. 描述疾病的分布特征　　　　　　　B. 探索病因

C. 提出预防疾病的措施　　　　　　　D. 对病人提供个体化的治疗

（3）疾病的时间分布特征不包括（　　　）

A. 流行　　　　　B. 暴发　　　　　C. 周期性　　　　　D. 季节性

(4) 综合地进行描述疾病三间分布的经典流行病学方法是（   ）
A. 出生队列研究　　　　　　　　B. 横断面研究
C. 移民流行病学研究　　　　　　D. 遗传流行病学研究
(5) 疾病的流行强度包括（   ）
A. 散发、暴发、流行　　　　　　B. 流行、暴发、续发
C. 暴发、继发、流行　　　　　　D. 续发、继发、散发

Experiment 9　Cross-sectional Study

Ⅰ. Objectives

To master the basic contents of the cross-sectional study design, and to understand the design principles, sampling methods, and main uses of the cross-sectional study in epidemiological research.

Ⅱ. Principles

(1) Cross-sectional survey: It is the collection and description of data on the distribution of diseases or health conditions and related factors in a specific time point (or period) in a specific range of population, to provide etiological clues for further study. As the study collects the data of a specific time section, it is also known as cross-sectional study. Since the frequency indicators obtained in the study are generally the prevalence rates of the investigated population in a specific time period, it is also called prevalence study.

(2) Cross-sectional study's characteristics: A cross-sectional study generally does not set up a control group at the study design stage; A cross-sectional study generally focuses on the relationship between exposure and disease in a group at a specific time point or period; A cross-sectional study generally cannot make causal inference (except for some fixed exposure factors such as gender, race, blood group, genotype, etc); Information on incidence rates can be obtained from periodic repetition of a cross-sectional study.

(3) The main uses of a cross-sectional survey are to identify high-risk groups and to evaluate the effectiveness of prevention programs, such as health education/promotion and vaccination.

(4) The cross-sectional study can be divided into census and sampling survey based on of the study subjects involved.

(5) Census survey, or population survey, refers to a survey that covers the whole population that targeted at a specific time point or period, such as a physical examination of all children under age 14 in a specific location.

(6) Sampling survey, through random sampling method, to investigate a representative sample of the population at a specific time point and within a specific range, and to estimate the

range of overall parameters with the statistics of the sample. It is a relatively common research method compare to census survey. The result from sampling survey is often used to infer the overall situation of the population which the samples were drawn.

(7) Random sampling is a sampling process follows the principle of randomization to ensure each object with non-zero probability is selected as the research object, in order to ensure the study samples have full representativeness of the whole population in target.

(8) The commonly used random sampling methods in cross-sectional studies include simple random sampling, systematic sampling, stratified sampling, cluster sampling, and multistage sampling.

(9) Simple random sampling is the simplest and most basic sampling method. From the population of N objects, n objects are selected by drawing dice or other random methods (such as random numbers) to form a sample. The important principle is that each object in the population has an equal probability of being drawn (all n/N).

(10) Systematic sampling, also known as mechanical sampling, is a sampling method in which units are mechanically sampled at intervals of several units in a certain order. The specific sampling method is as follows: Assuming the population unit number is N and the sample size to be investigated is n, then the sampling ratio is n/N and the sampling interval $K = N/n$. Each K units is a group, and then a starting number is determined in the first group by simple random method. From the starting point, one unit is selected from every K units as the study object, constituting the study sample.

(11) Stratified sampling, the population is firstly divided into several layers according to certain characteristics, and then simple random sampling is performed from each layer to form a sample. The smaller the individual variation within each layer, the better, while the greater the inter-layer variation, the better. Stratified sampling is more accurate than simple random sampling, which is convenient for organization and management, and it can ensure that individuals are drawn from each layer in the population. Stratified sampling is commonly used in cross-sectional studies.

(12) Cluster sampling is to divide the population into several groups, and select some of the groups as the observation unit to form a sample. This sampling method is called cluster sampling. Cluster sampling is easy to organize and implement, and can save manpower and material resources, but the sampling error can be large.

(13) Multistage sampling, which refers to phasing the sampling process, often uses different sampling methods at each stage, that is, the combination of the above methods is commonly used in large epidemiological surveys.

III. Materials

Osteoporosis less muscle obesity (osteosarcopenic obesity, OSO) is a complex systemic disease that includes three typical body damages, i.e. bone mass reduction or osteoporosis, sarcopenia and obesity. This group of people easily leads to fractures and blood lipid abnormalities, which are caused by related cardiovascular diseases, in middle-aged and older adults. The research data from South Korea and the United States shows that the prevalence of OSO among middle-aged and older women is 5.4% and 12.4%, respectively. However, there are few studies about OSO among Chinese people, especially ethnic minority groups. In the study presented below, five ethnic minority groups (Jing, Maonan, Miao, Mulao and Yao) were selected in Guangxi Zhuang Autonomous Region to investigate the distribution characteristics of osteoporosis and less muscle obesity among different ethnic groups and genders.

Question 1: What kind of epidemiological investigation is this? Is it a census or a sampling survey? Is it descriptive or analytical epidemiological study design?

Question 2: What are the characteristics of this research method? What are the main uses of this research method?

From August 2012 to August 2017, 2369 middle-aged and older adults were selected in Dongxing City, Maonan Autonomous County, Luocheng Yan Autonomous County, Meltwater Miao Autonomous County and Dahua Yi Autonomous County of Guangxi Zhuang Autonomous Region, by using random cluster sampling method. The basic demographic information was collected through a questionnaire. The BMI and muscle mass were measured using body component analyzer. The bone mineral density of right heel was measured using ultrasonic absorptiometry. Based on the measurement parameters, those patients with osteoporosis, sarcopenia, and obesity were diagnosed as the OSO patients.

Question 3: What are the methods of random sampling for cross-sectional study?

Question 4: What are the advantages and disadvantages of sampling methods in this study?

A total of 2369 subjects were enrolled with a mean age of 66.97 (±9.38) years, including 1361 females (mean age 66.36 ± 9.57 years). The distribution of gender and ethnicity of the study population is shown in Table 9 – 1.

Table 9 – 1 Comparison of OSO diseases by sex and ethnic group

Variables	Total number	OSO cases	Disease rate	x^2 value	P value
Gender					
Male	1008	68			
Female	1361	161			
Ethnic group				57.57	<0.001
Jing	466	64			
Maonan	520	79			
Miao	536	51			
Mulao	413	21			
Yao	434	14			

Question 5: What are the disease frequency indicators that can be calculated by cross-

sectional study design?

Question 6: Complete the calculation of Table 9 – 1 and interpret the results.

Question 7: What dimensions of the three-dimension distributions of disease are shown in Table 9 – 1?

Ⅳ. Exercises

(1) If you want to investigate the HBsAg carrying situation in Hainan Province, which of the following survey methods can be used (　　)

　　A. Case study　　　　　　　　　　B. Outbreak survey
　　C. Prospective survey　　　　　　　D. Sampling survey

(2) The main analytical indicator of the cross-sectional study is (　　)

　　A. Death composition ratio　　　　　B. Incidence of a disease
　　C. Prevalence of a disease　　　　　D. Mortality of a disease

(3) Which of the following sampling methods has the greatest sampling error in a sampling survey? (　　)

　　A. Simple random sampling　　　　　B. Systematic sampling
　　C. Stratified sampling　　　　　　　D. Cluster sampling

(4) What is the main purpose of cross-sectional study for a disease whose cause is unknown? (　　)

　　A. Determining the cause　　　　　　B. Verify the cause
　　C. Looking for clues to the cause　　D. Causal inference

(5) To investigate the prevalence of myopia in a primary school. Firstly, stratified according to grades, and then randomly selected 100 students from each level to participate in the survey. This sampling method is called (　　)

　　A. Simple random sampling　　　　　B. Systematic sampling
　　C. Stratified sampling　　　　　　　D. Cluster sampling

实验九　现况研究

一、实验目的

掌握现况研究设计的基本内容，理解现况研究的设计原理、抽样方法及主要用途。

二、实验原理

(1) 现况调查定义：是通过对特定时点（或时期）和特定范围内人群中的疾病或健康状况和有关因素的分布状况的资料收集、描述，从而为进一步的研究提供病因线索。从时间上来说，现况研究收集的是某特定的时间断面的资料，故又称为横断面研究。从观察分析指标来说，由于该种研究所得到的频率指标一般为特定时间内调查群体的患病率，故也称为患病率研究。

（2）现况调查的特点：现况调查在研究设计阶段一般不设立对照组；现况调查关注的一般是某一特定时点或时期内某一群体中暴露与疾病的关联；现况调查结果一般不能做因果关系推论（除去某些固定暴露因素如性别、种族、血型、基因型等）；现况调查定期重复进行可以获得发病率的资料。

（3）现况调查的主要用途为：确定高危人群；评价疾病监测、预防接种等防制措施的效果。

（4）现况调查根据涉及研究对象的范围可分为普查和抽样调查。

（5）普查，即全面调查，是指在特定时点或时间内，以特定范围内的全部人群（总体）作为研究对象的调查，如对某地全部儿童（≤14岁）进行体格检查。

（6）抽样调查，是指通过随机抽样的方法，对特定时点、特定范围内人群的一个代表性样本进行调查，以样本的统计量来估计总体参数所在范围。它相对于普查是一种比较常用的现况研究方法。抽样调查是以样本的调查结果来推论总体的情况。

（7）随机抽样，是指抽样过程遵循随机化原则，保证总体中每一个对象都有已知的非零的概率被选为研究对象，以保证样本的代表性。

（8）现况调查常用的随机抽样方法有：单纯随机抽样、系统抽样、分层抽样、整群抽样、多阶段抽样。

（9）单纯随机抽样，也称简单随机抽样，是最简单、最基本的抽样方法。从总体 N 个对象中，利用抽签或其他随机方法（如随机数字）抽取 n 个，构成一个样本。它的重要原则是总体中每个对象被抽到的概率相等（均为 n/N）。

（10）系统抽样，又称机械抽样，是按照一定顺序，机械地每隔若干单位抽取一个单位的抽样方法。具体抽样方法如下：假设总体单位数为 N，需要调查的样本数为 n，则抽样比为 n/N，抽样间隔 $K=N/n$。每 K 个单位为一组，然后用单纯随机方法在第一组中确定一个起始号，从此起始点开始，每隔 K 个单位抽取一个作为研究对象，构成研究样本。

（11）分层抽样，是指先将总体按照某种特征分为若干层，然后再从每一层内进行单纯随机抽样，组成一个样本。每一层内个体变异越小越好，层间变异则越大越好。分层抽样比单纯随机抽样所得到的结果精确度更高，组织管理方便，而且它能保证总体中每一层都有个体被抽到。现况调查中常用到分层抽样。

（12）整群抽样，是将总体分成若干群组，抽取其中部分群组作为观察单位组成样本，这种抽样方法称为整群抽样。整群抽样易于组织、实施方便，可以节省人力、物力，但是抽样误差较大。

（13）多阶段抽样，是指将抽样过程分阶段进行，每个阶段使用的抽样方法往往不同，即将上述方法结合使用，在大型流行病学调查中常用。

三、实验材料

骨质疏松性少肌性肥胖（osteosarcopenic obesity，OSO）是一种复杂的全身性疾病，包含3种典型的机体受损情况，即骨量减少或骨质疏松、少肌症及肥胖。该类人群极易导致骨折和血脂异常引发的相关心脑血管疾病，常见于中老年群体。韩国和美国的研究数据显示，中老年女性人群 OSO 患病率分别为 5.4% 和 12.4%。但关于国内人群 OSO 的报道较少，尤其是少数民族群体。本研究在广西壮族自治区选取 5 个少数民族人群（京族、毛南族、苗族、仫佬族和瑶族）开展调查，了解骨质疏松性少肌性肥胖症在不同民族、不同性别间的分布特点。

问题 1：这是一种什么性质的流行病学调查，是普查还是抽样调查，是描述性的还是分析性的？

问题 2：该种研究方法有何特点？其应用范围包括哪些方面？

2012 年 8 月至 2017 年 8 月期间，在广西壮族自治区的东兴市江平镇、环江毛南族自治县、罗城仫佬族自治县、融水苗族自治县和大化瑶族自治县随机整群抽取 2369 例中老年人作为研究对象。通过问卷调查其基本信息。采用人体体成分分析仪测量 BMI 及肌肉量，超声骨密度仪测量右脚跟骨骨密度，根据相应测量值同时满足骨质疏松、少肌症及肥胖则诊断为 OSO 患者。

问题 3：随机抽样调查的方法有哪些？

问题 4：本研究抽样方法的优缺点是什么？

该研究共纳入 2369 名受试者，平均年龄（66.97±9.38）岁，女性 1361 名，平均年龄（66.36±9.57）岁。性别、年龄、民族分布情况见表 9-1。

表 9-1 不同性别、民族 OSO 疾病情况比较

变量	人数	OSO 例数	疾病指标	x^2 值	P 值
性别					
男性	1008	68			
女性	1361	161			
民族				57.57	<0.001
京族	466	64			
毛南族	520	79			
苗族	536	51			
仫佬族	413	21			
瑶族	434	14			

问题 5：本研究方法能计算的疾病频率指标是什么？

问题 6：完成表 9-1 的计算，并对结果进行解释。

问题 7：上述数据是展示疾病三间分布中什么维度的分布特征？

四、课后习题

（1）若想调查海南省 HBsAg 携带情况，可采用（　　）

A. 个案调查　　　B. 暴发调查　　　C. 前瞻性调查　　　D. 抽样调查

（2）现况调查主要分析指标是（　　）

A. 死亡构成比　　　B. 某病的发病率　　　C. 某病的患病率　　　D. 某病的死亡率

（3）在抽样调查中，下列哪种抽样方法的抽样误差最大？（　　）

A. 单纯随机抽样　　B. 系统抽样　　　　C. 分层抽样　　　　D. 整群抽样

（4）对于病因未明的疾病，现况调查的主要目的是（　　）

A. 确定病因　　　　B. 验证病因　　　　C. 寻找病因线索　　　D. 进行因果推断

（5）为了解某小学近视现患率，按照年级分层，再在每一层中随机抽取100名学生参与调查，该抽样方法称为（　　）

A. 单纯随机抽样　　B. 系统抽样　　　　C. 分层抽样　　　　D. 整群抽样

Experiment 10　Case-control Study

Ⅰ. Objectives

The objectives of this chapter are, through some cases, to master the principles of case-control study design, data compilation, statistical analysis methods, and interpretation of statistical results, and to understand the implementation procedures of case-control studies.

Ⅱ. Principles

(1) The basic principle of case-control studies is to select people with and without a particular disease as case group and control group respectively. It is an observational research method investigates the proportion or level of exposure to certain or certain suspected risk factors in each group in the past, and then compares the differences in the proportion or level of exposure between each group to determine whether the exposure factors are associated with the disease studies, and to what extent the degree of association is.

(2) Exposure meaning: it means that the study subjects have been exposed to certain factors or has certain characteristics, such as exposure to certain chemical substances or with characteristics such as gender, age, race or occupation, etc.

(3) Types of case-control study: unmatched case-control study; matched case-control study (frequency matching and individual matching).

(4) Matching meaning: it requires the control to be consistent with the case in some features or factors, to ensure the exchangeability between the control and the case, in order to eliminate the interference of matching factors.

(5) Features of case-control study: it is an observational study; the subjects are divided into case group and control group; from "effect" to "cause"; causal argument is less strong than cohort studies and randomized control trails.

(6) Cautions in case selection: firstly, all cases (those with a disease) should meet the

unified diagnostic criteria; secondly, cases can be new cases, existing cases, and disease-caused death, however, new cases are most desirable; thirdly, cases can originally selected from hospitals and communities.

(7) Cautions in control selection: controls (those without a disease) must be selected using the same diagnostic criteria as the cases'; controls should be representative of the population from which the case originated; controls can also be originated in hospitals and communities.

(8) OR value: the odds ratio, is the ratio of the exposure between the case group and the control group, reflecting the strength of the association between exposure and disease. It indicates the risk of disease of the exposed group is many times that of the non-exposed group.

(9) Bias of case-control study: selection bias includes admission rate bias, prevalence and incidence bias, and detected symptoms bias; information bias includes recall bias, investigation bias and report bias; confounding bias.

III. Materials

Non-alcoholic fatty liver disease (NAFLD) refers to a clinicopathological syndrome characterized by diffuse bullae fat of liver cells caused by alcohol and other liver damage factors, and is considered to be the manifestation of liver metabolic syndrome. There are many factors can cause NAFLD. Dietary play an important role in the occurrence and development of NAFLD due to its long-term exposure characteristics. Eggs are one of the major sources of dietary cholesterol, despite its benefits on blood lipids, it may also damage glucose metabolism and promote inflammation and thus increases the risk of diabetes and cardiovascular disease. Previous studies have suggested that egg intake may play a role in NAFLD. This study explores the relationship between egg intake and the risk of NAFLD, to provides epidemiological evidence for the development of dietary guidelines on egg consumption in China.

In this study, a case-control study was used to recruit the subjects who underwent a physical examination at the Physical Examination Center of the First Hospital of Nanping, Fujian Medical University, from April 2015 to August 2017. The subjects were divided into the case and control group with 541 subjects in each group according to the imaging diagnosis in the *Guidelines for the Diagnosis and Treatment of Nonalcoholic Fatty Liver Disease in China* (2010 *Revised Edition*). Egg intake was measured by a semi-quantitative food frequency questionnaire. The general demographic characteristics of the subjects are listed in Table 10 – 1. It shows that among 541 NAFLD patients, 199 consumed eggs daily, compared with 225 consumed eggs daily among 541 controls. In addition to daily consumption of eggs, the other characteristics of cases and controls are shown in Table 10 – 2.

Table 10-1 General demographic characteristics of case-control studies

Variable	Case ($n=541$)	Control ($n=541$)	χ^2/Z	P value
Age [Years, ($P25$, $P75$)]	48 (39, 54)	48 (39, 54)	-0.024	0.981
Gender			<0.001	1.000
Male	369 (68.21)	369 (68.21)		
Female	172 (31.79)	172 (31.79)		
Education			3.636	0.162
Illiteracy and primary school	42 (7.76)	53 (9.80)		
Junior and Senior Secondary School	226 (41.78)	198 (36.60)		
College degree or above	273 (50.46)	290 (53.60)		
Occupation			5.786	0.055
Mental worker	157 (29.02)	150 (27.73)		
Manual worker	162 (29.94)	198 (36.60)		
Other	222 (41.04)	193 (35.67)		
Income (Yuan/Month)			1.28	0.527
<2000	33 (6.10)	36 (6.65)		
2000~2999	160 (29.57)	175 (32.35)		
≥3000	348 (64.33)	330 (61.00)		
BMI (kg/m^2)			214.8	<0.001
<18.5	3 (0.55)	19 (3.51)		
18.5~23.9	172 (31.80)	387 (71.54)		
24.0~27.9	289 (53.42)	128 (23.66)		
≥28	77 (14.23)	7 (1.29)		
Smoking			0.179	0.672
Yes	136 (25.14)	130 (24.03)		
No	405 (74.86)	411 (75.97)		
Drinking			0.018	0.894
Yes	162 (29.94)	160 (29.57)		
No	379 (70.06)	381 (70.43)		

Table 10-2 Egg consumption frequency in cases and controls

Frequency of egg consumption	Case ($n=541$)	Control ($n=541$)	OR (95% CI)
≥7 times per week	199	225	1.00
4~6 times per week	172	150	0.55 (0.22~1.38)
1~3 times per week	121	105	1.56 (0.79~3.09)

续表 10-2

Frequency of egg consumption	Case ($n=541$)	Control ($n=541$)	OR (95% CI)
1～3 times per month	38	45	1.65 (0.93～2.94)
0 time per month	11	16	1.86 (1.10～3.15)

The *OR* values were adjusted for gender, age, education, occupation, income, BMI, smoking, alcohol consumption, etc. *P*-trend <0.05.

Question1: Please list a four-grid table of daily egg consumption exposure in NAFLD cases and control groups based on the main results in the tables.

Question2: Calculate the exposure of NAFLD cases and the control group with daily egg consumption. Are there any differences between the two groups? What is the value of *OR* and 95% CI? What does the calculation tell us? What does the *OR* value tell us that χ^2 and *P* values don't?

Question3. What is the purpose of Table 10-1 in comparing the various characteristics between the case and control groups?

Question4: Table 10-1 shows that there was a statistically significant difference in BMI between the two groups. What should be done next?

Question5: What can be explained by the adjusted *OR* value and the linear trend test results (*P-trend* <0.05) in Table 10-2?

IV. Exercises

(1) The limitation of case-control study is (   )

A. Multiple suspected causes cannot be investigated

B. The relative risk cannot be estimated

C. It is easy to be biased when recalling

D. The sample size is very large

(2) The most likely bias in case-control study is (   )

A. Admission rate bias   B. Current cases-new cases bias

C. Confounding bias   D. Recall bias

(3) What is the maximum number of matching factors for a case-control study using an individual matching design? (   )

A. 1   B. 2   C. 3   D. 4

(4) In a case-control study on the relationship between pancreatic cancer and smoking, 60 out of 100 patients with pancreatic cancer smoked, and 20 out of 100 controls smoked. What is the strength of the association between smoking and pancreatic cancer? (   )

A. *OR* = 6.0   B. *OR* = 5.5   C. *RR* = 6.0   D. *RR* = 5.5

(5) In a case-control study, 100 out of 200 patients had a history of exposure, and 50 out of 200 controls had a history of exposure. What is the incidence rate among those with a history of exposure? (   )

A. 100%
B. 80%
C. 40%
D. It cannot be calculated

 实验十　病例对照研究

一、实验目的

通过案例分析，掌握病例对照研究的设计要点、资料整理和统计分析方法及统计结果的解释。熟悉病例对照研究实施步骤。

二、实验原理

（1）病例对照研究的定义：选择患有和未患有某特定疾病的人群分别作为病例组和对照组，调查各组人群过去暴露于某种或某些可疑危险因素的比例或水平，通过比较各组之间暴露比例或水平的差异，判断暴露因素是否与研究疾病有关联及关联程度大小的一种观察性研究方法。

（2）暴露含义：是指研究对象曾经接触过某些因素或具备某些特征，如接触过某种化学物质或具备的性别、年龄、种族或职业等特征。

（3）病例对照研究的类型：非匹配型病例对照研究；匹配型病例对照研究（频数匹配和个体匹配）。

（4）匹配含义：又称配比，要求对照在某些特征或因素上与病例保持一致，保证对照与病例具有可比性，从而排除匹配因素的干扰。

（5）病例对照研究特点：属于观察性研究；研究对象分为病例组和对照组；由"果"溯"因"；因果论证强度不高。

（6）病例选择注意事项：首先，病例要符合统一、明确的疾病诊断标准；其次，病例种类有新发病例、现患病例、死亡病例，优先选择新发病例；最后，病例可来源于医院和社区。

（7）对照选择注意事项：对照必须是与病例相同诊断标准确认不患所研究疾病的人；对照应该能代表产生病例的源人群；对照可来源于医院和社区。

（8）OR值：比值比又称优势比，为病例组与对照组两组暴露比值之比，反映暴露与疾病关联强度，暴露者疾病的危险性是非暴露者的多少倍。

（9）病例对照研究易产生的偏倚：选择偏倚（包括入院率偏倚、现患病例－新发病例偏倚、检出症候偏倚）；信息偏倚（包括回忆偏倚、调查偏倚、报告偏倚）；混杂偏倚。

三、实验材料

非酒精性脂肪肝病（non-alcoholic fatty liver disease，NAFLD）是指除酒精和其他明确的损肝因素所致的，以弥漫性肝细胞大泡性脂肪变为主要特征的临床病理综合征，被认为是肝脏代谢综合征的表现。引发 NAFLD 的因素有很多，其中膳食因素由于其长期暴露特征在该病的发生发展过程中起着重要作用。鸡蛋是膳食胆固醇的主要来源之一,而胆固醇除了对血脂的影响外,可能还会损害葡萄糖代谢、促进炎症,从而增加糖尿病、心血管疾病的风险。既往研究提示鸡蛋摄入也可能与 NAFLD 发生有关。本研究在探讨鸡蛋摄入与 NAFLD 患病风险之间的关系,为中国制定有关鸡蛋摄入的饮食指南提供流行病学证据。

本研究采用病例对照研究的方法,招募于 2015 年 4 月至 2017 年 8 月在福建医科大学附属南平市第一医院体检中心进行体检的人为研究对象。参照《中国非酒精性脂肪肝病诊疗指南》(2010 年修订版)中的影像学诊断将研究对象分为病例组和对照组,各 541 人。鸡蛋摄入采用半定量食物频率问卷调查。研究对象的一般人口学特征信息比较详见表 10-1。结果在 541 名 NAFLD 病人中每天都有鸡蛋摄入的人有 199 人,对照 541 人中每天都有摄入鸡蛋的是 225 人,其余人员未能达到每天都有鸡蛋摄入。除了每天都摄入鸡蛋外,其他摄入频率详见表 10-2。

表 10-1 病例对照研究的一般人口学特征

变量	病例组 ($n=541$)	对照组 ($n=541$)	χ^2/Z 值	P 值
年龄 [岁,(P_{25},P_{75})]	48(39,54)	48(39,54)	-0.024	0.981
性别			<0.001	1.000
男性	369(68.21)	369(68.21)		
女性	172(31.79)	172(31.79)		
教育程度			3.636	0.162
文盲及小学	42(7.76)	53(9.80)		
初中及高中	226(41.78)	198(36.60)		
大专以上	273(50.46)	290(53.60)		
职业			5.786	0.055
脑力劳动者	157(29.02)	150(27.73)		
体力劳动者	162(29.94)	198(36.60)		
其他	222(41.04)	193(35.67)		
收入(元/月)			1.28	0.527
<2000	33(6.10)	36(6.65)		
2000~2999	160(29.57)	175(32.35)		
≥3000	348(64.33)	330(61.00)		
BMI(kg/m^2)			214.8	<0.001
<18.5	3(0.55)	19(3.51)		
18.5~23.9	172(31.80)	387(71.54)		
24.0~27.9	289(53.42)	128(23.66)		
≥28	77(14.23)	7(1.29)		

续表10-1

变量	病例组（n=541）	对照组（n=541）	χ^2/Z 值	P 值
吸烟			0.179	0.672
是	136（25.14）	130（24.03）		
否	405（74.86）	411（75.97）		
饮酒			0.018	0.894
是	162（29.94）	160（29.57）		
否	379（70.06）	381（70.43）		

表10-2　病例对照组鸡蛋摄入频率

鸡蛋摄入频率	病例组（n=541）	对照组（n=541）	OR（95% CI）
≥7 次/周	199	225	1.00
4～6 次/周	172	150	0.55（0.22～1.38）
1～3 次/周	121	105	1.56（0.79～3.09）
1～3 次/月	38	45	1.65（0.93～2.94）
0 次/月	11	16	1.86（1.10～3.15）

注：OR 值调整性别、年龄、教育程度、职业、收入、BMI、吸烟、饮酒等；P-trend<0.05。

问题1：请根据文中主要结果列出 NAFLD 病例和对照组每天都有摄入鸡蛋的暴露情况四格表。

问题2：计算 NAFLD 病例和对照组每天都有摄入鸡蛋的暴露情况两组间有无差别？OR 值及 95% CI 是多少？计算结果能说明什么问题？OR 值能提供哪些 χ^2 值和 P 值不能提供的信息？

问题3：表10-1 比较病例和对照组间各种特征的目的是什么？

问题4：表10-1 中发现 BMI 在两组间差异有统计学意义，下一步应该怎么处理？

问题5：表10-2 中经过校正后的 OR 值及线性趋势检验结果（P-trend<0.05）能说明什么问题？

四、课后练习

（1）病例对照研究的缺点是（　　）
A. 不能调查多种可疑病因　　　　B. 不能估计相对危险度
C. 回忆时易产生偏倚　　　　　　D. 样本量要求很大

（2）病例对照研究最容易产生的偏倚是（　　）
A. 入院率偏倚　　　　　　　　　B. 现患-新发病例偏倚
C. 混杂偏倚　　　　　　　　　　D. 回忆偏倚

（3）采用个体匹配设计的病例对照研究，匹配因素最好不要超过多少个？（　　）
A. 1 个　　　　B. 2 个　　　　C. 3 个　　　　D. 4 个

（4）在一个胰腺癌与吸烟关系的病例对照研究中，100 例胰腺癌患者中有 60 人吸烟，100 例对照中有 20 人吸烟，吸烟与胰腺癌的关联强度是（　　）

A. $OR = 6.0$　　　B. $OR = 5.5$　　　C. $RR = 6.0$　　　D. $RR = 5.5$

（5）在某项病例对照研究中，200 名病例中有暴露史者 100 人，200 名对照中有暴露史者 50 人，有暴露史者中发病率为（　　）

A. 100%　　　B. 80%　　　C. 40%　　　D. 无法计算

Experiment 11　Cohort Study

Ⅰ. Objectives

The objectives of this chapter, through analyzing some research examples, the basic principles, research characteristics, data collation methods, calculation and application of cohort study, are mastered. Students should be familiar with the basic cohort study design and real-life implications.

Ⅱ. Principles

(1) Definition of cohort study: an observational research method in which people are divided into different groups according to whether they are exposed to a suspicious factor and the degree of exposure, the outcomes of each group are tracked, and the difference in outcome frequency between different groups is compared, so as to determine whether there is a causal correlation between exposure factors and outcomes and the size of the correlation.

(2) Features of cohort study: observational method; reference group is set up; from "cause" to "effect"; the ability to test the causal relationship between exposure and outcome is strong.

(3) Type of cohort study: prospective cohort study; retrospective cohort study; bidirectional cohort study.

(4) Source of exposed population: can be occupational population, people with special experiences (fx. nuclear radiation exposure), general population, an organized group of people (fx. school or military unit), and etc.

(5) Source of control population: internal control; outside control; population control.

(6) Cumulative incidence rate: the cumulative incidence rate calculated by the number of people at the beginning of observation as the denominator and the number of cases (or deaths) during the whole observation period as the numerator, which is suitable for large and stable follow-up population.

(7) Incidence density: the incidence rate calculated by the total observed person-time as the denominator and the number of cases (or deaths) during the whole observation period as the

numerator which has the property of instantaneous frequency. It is suitable for the dynamic cohort where the personnel are constantly changing during the follow-up period.

(8) Relative risk (RR), is an indicator reflecting the strength of the association between exposure and outcome (fx. cancer or death). It reflects how many times the risk of outcome (fx. cancer or death) in the exposure group is compared with the non-exposure group.

(9) Attributable risk (AR), is the absolute difference in incidence of outcome between the exposure group and the non-exposure group. It represents the degree to which the risk is specific to the exposure factors.

(10) Attribution risk percentage (AR%), is the percentage of the total outcome (fx. mortality) in the exposed population attributable to the exposure.

(11) Population-attributable risk (PAR), is the portion of the total population incidence of outcome attributable to exposure.

(12) Population-attributable risk percentage (PAR%), is the percentage of the total outcome in the total population attributable to exposure.

Ⅲ. Materials

Since the 1940s, more and more people in the United States died of cardiovascular disease (CVDs), which gradually attracted the attention of the United States health department. In order to explore the etiology of chronic lifestyle diseases such as CVDs, epidemiological research methods should be used to find the pathogenic factors.

In 1948, the US National Institutes of Health (NIH) initiated a cardiovascular study in Framingham, Massachusetts, to understand the disease characteristics and determinants of coronary heart disease in the general population. Framingham's proximity to several medical centers in Boston, a city with low unemployment rate, stable population, and easy to collaborate with local physicians, make it a good place for being able to follow the residents over a long period of time. A total of 5,209 residents aged 28 to 62 in the town were enrolled in the Framingham initial cohort and were followed every two years. The Offspring study was started in 1971 with 5,124 offspring and spouses in the initial cohort and was followed every three years. The Omni study began in 1995, merged with Asian, African, and Latino origins to investigate the similarities and differences in CVDs.

Question 1: What epidemiological method is used in this study?

Question 2: What are the features of this research method?

Question 3: Could Framingham's original subjects have CVD disease?

Question 4: What is the origin of the exposure group in this study?

Question 5: What type of reference population was included in this study?

The researchers defined the study outcome as a diagnosis of CVD, with the following criteria for diagnosis:

(1) There is historical and/or present clear eletrocardiogram evidence of myocardial

infarction.

(2) Clear angina pectoris.

(3) Sudden death due to heart disease.

The Framingham study selected a number of simple biological indicators for follow-up, such as blood pressure, BMI, smoking, alcohol consumption, educational level, etc.

Question 6: What is the study outcome? What are the requirements of outcome for cohort study?

Since 1948, the Framingham researchers have invited the subjects to the detailed physical examinations, laboratory tests, and questionnaire surveys every two years. Until the subsequent offspring studies, this cohort has maintained a relative excellent follow-up record, with a loss of follow-up rate of less than 4% for decades, which has ensured the quality of this study.

Question 7: What is lost follow-up? What are the reasons for the loss of follow-up? What effect does loss of follow-up have on cohort study?

Question 8: How to control loss of follow-up?

To investigate whether parental intermittent claudication is a risk factor for offspring claudication, the researchers used data from three 12-year follow-up studies from the offspring cohort studied in Framingham. Participants underwent physical examinations and questionnaires every three years. Table 11 – 1 shows the incidence of disease among 6306 participants following up for 12 years.

Table 11 – 1 12-year follow-up of 6306 participants

Queue time (years)	The number of observed	The number of lost to follow-up	Number of new claudication
1971 – 1975	2039	68	35
1983 – 1987	2242	156	36
1995 – 1998	2025	284	30

Question 9: It was assumed that the average follow-up time of all the lost subjects was 6 years. Please calculate the total number of person-times for all observers and calculate the incidence density of claudication.

Question 10: If the total number of people observed was used as the denominator without considering the loss of follow-up, please calculate the cumulative incidence rate of claudication in the above-mentioned population after 12 years of follow-up.

Question 11: What is the difference between cumulative incidence rate and incidence density in cohort study?

In 1950, 1307 healthy men aged 45 to 62 years of age in Framingham's initial cohort were surveyed for their smoking status. They were divided into four groups according to their smoking status. With a follow-up of 6 years, the incidence of CVDs among the groups was recorded in table

11 − 2.

Table 11 − 2 CVDs incidence in men aged 45 to 62 years with different smoking status

Smoking history	The number of observed	The number of cases
Never smoking	141	14
Past smoking	115	8
Smoke cigars or pipes	177	14
Smoke paper cigarettes	594	57
Total	1027	94

Question 12: What type of cohort study does this cohort study belong to?

Question 13: Using the never smoking group as the control group, please calculate the RR, AR and AR% of each exposure group separately and explain the meaning of each indicator.

IV. Exercises

(1) Which of the following observational studies is most effective in examining the causal association between a factor and a disease? (   )

　　A. The cross-sectional study　　　　B. Case-control study

　　C. Ecological study　　　　　　　　D. Cohort study

(2) The greatest advantage of cohort studies is that (   )

　　A. More people were followed up for longer periods of time

　　B. Less chance of bias

　　C. More directly verify the causal relationship between exposure and disease

　　D. It is suitable for research on rare diseases

(3) To evaluate the public health significance of a pathogenic factor, we should choose (   )

　　A. Absolute risk　　　　　　　　　B. Relative risk

　　C. The sensitivity　　　　　　　　　D. Attributed risk percentage

(4) At the start of the prospective cohort study, the subjects were (   )

　　A. People who suffer from the disease

　　B. People who don't have the disease

　　C. People with the exposure factors

　　D. People with a family history of a disease

(5) In a cohort study, 100 people in the smoking group died after 5 years of follow-up among 500 people, and 100 people in the non-smoking group died after the same 5 years of follow-up among 1000 people. The relative risk of death for smokers in this study is (   )

　　A. 1.00　　　　B. 1.50　　　　C. 2.00　　　　D. 2.50

实验十一 队列研究

一、实验目的

通过研究实例分析,掌握队列研究的基本原理、研究特点、资料整理方法及常用指标的计算与应用。熟悉队列研究的设计基本步骤,并注意实施过程中细节的把握。

二、实验原理

(1)队列研究定义:将人群按是否暴露于某可疑因素及其暴露程度分为不同组,追踪其各组的结局,比较不同组之间结局频率的差异,从而判定暴露因素与结局之间有无因果关联及关联大小的一种观察性研究方法。

(2)队列研究特点:属于观察法;设立对照组;由"因"及"果";检验暴露与结局的因果联系能力较强。

(3)队列研究类型:前瞻性队列研究;历史性队列研究;双向性队列研究。

(4)暴露人群来源:职业人群;特殊经历人群(如接受过核辐射);一般人群;有组织的人群团体(如学校或部队)。

(5)对照人群来源:内对照;外对照;总人口对照。

(6)累积发病率:以观察开始时的人口数作分母,以整个观察期内的发病(或死亡)人数为分子,计算的发病率叫作累积发病率,适用于研究人群较大且比较稳定的随访人群。

(7)发病密度:以观察人时为分母,以用整个观察期内的发病(或死亡)人数为分子,人时为单位计算出来的发病率带有瞬时频率性质叫作发病密度,适用于动态队列,随访期间人员在不断变动的队列。

(8)相对危险度(RR):反映暴露与发病(死亡)关联强度的指标,反映暴露组发病或死亡风险是对照组的多少倍。

(9)归因危险度(AR):暴露组发病率与对照组发病率相差的绝对值,表示危险特异的归因于暴露因素的程度。

(10)归因危险度百分比(AR%):暴露人群中的发病或死亡归因于暴露的部分占全部发病或死亡的百分比。

(11)人群归因危险度(PAR):总人群发病率归因于暴露的部分。

(12)人群归因危险度百分比(PAR%):总人群中发病或死亡归因于暴露部分占总人群全部发病或死亡的百分比。

三、实验材料

20世纪40年代开始,美国死于心血管疾病(cardiovascular disease,CVD)的人越来越多,逐渐引起美国卫生部门的重视。针对CVD这类慢性生活方式疾病病因探讨,须采用流行病学研究方法寻找致病因素。

1948年，美国国立卫生研究院（National Institutes of Health，NIH）在马萨诸塞州Framingham小镇启动了一项心血管病研究，目的是了解一般人群中冠心病的疾病特征和决定因素。Framingham小镇临近波士顿的几个医学中心，小镇居民失业率低，人口稳定，当地医生也较为配合，这些都有利于长期随访该地居民。该镇5209名28～62岁的居民均纳入Framingham初始队列，每2年随访一次。1971年开始OFFSPRING研究，对象为初始队列的子女和配偶，共计5124人，每3年随访一次。1995年开始Omni研究，观察拉丁裔与亚裔、非裔、美裔人群新发CVD的异同。

问题1：该研究属于哪种流行病学研究方法？
问题2：该种研究方法有什么特点？
问题3：Framingham初始研究对象能否患有CVD？
问题4：本研究的暴露组人群来源于什么群体？
问题5：本研究的对照组人群是什么类型的对照？

研究者定义研究结局为确诊CVD，确诊标准如下：
（1）有历史和（或）现在明确的心电图证据显示心肌梗死；
（2）明确的心绞痛；
（3）由心脏疾病引起的突然死亡。

Framingham研究选择一些简便易行的生物学指标进行随访，如血压、BMI、吸烟、饮酒、文化程度等。

问题6：什么是研究结局？队列研究对研究结局有何要求？

自1948年开始，Framingham研究工作者对研究对象每两年进行一次详细的体格检查、实验室检查和问卷调查。直至后面的子代研究，该队列研究一直都维持很好的随访记录，数十年来维持着低于4%的失访率，提高了本研究质量。

问题7：什么是失访？失访的原因有哪些？失访会对队列研究产生什么影响？
问题8：如何控制失访？

为了研究父母患有间歇性跛行是否是子代跛行的危险因素，研究者在Framingham研究的Offspring队列中选取了3次12年随访研究数据，参与者每3年接受一次体检和问卷调查。表11-1为6306名参与者随访12年的发病情况。

表11-1　6306名参与者12年的随访情况

进入队列时间/年	观察人数	失访人数	新发跛行人数
1971—1975	2039	68	35
1983—1987	2242	156	36
1995—1998	2025	284	30

问题9：假设所有失访人群平均随访时间均为6年，请计算所有观察者的总人时数，并计算跛行的发病密度。

问题10：如果不考虑失访，将观察总人数作为分母，请计算上述人群随访12年跛行的累积发病率。

问题11：累积发病率和发病密度有何区别？

1950年，研究者调查了Framingham初始队列中1307名45～62岁健康男性的吸烟状况，并根据吸烟状况分四组，研究者对他们随访6年并记录下CVD的发生情况，相关数据见表11-2。

表11-2 45～62岁男性不同吸烟状况的CVD发病情况

吸烟史	观察人数	病例数
从不吸烟	141	14
过去吸烟	115	8
抽雪茄或烟斗	177	14
吸纸烟	594	57
合计	1027	94

问题12：该队列研究属于哪一类型的队列研究？

问题13：以从不吸烟组为参照组，分别计算各暴露组的RR、AR及AR%，并解释各指标含义。

四、课后练习

(1) 在检验某因素与某疾病的因果关联时，下列哪种观察法最有效？（   ）
　A. 现况调查　　　　　　　　　　B. 病例对照研究
　C. 生态学研究　　　　　　　　　D. 队列研究

(2) 队列研究最大的优点是（   ）
　A. 对较多人进行较长时间的随访　　B. 发生偏倚的机会少
　C. 较为直接地验证病因与疾病的因果关系　D. 适用于罕见疾病研究

(3) 评价一个致病因子的公共卫生学意义，宜选用（   ）
　A. 绝对危险度　　　　　　　　　B. 相对危险度
　C. 灵敏度　　　　　　　　　　　D. 归因危险度百分比

(4) 前瞻性队列研究开始时，研究对象为（   ）
　A. 患该病的人　　　　　　　　　B. 未患该病的人
　C. 具有研究暴露因素的人　　　　D. 具有某病家族史的人

(5) 某项队列研究吸烟组500人随访5年后100人死亡，非吸烟组1000人相同随访5年后死亡100人，请问该研究中吸烟者死亡的相对危险度是（   ）
　A. 1.00　　　　B. 1.50　　　　C. 2.00　　　　D. 2.50

Experiment 12 Experimental Epidemiological Study

Ⅰ. Objectives

Through material analysis, master the basic concept, features and types of experimental epidemiology as well as the basic principles and steps of field trial design, and be familiar with the collation and basic statistical analysis of experimental study data.

Ⅱ. Principles

(1) Rationale of experimental epidemiology: according to the study purpose, the investigators randomly assign the study subjects to the experimental group and the control group according to the predetermined study protocol, artificially apply or reduce a certain treatment factor, then track and observe the effect results of treatment factors, compare and analyze the outcomes of the two groups, to assess the effect of treatment factors.

(2) Basic characteristics of experimental epidemiology: it's considered as prospective study; human intervention; random grouping (randomization); with balanced and comparable controls.

(3) Main study types: clinical trial (taking patient as the study subject and implementing the intervention measures to the individual); field trial (taking non-patient as the study subject and implementing the intervention measures to the individual); community trial (taking non-patient as the study subject and implementing the intervention to the group).

(4) Randomized clinical trial (RCT): this method is a prospective study in which clinical patients are randomly divided into the trial and control group, the trial group is given an intervention, and the control group is given control measures (receive no intervention). The effect of intervention is evaluated by comparing the difference in the effects of each group. It is a typical study type designed according to the four basic principles of experimental research, with the highest causality power.

(5) The basic principles of research object selection: select the population that is effective for the intervention measures; select the population with expected higher incidence rate; select the population that is harmless to the intervention; select the population that can persist the trial to the end; select the population with good compliance.

(6) Methods of experimental study randomization include simple randomization, block randomization, stratified randomization, and cluster randomization.

(7) Control types of experimental study include standard control, placebo control, parallel control, cross control, self-control, historical control, blank control, and etc.

(8) Application of blind method in experimental study: single-blind, the study participants do not know whether they are belong to the experimental group or the control group; double-blind,

neither the study participants nor the implementers know the experimental grouping; triple-blind, none of the study participants, implementers, and data collection and analysis personnel know the experimental grouping.

(9) Analysis methods of experimental research data include intention to treat analysis, compliance analysis, and treatment received analysis.

(10) Main evaluation indicators of experimental study data analysis: Main evaluation indicators of treatment effect include effective rate, cure rate, N-year survival rate, etc.; Main evaluation indicators of preventive measures effect include protective rate, index of effectiveness.

(11) Calculation method of protective rate:

$$\text{Protective rate} = \frac{\text{Incidence rate of control group} - \text{Incidence rate of trial group}}{\text{Incidence rate of control group}} \times 100\% \quad (\text{Formula } 12-1)$$

(12) Calculation method of index of effectiveness:

$$\text{Index of effectiveness} = \frac{\text{Incidence rate of control group}}{\text{Incidence rate of trial group}} \quad (\text{Formula } 12-2)$$

(13) Number needed to treat (NNT): The number of patients in the same category who need to be treated to prevent one adverse event. This index can quantitatively express the efficacy to help doctors and patients to make clinical decisions. The smaller the NNT, the better the effect.

(14) Calculation method of NNT:

$$\text{NNT} = \frac{1}{\text{Incidence rate of control group} - \text{Incidence rate of trial group}} \quad (\text{Formula } 12-3)$$

III. Materials

Effect of outdoor activity time on myopia in children: a randomized experimental study

1. Study background

The global myopia rate is gradually increasing, especially in urban areas of East Asia and Southeast Asia. 80% – 90% of high school students in these places have different degrees of Myopia brings inconvenience and certain degrees of burden to the individuals and society, and the current trend of myopia gradual juvenile is also more obvious. Premature myopia may lead to high myopia. If it develops into pathological changes such as macular degeneration, it will bring serious burden to personal physical and mental health and treatment costs. So far, there is no effective interventions to prevent myopia. Although low-dose atropine eye drops and the use of corrective lenses can delay the progression of myopia, their effects are weak.

Studies have suggested in recent years that outdoor activities have the potential to prevent the occurrence of myopia, but there is a lack of high-quality randomized clinical trials to provide evidence for the development of health policies. On September 15, 2015, JAMA published a study to assess the effect of increasing outdoor activity time at school on preventing myopia. This study was a cluster randomized trial with first-year students from 12 primary schools in Guangzhou,

China, from October 2010 to October 2013.

2. Study Design

This study was conducted in Guangzhou, China. The schools were selected as the intervention location and the first-year students were designed as the study participants. Using a cluster randomized trial design method to carry out a 3-year experimental study to assess the effect of increasing outdoor activity time in school on the prevention of myopia. The study was reviewed by the Ethics Committee, and informed consent was obtained from the study participants.

Since 1987, the Guangzhou Institute of Health Education has begun to perform annual visual acuity examinations for students in all grades of 30 different public primary schools in six districts. In early 2009, this study began to invite these 30 primary schools, excluding one of the primary schools with incomplete visual acuity examination data, and the remaining 29 primary schools were divided into six layers according to the proportion of all students with normal vision in grades 1 to 6 in 2008, including five schools in each of the five layers and four schools in the remaining one layer. Two more schools were randomly selected in each layer, one into the intervention group and one into the control group. The intervention and control group come from the same layer and match the confounding effect of the factors of longitudinal vision loss (vision loss in the child group over time) in children, which is closely related to myopia in children. Randomization was performed using SAS9.2 for simple random sampling.

Children entered first grade for baseline data collection and were followed annually for 3 years until the end of the fourth grade study.

With a total of 952 first-grade students in the six intervention schools, the intervention was to add one 40-minute outdoor activity class to each teaching day and encouraged parents to have their children participate in outdoor activities after school, especially weekends and holidays. There were a total of 951 first-grade students in the six control schools, and parents and children maintained their daily activity patterns as usual.

The primary outcome was the 3-year cumulative incidence rate of myopia (defined as children's refractive error spherical equivalent $\leqslant -0.5$ diopters [D]) in students without myopia at baseline. Secondary outcomes were changes in spherical equivalent refractive index and axial length for all students, analyzed using the intention to treat principle. Right eye data were used for analysis.

Question 1: Which type of epidemiological experimental studies does this study belong to?

Question 2: Is it appropriate to select the trial locations and study participants for this study?

Question 3: What is the sampling method for the study participants in this study?

Question 4: What is the randomization method in this study?

Question 5: How is the blind method of this study considered?

3. Study process

The study flow chart is shown in Figure 12-1.

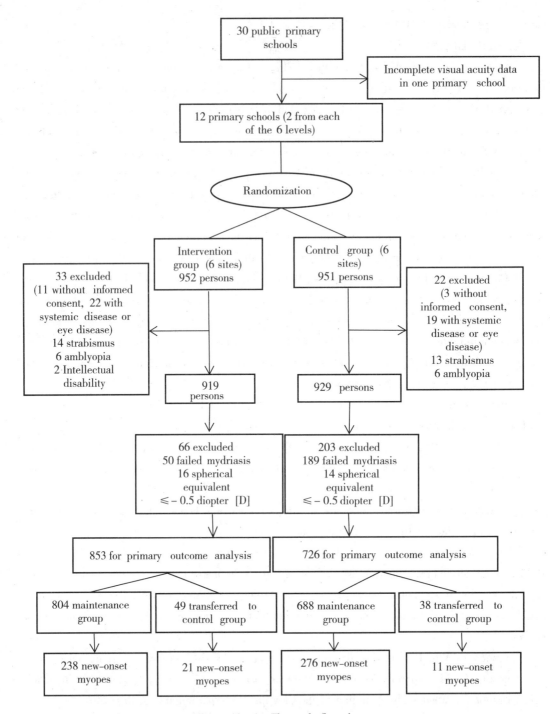

Figure 12-1 The study flow chart

4. Study population

The baseline characteristics of the study participants are listed in Table 12-1.

Table 12 – 1 Baseline characteristics of participants in the Guangzhou outdoor activity longitudinal trial

	Intervention Group ($n = 919$)[a]	Control Group ($n = 929$)[a]	P Value
Age, mean (SD), y	6.61 (0.33)	6.57 (0.32)	0.01
Boys, No. (%)	489 (52.58)	509 (54.61)	0.38
Height, mean (SD), cm	120.29 (0.17)	120.51 (0.16)	0.36
Weight, mean (SD), kg	22.54 (0.15)	22.56 (0.14)	0.93
Body mass index, mean (SD)[b]	15.48 (0.07)	15.45 (0.07)	0.71
Wearing glasses, No. (%)	47 (5.11)	40 (4.31)	0.41
Uncorrected visual acuity, median (IQR)	0.80 (0.80 – 0.80)	0.80 (0.80 – 1.00)	0.16
Spherical equivalent refraction, mean (SD), D[c]	1.30 (0.97)	1.26 (0.81)	0.42
Prevalence of myopia, No./total (%)[c]	16/869 (1.84)	14/740 (1.89)	0.94
Axial length, mean (SD), mm	22.60 (0.71)	22.66 (0.70)	0.05
Corneal radius of curvature, mean (SD), D	43.54 (1.64)	44.42 (1.40)	0.08
Time spent outdoors outside of school hours, median (IQR), min/d	46.1 (30.00 – 68.04)	46.07 (30.00 – 67.50)	0.34
Parental myopia, No. (%)			0.001
0	376 (46.36)	273 (40.21)	
1	306 (37.73)	245 (36.08)	
Both	129 (15.91)	161 (23.71)	

Note: a. Right eye data for students who had informed consent and completed baseline examination.

b. Calculated as weight in kilograms divided by height in meters squared.

c. Right eye data for children with cycloplegic refraction only.

Question 6: Are you satisfied with the comparability data of intervention and control group in Table 12 – 1? If you are, please explain your reasons.

Question 7: In the experimental epidemiological study, is there any difference or no difference in the requirements for the experimental group and the control group in the baseline data?

5. Results

There were a total of 952 children in the intervention group and 951 children in the control group, with a mean age of 6.6 ($SD = 0.34$) years. Excluding the cases of failure to obtain parental informed consent, systemic or ocular pathological changes at baseline, and mydriasis failure, 853 patients in the intervention group and 726 patients in the control group were eligible for analysis. Notably 49 students in the intervention group were transferred to the control group, and 38 students in the control group schools were transferred to the intervention group during the intervention period. The number of students developed myopes at 3 years of follow-up in both groups is shown in Fig12 – 1. Table 12 – 2 shows an overview of the main outcomes at 3 years follow-up. Please calculate the cumulative incidence of myopia in the two groups according to the data in Figure 12 – 1. Please compare whether the difference between the two groups is statistically significant. Please fill the results in table12 – 2.

Table 12 – 2 Refractive and biometric outcomes at 3-year follow-up of the Guangzhou outdoor activity longitudinal trial [a]

	Intervention Group	Control Group	P Value
Cumulative incidence rate of myopia			
Cumulative change, mean (95% CI)[b]			
Spherical equivalent refraction, D	– 1.42 (– 1.58 to – 1.27)	– 1.59 (– 1.76 to – 1.43)	0.04
Axial length, mm	0.95 (0.91 to 1.00)	0.98 (0.94 to 1.03)	0.07

Note: a. The calculation on all outcomes was based on right eye data only.

b. Cumulative number of cases of incident myopia/number of analyzed participants (%).

Question 8: This study uses intention to treat analysis. Please answer the idea and characteristics of this analysis.

Question 9: According to the intention-to-treat analysis method, please calculate the cumulative incidence of myopia between the intervention group and the control group at 3 years. Please compare whether there is a statistical difference between the two groups. Please fill the results in Table 12 – 2.

Question 10: What conclusions can be drawn from the study results in Table 12 – 2?

Question 11: Please summarize the characteristics of this type of experimental study.

IV. Exercises

(1) Which of the following is not an experimental epidemiology study? (　　)

A. Observational trial　　B. Clinical trial　　C. Field trial　　D. Community trial

(2) After COVID-19 vaccination, the core indicator for evaluating the vaccination effect of the population is (　　)

A. Post-vaccination response rate　　　　B. Safety

C. Protective rate D. Clinical manifestations

（3）The most obvious characteristic of experimental studies compared with observational studies is（　　）

A. Prospective B. Intervention
C. Randomness D. Comparative

（4）The largest difference between the intervention and control group in epidemiological field trial is（　　）

A. Different observation indicator B. Different follow-up method
C. Different selection criteria D. Different intervention method

（5）Which of the following is not a disadvantage of experimental epidemiology?（　　）

A. Strict design, complex implementation and high cost of follow-up observation
B. Easily cause medical ethics or ethical problems
C. Randomization to control for bias
D. Blind methods not easy to implement

实验十二　实验流行病学研究

一、实验目的

通过材料分析，掌握实验流行病学的基本含义、特点、类型以及现场试验设计的基本原则和步骤，熟悉试验研究数据资料的整理及基本统计分析。

二、实验原理

（1）实验流行病学的基本原理：研究者根据研究目的，按照预先确定的研究方案将研究对象随机分配到实验组和对照组，人为地施加或减少某种处理因素，然后追踪观察处理因素的作用结果，比较和分析两组人群的结局，从而判断处理因素的效果。

（2）实验流行病学的基本特征：属于前瞻性研究；有人为干预；随机分组；有均衡可比的对照。

（3）主要研究类型：临床试验（以患者为研究对象且干预措施落实到个人）；现场试验（以非患者为研究对象且干预措施落实到个人）；社区试验（以非患者为研究对象且干预措施落实到群体）。

（4）随机临床试验研究（RCT）：该方法是将临床患者随机分为试验组与对照组，试验组给予干预措施，对照组给予对照措施，通过比较各组效应差别而判断干预措施效果的一种前瞻性研究。它是典型的按照实验研究的4个基本原则设计的研究类型，研究效力最高。

（5）研究对象选择的基本原则：选择对干预措施有效的人群；选择预期发病率较高的人群；选择干预对其无害的人群；选择能将试验坚持到底的人群；选择依从性好的人群。

(6) 实验研究随机分组的方法：简单随机分组、区组随机分组、分层随机分组、整群随机分组。

(7) 实验研究对照类型：标准对照、安慰剂对照、平行对照、交叉对照、自身对照、历史对照、空白对照等。

(8) 实验研究盲法的应用：单盲，研究对象不清楚自己是实验组还是对照组；双盲，研究对象和研究实施者均不知道实验分组情况；三盲，研究对象、研究实施者和资料收集分析人员也不知道实验分组情况。

(9) 实验研究资料分析方法：意向治疗分析、依从者分析、接受治疗分析。

(10) 实验研究数据分析主要评价指标：评价治疗效果主要指标（有效率、治愈率、N 年生存率等）；评价预防措施效果主要指标（保护率、效果指数）。

(11) 保护率计算方法。

保护率 =（对照组发病率 − 实验组发病率）/对照组发病率 × 100%　　（公式12 − 1）

(12) 效果指数计算方法。

效果指数 = 对照组发病率/实验组发病率　　（公式12 − 2）

(13) 需要治疗人数（NNT）：为预防 1 例不良事件发生，需要治疗同类病人的人数。该指标可以定量表述疗效大小，有助于医生和病人做临床决策，NNT 越小效果越好。

(14) NNT 计算方法。

NNT = 1/（对照组发病率 − 实验组发病率）　　（公式12 − 3）

三、实验材料

在学校室外活动时间对儿童近视的影响：一项随机实验研究

1. 研究背景

当前全球近视率呈现逐渐上升趋势，尤其是在东亚和东南亚城市地区。这些地方的高中生 80%～90% 都有不同程度的近视，其中约 20% 为高度近视。近视会给个人和社会带来不便及沉重负担，且当前近视逐渐幼年化趋势亦较为明显。早发近视可能导致高度近视，如果发展成为黄斑变性等病理性改变，将给个人身心健康及治疗费用带来沉重负担。目前尚没有预防近视的有效干预措施。尽管低剂量阿托品滴眼、使用矫正镜片能够延缓近视的进程，但是其作用较微弱。

今年来有研究提示室外活动有可能预防近视的发生，但是缺乏高质量的随机临床试验为卫生政策的制定提供证据。2015 年 9 月 15 日，《美国医学会杂志》（JAMA）发表了一项研究，旨在评估增加学校室外活动时间对预防近视的效果。本研究于 2010 年 10 月至 2013 年 10 月对中国广州 12 所小学的一年级学生进行整群随机试验。

2. 研究设计

本研究在中国广州开展，以学校为研究单位，采用整群随机试验设计方法，以小学一年级学生为研究对象，开展为期 3 年的试验研究，旨在验证在校增加室外活动时间对于预防近视的效果。该研究通过伦理委员会的审核，获得研究对象的知情同意。

从 1987 年开始，广州市健康教育研究所就开始每年对 6 个区 30 所不同公立小学所有年级的学生进行视力检查。2009 年初，本研究开始对这 30 所小学发出邀请，排除其中一所视力检查数据不完整的小学，剩余 29 所小学根据 2008 年 1～6 年级所有学生正常视力者所占比例，将这些小学分为 6 层，其中 5 层各 5 所学校，剩余 1 层 4 所学校。每层中再随机选取 2 所学校，一所进入干预组，一所进入对照组。干预组和对照组来自同一层，匹配掉儿童纵向视力减退（随着时间减退，儿童群体视力亦减退）因素的混杂作用，该因素与儿童近视有密切关系。随机化采用 SAS9.2 进行简单随机抽样。

儿童进入一年级时进行基线数据收集，每年随访一次，随访 3 年，直到四年级研究结束。

6 所干预学校一年级学生共 952 人，干预措施为每个教学日增加 1 节 40 分钟的室外活动课，并鼓励家长在放学后让孩子们参加室外活动，尤其是周末和节假日。6 所对照学校一年级学生共 951 人，家长和儿童维持其日常活动模式。

主要结局是基线无近视的学生 3 年累积近视发生率（定义为儿童屈光不正等效球镜 ≤ -0.5 屈光度 [D]）。次要结局是所有学生的球面等效折射率和轴向长度的变化，使用意向治疗原则进行分析。右眼数据用于分析。

问题 1：本研究属于哪种类型的流行病学实验研究？
问题 2：本研究选择试验现场及研究对象是否合适？
问题 3：本研究研究对象的抽样方法是什么？
问题 4：本研究采用的随机分组方法是哪一种？
问题 5：本研究的盲法是如何考虑的？

3. 研究流程

研究流程如图 12-1 所示。

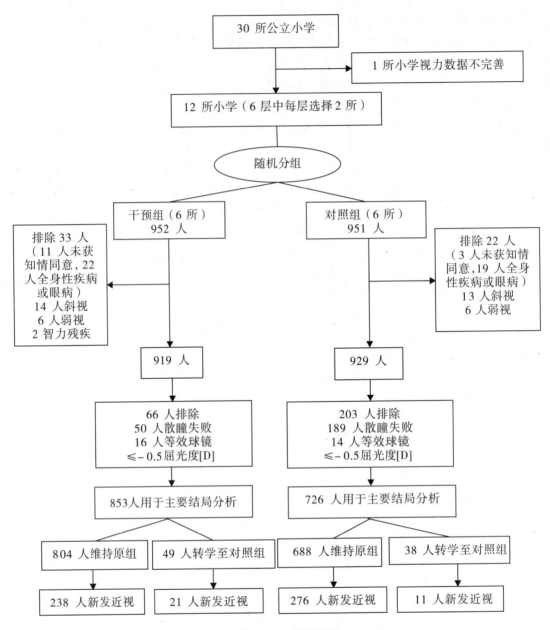

图 12-1 研究流程

4. 研究人群

研究人群基本特征见表 12-1。

表 12-1　干预组和对照组研究人群基线构成比较

	干预组 ($n=919$)[a]	对照组 ($n=929$)[a]	P 值
年龄，均数（s）/岁	6.61 (0.33)	6.57 (0.32)	0.01
男孩，人数（比例）/%	489 (52.58)	509 (54.61)	0.38
身高，均数（s）/cm	120.29 (0.17)	120.51 (0.16)	0.36
体重，均数（s）/kg	22.54 (0.15)	22.56 (0.14)	0.93
体质指数，均数（s）[b]	15.48 (0.07)	15.45 (0.07)	0.71
佩戴眼镜，人数（比例）/%	47 (5.11)	40 (4.31)	0.41
未矫正视力，中位数（IQR）	0.80 (0.80-0.80)	0.80 (0.80-1.00)	0.16
等效球镜，(s)，(D)[c]	1.30 (0.97)	1.26 (0.81)	0.42
近视患病率，近视人数/总人数/%[c]	16/869 (1.84)	14/740 (1.89)	0.94
轴向长度，均数（s）/mm	22.60 (0.71)	22.66 (0.70)	0.05
角膜曲率半径，(s)，(D)	43.54 (1.64)	44.42 (1.40)	0.08
校外室外活动时间，中位数（IQR），（分钟/天）	46.1 (30.00-68.04)	46.07 (30.00-67.50)	0.34
父母亲近视，人数（比例）/%			0.001
父母均无近视	376 (46.36)	273 (40.21)	
一方近视	306 (37.73)	245 (36.08)	
双方近视	129 (15.91)	161 (23.71)	

注：s 为标准差，IQR 为四分位数间距。

a：获得知情同意并完成基线检查的学生右眼数据。

b：BMI = 体重（kg）/［身高（m）］^{2}。

c：仅来源于散瞳验光的学生右眼数据。

问题 6：你对表 12-1 中干预组和对照组可比性资料是否满意，为什么？

问题 7：实验流行病学研究中，基线资料实验组和对照组是要求有差异还是无差异？

5. 研究结果

干预组总共 952 名儿童，对照组 951 名儿童，平均年龄 6.6（0.34）岁。排除掉未获得父母知情同意、基线有全身或眼部病理性改变、散瞳失败等情况，最终用于分析的人数干预组 853 人，对照组为 726 人，其中干预组 49 人在实验期间转学至对照组学校，对照组 38 人在实验期间转学至干预组学校。两组 3 年后新发生近视人数见图 12-1。表 12-2 为 3 年随访后主要结局概况。请根据图 12-1 的数据计算两组累积近视发病率，并比较两组差异是否具有统计学差异，并将结果填入表 12-2 中。

表 12-2 3 年随访后结局概况[a]

	干预组	对照组	P 值
近视累计发病率[b]			
累计改变，均数（95% CI）			
等效球镜，D	-1.42（-1.58～-1.27）	-1.59（-1.76～-1.43）	0.04
轴向长度，mm	0.95（0.91～1.00）	0.98（0.94～1.03）	0.07

注：a：所有结局均以右眼为基础计算。

b：累积发病率为新发累积近视病例数/参与分析的总人数。

问题8：本研究使用意向治疗分析，请回答其分析思路和特点。

问题9：根据意向性分析方法，请计算3年后干预组与对照组的累积近视发病率，并比较两组间差异是否有统计学差异，并将结果填入表12-2中。

问题10：根据表12-2的研究结果可以得出哪些结论？

问题11：请总结该类试验研究的特点。

四、课后练习

（1）下列哪项试验不属于实验流行病学研究？（　　）

A. 观察性试验　　　B. 临床试验　　　C. 现场试验　　　D. 社区试验

（2）新冠肺炎疫苗接种后，评价人群疫苗接种效果的核心指标是（　　）

A. 接种后反应率　　B. 安全性　　　C. 保护率　　　D. 临床表现

（3）实验研究相较于观察性研究最明显的特点是（　　）

A. 前瞻性　　　B. 干预性　　　C. 随机性　　　D. 对比性

（4）流行病学现场试验中实验组与对照组最大的区别是（　　）

A. 观察指标不同　　B. 随访方式不同　　C. 选择标准不同　　D. 干预措施不同

（5）以下哪一条不是实验流行病学的缺点？（　　）

A. 设计严格，实施复杂且随访观察费用较大

B. 容易引起医学伦理或道德的问题

C. 随机分组很难控制偏倚

D. 盲法不容易实施

Experiment 13　Screening Evaluation

Ⅰ. Objectives

Through case analysis, master the basic principle of screening test, the basic method, indexes and calculation methods of screening test evaluation design, and be familiar with the relationship between validity indexes, prevalence rate and predictive values.

Ⅱ. Principles

(1) Definition of screening: screening is a series of medical and health services aimed at preclinical, or early stages of disease, using quick and easy tests, examinations, or other methods to distinguish between individuals who may have a disease, but who appear to be healthy, from those who do not have said disease.

(2) The roles of screening: screening can be used to detect hidden cases, identify high-risk groups, and understand the natural progression history of the disease.

(3) Principles for screening of diseases: the screened diseases, or related health states should pose a public health problem in the region at present stage; the natural history of target diseases should be clear, with sufficiently long preclinical and identifiable disease identification; there needs to be a clear understanding of the intervention effect and adverse reactions at different stages of the diseases.

(4) Characteristics of the screening test: simplicity, inexpensiveness, rapidity, safety, acceptability.

(5) The validity of screening test: also called as accuracy, refers to the degree of coincidence between measured value and actual value.

(6) Indicators for evaluating the validity of screening test: sensitivity and false negative rate, specificity and false positive rate, correct index (Youden index), and likelihood ratio.

(7) Sensitivity: also known as true positive rate, is the percentage of patients who are actually ill and are accurately tested/detected positive by the screening test criteria, which reflects the ability of the screening test to detect/diagnosis patients.

(8) False negative rate: also known as missed diagnosis rate, refers to the percentage of patients who actually have the disease but are tested negative, reflecting the situation of patients missed by screening tests.

(9) Specificity: also known as true negative rate, refers to the percentage of patients who are actually disease-free and tested negative, which reflects the ability of screening test to exclude patients.

(10) False positive rate: also known as misdiagnosis rate, i.e., the percentage of patients who are actually disease-free but tested positive, reflecting the situation of patients misdiagnosed by screening test.

(11) Correct index: also known as Youden index, is the sum of sensitivity and specificity minus 1, indicating the total ability of screening test to identify patients and non-patients. The correct index ranges from 0 to 1. The larger the correct index is, the higher the validity of the screening test is.

(12) Likelihood ratio: is a comprehensive index reflecting both sensitivity and specificity, and is divided into positive likelihood ratio and negative likelihood ratio.

(13) Positive likelihood ratio is the ratio of the true positive rate to the false positive rate of the screening results. The higher the ratio is, the greater the probability that the positive result of the screening test is true positive.

(14) Negative likelihood ratio is the ratio of false negative rate to true negative rate of screening test results. The smaller the ratio is, the greater the probability that the negative result of the screening test is true negative.

(15) Reliability: also called repeatability and precision, refers to the consistency of the results when a certain screening test method is used to repeatedly measure the same subjects under the same conditions.

(16) The reliability indexes for evaluating continuous measurement data are: standard deviation and coefficient of variation or correlation coefficient; the reliability indexes for evaluating classified measurement data are: agreement rate and kappa value.

(17) Predictive values: indicators that use the positive and negative screening results to estimate the possibility that the subject is a patient and a non-patient, including the positive predictive value and the negative predictive value.

(18) Positive predictive value: the proportion of people with the target disease among those who are screened positive.

(19) Negative predictive value: the proportion of people who do not suffer from the target disease among those who are screened negative.

(20) Combined tests: in the implementation of screening test, two or more screening tests can be used to examine the same subject, to improve the sensitivity or specificity of screening and to increase the benefits of the screening tests, including serial test and parallel test.

(21) Serial tests: a group of screening tests are connected in a certain order, i.e., those who are positive in the initial screening enter the next round of screening, and all the screening test results are positive are defined as positive. The serial tests can improve the screening specificity, but it will reduce the sensitivity.

(22) Parallel tests: all screening tests are conducted in parallel at the same time, and any positive screening test result is judged as positive. This method can improve the sensitivity of screening, but it will reduce the specificity.

Ⅲ. Materials

Material Ⅰ

Colorectal cancer is one of the most common malignant tumors in China. Nationwide colorectal cancer screening can effectively reduce the incidence and mortality due to colorectal cancers. A city intended to carry out the method evaluation of fecal occult blood test (OB) screening for colorectal cancers in the population. The researchers carried out a screening study in residents with household registration aged 40~74 years. The gold standard for the diagnosis of colorectal cancer is microscopic examination and histopathological examination. The screening process and the corresponding number of people screened are shown in Figure 13-1.

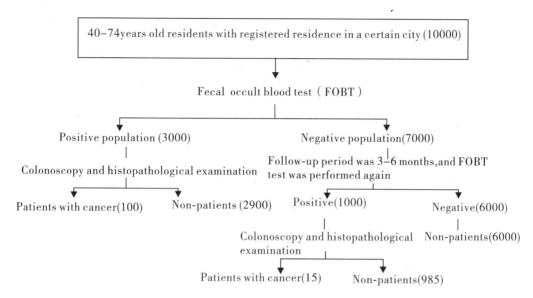

Figure 13-1 Screening process and number of colorectal cancer patients

Question 1: What is the rationale for screening?

Question 2: What are the objectives of screening?

Question 3: What principles should be followed when carrying out screening test?

Question 4: What is the gold standard for the evaluation of this screening test according to the positive and negative population in the primary screening? Please specify whether the judgment process for patients with negative by preliminary screening is appropriate.

Question 5: Please arrange the four-grid table of screening test evaluation according to Figure 13-1.

Question 6: What are the indicators to evaluate the validity of screening test? According to the listed four-grid table, calculate the values of various validity evaluation indicators.

Question 7: What are the reliability indicators for evaluation of screening test? What reliability values can be calculated in this case.

Question 8: Calculate the negative predictive value and positive predictive value of fecal occult blood screening test (FOBT) for colorectal cancer in this case.

Material II

In the implementation of screening test, two or more screening tests can be used to examine the same subject, to improve the sensitivity or specificity of screening and increase the screening benefits. This way is called combined test, including serial test and parallel test. Serial test, also known as series tests, that is, a group of screening tests are connected in a certain order, those who are positive in the initial screening enter the next round of screening, and all screening test results are positive are defined as positive. Parallel test, that is, all screening tests are conducted in parallel at the same time, and a positive result of any screening test is judged as positive. In order to evaluate the application value of fecal occult blood test (FOBT) and fecal cryptoprotein test (FCPT) in colorectal cancer screening, 165 patients who visited the doctor were selected for FCPT and FOBT combined test screening, including 75 patients with colorectal cancer and 90 non-patients. The results of combined test are shown in Table 13 – 1.

Table 13 – 1 Results of screening for colorectal cancer in the combined FOBT and FCPT trial

Screening test		Patients with colorectal cancer	Colorectal cancer non-patient
FOBT	FCPT		
+	−	20	63
−	+	36	42
+	+	140	9
−	−	4	186
Total		200	300

Question 1: Please calculate the sensitivity and specificity of screening test for simple FOBT and FCPT, respectively, and calculate the sensitivity and specificity of parallel test and serial test, respectively.

Question 2: How does the sensitivity and specificity of the combined test change compared to a single screening test?

Question 3: Do you think colorectal cancer screening should be done in a single trial or in a combined trial? Why is that?

IV. Exercises

(1) Regarding screening, which of the following statements is incorrect? (　　)

A. The disease screened should be a major health problem that endangers the population health to certain degrees

B. For those who screen positive, there should be clear diagnostic and therapeutic measures in the subsequent period

C. Screening is to detect rare cases

D. Screening tests should be conducted in a manner that does not cause serious physical or mental harm to subjects

(2) Which of the following diseases are suitable for large-scale screening? (　　)

A. Cervical carcinoma in situ　　　　　　B. National examination of HBsAg

C. AIDS　　　　　　　　　　　　　　　D. Influenza

(3) Subjects are actually sick, the ability to accurately judge as positive by screening test is called (　　)

A. Sensitivity   B. Specificity

C. Positive likelihood ratio   D. Correct Index

（4）The correct method to improve the benefits of screening tests is（　　）

A. Screening of high-risk population

B. Reduce sensitivity of screening test

C. Improve the specificity of screening test

D. Screening in a population with low prevalence

（5）To improve the specificity of the screening test, several independent tests can be used by（　　）

A. Serial tests   B. Parallel tests

C. Serial first and then parallel tests   D. Parallel first and then serial tests

实验十三　筛检评价

一、实验目的

通过案例分析，掌握筛检试验的基本原理、筛检试验评价设计的基本方法、指标及计算方法，熟悉真实性指标、患病率与预测值之间的相互关系。

二、实验原理

（1）筛检定义：筛检或筛查是针对临床前期或早期的疾病阶段，运用快速、简便的试验、检查或其他方法，将人群中那些可能有病但表面健康的个体同那些可能无病者鉴别开来的一系列医疗卫生服务措施。

（2）筛检的作用：发现隐匿的病例，发现高危人群，了解疾病自然史，等等。

（3）筛检的疾病原则：所筛检的疾病或相关健康状态应该是该地区现阶段重大的公共卫生问题；目标疾病的自然史清晰，有足够长的临床前期和可被识别的疾病标识；对疾病不同阶段的干预效果及不良反应有清楚的认识。

（4）筛检试验的特征：简单性、廉价性、快速性、安全性、可接受性。

（5）筛检试验真实性：也叫作效度，是指测量值与实际值相符合程度，也可叫准确性。

（6）评价筛检试验真实性的指标：灵敏度与假阴性率，特异度与假阳性率，正确指数，似然比。

（7）灵敏度：又叫作真阳性率，是实际患病且被筛检试验标准准确地判断为阳性的百分比，反映了筛检试验发现病人的能力。

（8）假阴性率：又称漏诊率，指实际患病但被筛检试验确定为阴性的百分比，反映筛检试验漏诊病人的情况。

（9）特异度：又称真阴性率，指实际无病且被筛检试验标准判断为阴性的百分比，反映筛检试验排除病人的能力。

（10）假阳性率：又称误诊率，即实际无病但被筛检试验判断为阳性的百分比，反映筛检试验误诊病人的情况。

（11）正确指数：也称约登指数，是灵敏度与特异度之和减去1，表示筛检试验识别病人和非病人的总能力。正确指数的范围在0～1之间，指数越大，真实性越高。

（12）似然比：是同时反映灵敏度和特异度的综合指标，分为阳性似然比和阴性似然比。

（13）阳性似然比：是筛检结果真阳性率与假阳性率之比。比值越大，试验结果阳性时为真阳性的可能性越大。

（14）阴性似然比：是筛检结果假阴性率与真阴性率之比。比值越小，试验结果阴性时为真阴性的可能性越大。

（15）可靠性：也称信度、精确度、可重复性，是指在相同条件下用某种筛检试验方法重复测量同一受试者时结果的一致程度。

（16）评价连续性测量资料的可靠性指标为：标准差和变异系数或相关系数。评价分类测量资料的可靠性指标为：符合率和kappa值。

（17）预测值：是应用筛检结果的阳性和阴性来估计受检者为病人和非病人的可能性的指标，包括阳性预测值和阴性预测值。

（18）阳性预测值：筛检发现阳性者中患目标疾病的人所占的比例。

（19）阴性预测值：筛检发现阴性者中不患目标疾病的人所占的比例。

（20）联合实验：在实施筛检时，可采用两种或两种以上筛检试验检查同一受试对象，以提高筛检的灵敏度或特异度，增加筛检收益，包括串联试验与并联试验。

（21）串联试验：也称系列试验，即一组筛检试验按一定顺序相连，初筛阳性者进入下一轮筛检，全部筛检试验结果均为阳性者才定为阳性。串联试验可以提高筛检特异度，但会降低灵敏度。

（22）并联试验：也称平行试验，即全部筛检试验同时平行开展，任何一项筛检试验结果阳性就判定为阳性。该方法可以提高筛检的灵敏度，但是会降低特异度。

三、实验材料

材料一

结直肠癌是我国常见恶性肿瘤之一。开展人群结直肠癌筛查能有效降低结直肠癌的发病率和死亡率。某市拟在人群中开展粪便潜血筛检试验（Fecal Occult Blood Test，FOBT）筛检结直肠癌的方法评价，研究者在40～74岁的户籍居民中开展了筛查研究，结直肠癌诊断的金标准为镜检及组织病理学检查。筛检流程及相应人数见图13-1。

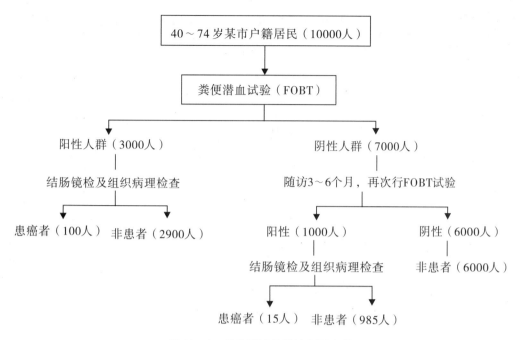

图 13-1 结直肠癌筛检流程及人数

问题 1：筛检的基本原理是什么？

问题 2：筛检的目的是什么？

问题 3：开展筛检时应遵循哪些原则？

问题 4：按照初筛的阳性人群和阴性人群说明本筛检试验评价的金标准是什么？请说明初筛阴性者的判断流程是否合适。

问题 5：根据图 13-1 整理筛检试验评价四格表。

问题 6：评价筛检试验真实性的指标有哪些？根据所列四格表，计算各真实性评价指标数值。

问题 7：评价筛检试验可靠性指标有哪些？本案例中可以计算哪些可靠性指标？

问题 8：计算本案例结直肠癌 FOBT 的阴性预测值、阳性预测值。

材料二

在实施筛检时，可采用两种或两种以上筛检试验检查同一受试对象，以提高筛检的灵敏度或特异度，增加筛检收益，这种方式叫作联合试验，包括串联试验与并联试验。串联试验，也称系列试验，即一组筛检试验按一定顺序相连，初筛阳性者进入下一轮筛检，全部筛检试验结果均为阳性者才定为阳性。并联试验，也称平行试验，即全部筛检试验同时平行开展，任何一项筛检试验结果阳性就判定为阳性。为评价 FOBT 及粪便隐蛋白试验（FCPT）对结直肠癌筛检的应用价值，某医生选择就诊的 165 名病人进行 FCPT 和 FOBT 联合试验筛检，其中结直肠癌患者 75 人，非患者 90 人，联合试验结果见表 13-1。

表 13-1 FOBT 和 FCPT 联合试验筛检结直肠癌结果

筛检试验		结直肠癌患者	结直肠癌非患者
FOBT	FCPT		
+	−	20	63
−	+	36	42
+	+	140	9
−	−	4	186
合计		200	300

问题 1：请分别计算单纯 FOBT、FCPT 的灵敏度和特异度，分别计算并联试验和串联试验的灵敏度和特异度。

问题 2：同单纯某一种筛检试验相比，联合试验的灵敏度和特异度有何改变？

问题 3：结直肠癌普查工作，你认为是采用某一项试验，还是联合试验中的某一组？为什么？

四、课后练习

（1）关于筛检，下列说法哪一项不正确？（   ）

A. 所筛检的疾病应该是危害人群健康的重大卫生问题

B. 对筛检阳性者，后续应该有明确的诊断和治疗措施

C. 筛检是为了发现罕见病例

D. 筛检试验的方法不应给受试者带来严重的身心伤害

（2）下列哪些疾病适合大规模筛检？（   ）

A. 原位子宫颈癌　　　B. 全民检查 HBsAg　　C. 艾滋病　　　　　D. 流行性感冒

（3）实际有病，用筛检试验准确地判断为阳性的能力称（   ）

A. 灵敏度　　　　　　B. 特异度　　　　　　C. 阳性似然比　　　　D. 正确指数

（4）提高筛检试验效益的方法正确的是（   ）

A. 对高危人群进行筛检

B. 降低筛检试验的灵敏度

C. 提高筛检试验的特异度

D. 在患病率低的人群中筛检

（5）为提高筛检试验的特异度，对几个独立的试验可使用（   ）

A. 串联试验　　　　　　　　　　　　　　　B. 并联试验

C. 先串联后并联　　　　　　　　　　　　　D. 先并联后串联

（曹文婷）

Chapter Three | Practical for Environmental Health

第三章 | 环境卫生学实验及案例

Chapter Three Practical for Environmental Health

Experiment 14 Determination of Particulate Matter in the Air

Particulate matter is the primary pollutant in most cities in China and the main cause of affecting urban air quality. The deposition of particulate matter in the air is related to its particle size. Air particles can generally be divided into the following categories by size: ① Total suspended particulates (TSP) refer to particulate matter smaller than or equal to 100 μm and include liquid, solid, or combined liquid and solid particles that are suspended in the air. ② Inhalable particles (IP, PM_{10}) are airborne particles with diameters less than or equal to 10 μm, named for their ability to enter the respiratory tract and suspended in the air. ③ Fine particulate matters ($PM_{2.5}$) are particles with the aerodynamic diameter $\leqslant 2.5$ μm. $PM_{2.5}$ are more likely to adsorb a variety of toxic organic and heavy metal elements, which are great harm to health. ④ Ultrafine particle matters ($PM_{0.1}$) are particles with an aerodynamic diameter $\leqslant 0.1$ μm.

Part 1 Determination of total suspended particulates in the air

Ⅰ. Objectives

To master the principle and operation of mass method for the determination of total suspended particulate matter in the air through practice.

Ⅱ. Experimental methods and procedures

1. Principle

When the air passes through the sampler, the total suspended particles are blocked on the filter film. The concentration of total suspended particles in the air are calculated according to the weight difference and sampling volume of the filter film before and after sampling.

2. Instruments

(1) Large-flow sampler: Flow range $1.1 - 1.7$ m^3/min, particle size $0.1 - 100.0$ μm.

(2) Barometer: The minimum fractional value is 2 hPa.

(3) Analytical balance: Sensitivity is 0.1 mg.

(4) Dryer: Filled with color-changing silica gel.

(5) Filter membrane: Ultrafine glass fiber filter membrane, the retention efficiency of 0.3 μm standard particles are no less than 99%, at the airflow velocity of 0.45 m/s, the single filter membrane resistance is no more than 3.5 kPa, under the same airflow velocity, the extraction of purified air by hePA filter for 5 h, 1 cm^2 filter membrane weight loss is no more than 0.012 mg.

(6) Forceps for bamboo or bone products.

(7) Filter storage box.

3. Methods

(1) Sampling.

The filter film was balanced in a dryer for 24 h and weighed to constant weight W_1 accurately. During sampling, place the filter film flat on the support network with forceps, the filter hair facing upwards, place it straight, smooth, press and fix it. Set the sampler at 3~5 m (relative height 1~1.5 m), turn on the power supply, and sample at a flow rate of 1.1~1.7 m³/min. The sampling time depends on the need. The temperature and pressure at the time of sampling were recorded simultaneously. After sampling, remove the filter film, put it in a dryer for balance for 24 h, and accurately weigh it to constant weight W_2. The weight difference of filter membrane before and after sampling is the weight of total suspended particulate matter.

(2) Calculation.

$$C = \frac{(W_2 - W_1) \times 1000}{V_0}$$

Note: C is the concentration of total suspended particulate matter (mg/m³).

W_1 is the weight of pre-filter membrane (g).

W_2 is the weight of the sampled filter membrane (g).

V_0 is the sampling volume (m³) converted to standard atmospheric pressure.

Conversion of sampling volume under standard state: since the volume of air changes with the change of temperature, pressure and other meteorological factors, it is necessary to convert the volume of air under standard state to make the data comparable.

$$V_0 = V_t \times \frac{T_0}{t} \times \frac{P}{P_0} = V_t \times \frac{273}{273+t} \times \frac{P}{101.3 \ (kPa)}$$

V_0 is the sampling volume (m³) converted to standard atmospheric pressure.

V_t is the actual sampling volume (L or m³).

T_0 is the absolute temperature in the standard state (273 K).

t is the Celsius temperature (℃) at the time of sampling.

P_0 is atmospheric pressure in standard state (101.325 kPa).

P is atmospheric pressure (kPa) at the time of sampling.

(3) Notes.

① Light inspection is required for each filter membrane before reuse, and no pinhole or any defective filter membrane sampling is allowed.

② If the BaP content in the total suspended particulate matters needs to be analyzed, the filter membrane should be baked in a muffle furnace at 550℃ for 30 min before sampling to remove organic impurities. If the content of heavy metals in total suspended particulate matter is determined, organic filtration membrane should be used.

③ If sampling time is too long or sampling in heavily polluted areas, too much dust on the filter film will affect the flow rate. Therefore, the filter membrane should be replaced in time and the flow rate should be adjusted and maintained.

④ Carefully remove the filter membrane with forceps after adoption, and place the sampling side of filter membrane in a dryer after half folding twice.

⑤ When the sampler is in use, the flow rate should be calibrated frequently, and the flow rate calibration error before and after sampling should be no more than 7%.

⑥ Always check the sampling head for air leakage. The panel gasket should be replaced when the boundary between the particles on the filter and the surrounding white edge becomes blurred.

⑦ The flow rate of the sampler still cannot meet the requirements except for factors such as insufficient voltage. At this time, the motor brush should be checked for wear. If it is worn, it should be replaced in time.

Part 2　Determination of inhalable particles in the air

Ⅰ. Objectives

To master the principle and operation of mass method for determination of inhalable particles in the air through practice.

Ⅱ. Experimental methods and procedures

1. Principle

Particles with aerodynamic equivalent diameter < 30 μm ($D_{50} = 10$ μm, geometric standard deviation is 1.5 μm) are collected on a constant weight filter by using a two-stage separation impact-type small flow sampler and sampling at the flow rate specified by the sampler. After sampling, the filter film is removed and weighed, and the concentration of inhalable particles in the air are calculated according to the quality difference of the filter film before and after sampling and the sampling volume.

2. Instruments

(1) PM_{10} sampler.

(2) Barometer: The minimum fractional value is 2 hPa.

(3) Analytical balance: Sensitivity is 0.1 mg.

(4) Dryer: Filled with color-changing silica gel.

(5) Filter membrane: Glass fiber filter membrane, the diameter of which is determined by the selected sampler.

(6) The forceps.

(7) Filter storage box.

3. Methods

(1) Sampling.

Place the constant weight filter (W_1), hair facing up, on the filter screen in the clean sampling clip. Operation in accordance with the selected sampler instructions, at the flow rate specified by the sampler, and extract gas for 8~24h. The temperature and pressure at the time of sampling were recorded simultaneously. After sampling, remove the filter, fold the dust side twice, and put it in the filter storage bag. Balance in a dryer for 24h and weigh to constant weight W_2. The difference of membrane quality before and after sampling is the weight of inhalable particles.

(2) Calculation.

$$C = \frac{(W_2 - W_1) \times 1000}{V_0}$$

C is the concentration of inhalable particles (mg/m^3).

W_1 is the weight of pre-filter membrane (g).

W_2 is the weight of the sampled filter membrane (g).

V_0 is the sampling volume (m^3) converted to standard atmospheric pressure.

(3) Notes.

① The flow rate should be kept constant during the sampling period. The soap membrane flowmeter should be used for calibration before using, and the error value should be less than 5%.

② Before sampling, the inside and outside surfaces of sampling head and grading nozzles should be carefully cleaned, and the filter membrane should be prevented from leakage and pressure loss during installation.

③ Quality control should be carried out on the weighing of sampling filter membrane. Specific operation method: 4~5 pieces of balanced and weighed filter membrane are randomly selected, each of which is repeatedly balanced and weighed more than 10 times, and the average quality of each membrane is calculated as the "standard filter membrane" for weighing quality control. Each time the blank filter and the sampled filter are weighed, the two "standard filter membrane" must be weighed simultaneously. When weighing with an analytical balance with a sensitivity of 0.1 mg, the difference between the mass of the so-called "standard filter membrane" and its mean value must be less than 0.45mg; otherwise, it should be weighed again after rebalancing.

Part 3 Determination of fine particulate matter in the air

Ⅰ. Objectives

To master the principle and operation of mass method for determination of fine particulate matter in the air through practice.

Ⅱ. Experimental methods and procedures

1. Principle

By means of a sampler with certain cutting characteristics, a certain volume of air is extracted at a constant speed, so that the fine particulate matters in the air are trapped on the filter film with constant weight. After sampling, remove the filter film, weigh it, and calculate the concentration of fine particulate matter in the air according to the weight difference and sampling volume of the filter film before and after sampling.

2. Instruments

(1) Medium-flow sampler: Flow range is 60 – 125 L/min.

(2) $PM_{2.5}$ cutter: Particle size $D_{50} = 2.5 \pm 0.2$ μm, geometric standard deviation 1.2 ± 0.1 μm.

(3) Analytical balance: Sensitivity is 0.1 mg.

(4) Dryer: Filled with color-changing silica gel.

(5) Filter film: Ultrafine glass fiber filter membrane, the diameter of which is determined by the sampler selected.

(6) Constant temperature and humidity box: The air temperature in the box is continuously adjustable within the range of 15 – 30℃, and the temperature control accuracy is ±1℃; Relative humidity is controlled at 50% ±5%.

(7) The tweezers.

(8) Filter storage bag.

3. Methods

(1) Sampling.

The constant weight filter (W_1), with the hair facing up, was placed flat on the filter screen in the clean sampling clip. Press the filter membrane firmly until there is no air leakage and stat sampling. The temperature and pressure at the time of sampling were recorded simultaneously. After sampling, remove the filter, fold the dust in half twice, and put it in the filter storage box. Balance in a constant temperature and humidity box for 24h and weigh accurately to constant weight W_2. The difference of membrane quality before and after sampling is the weight of fine particles.

(2) Calculation.

$$C = \frac{(W_2 - W_1) \times 1000}{V_0}$$

C is the concentration of fine particulate matter (mg/m³).

W_1 is the weight of pre-filter membrane (g).

W_2 is the weight of the sampled filter membrane (g).

V_0 is the sampling volume (m³) converted to standard atmospheric pressure.

(3) Notes.

① Flow calibration shall be carried out before each use of the sampler.

② Check the filter membrane: The filter membrane should be pervious to light before use to confirm that there is no pinhole or any other defect. The effect of static electricity should be eliminated when the filter membrane is weighed.

③ Check the sampling head for air leakage: When the filter membrane is placed correctly and the sampling system is free of air leakage, the boundary between the fine particles on the filter membrane and the surrounding white edge should be clear after sampling. If the boundary is blurred, the filter film sealing gasket should be replaced.

④ The same analytical balance should be used for the filter membrane weighing before and after sampling.

实验十四 大气中颗粒物的测定

颗粒物是我国大多数城市的首要污染物,是影响城市大气质量的主要原因。颗粒物在大气中的沉降与其粒径有关。按粒径大小,大气颗粒物一般可分为以下几类:①总悬浮颗粒物(total suspended particulates,TSP),指粒径≤100 μm 的颗粒物,包括液体、固体或者液体和固体结合存在的,悬浮于空气中的颗粒。②可吸入颗粒物(inhalable particle,IP,PM_{10}),指空气动力学直径≤10 μm 的颗粒物,因其能进入人体呼吸道而命名,又因其能长期飘浮在空气中,也被称为飘尘(suspended dusts)。③细颗粒物(fine particle,fine particulate matter,$PM_{2.5}$),指空气动力学直径≤2.5 μm 的细颗粒。$PM_{2.5}$ 更易于吸附各种有毒的有机物和重金属元素,对健康的危害极大。④超细颗粒物(ultrafine particle,ultrafine particulate matter,$PM_{0.1}$),指空气动力学直径≤0.1 μm 的颗粒物。

第一节 大气中总悬浮颗粒物(TSP)的测定

一、实验目的

通过实习掌握质量法测定大气中总悬浮颗粒物的原理和操作方法。

二、实验方法和步骤

1. 原理

将已恒重的滤膜装入大流量采样器的滤膜夹上,空气通过采样器时,总悬浮颗粒物被阻留在滤膜上,根据采样前后滤膜的质量差和采样体积来计算空气中总悬浮颗粒物的浓度。

2. 仪器

(1) 大流量采样器:流量范围 $1.1 \sim 1.7$ m^3/min,采集粒径 $0.1 \sim 100.0$ μm。

(2) 气压计:最小分度值为 2 hPa。

(3) 分析天平:感量为 0.1 mg。

(4) 干燥器:内盛变色硅胶。

(5) 滤膜:超细玻璃纤维滤膜,对 0.3 μm 标准粒子的阻留效率不低于 99%,在气流速度为 0.45 m/s 时,单张滤膜阻力不大于 3.5 kPa,在同样气流速度下,抽取经高效过滤器净化的空气 5 h,1 cm^2 滤膜失重不大于 0.012 mg。

(6) 竹制或骨制品的镊子。

(7) 滤膜贮存盒。

3. 方法

(1) 采样。

将滤膜放入干燥器中平衡 24 h,准确称量至恒重 W_1。采样时用镊子将滤膜平放于支持网上,滤膜毛面向上,放正、铺平、压紧、固定。置采样器于 3~5 m(相对高度 1~1.5 m)处,接通电源,以 1.1~1.7 m³/min 流量采样。采样时间根据需要而定。同时记录采样时的气温和气压。采样后,取下滤膜,放入干燥器中平衡 24 h,准确称量至恒重 W_2。采样前后滤膜称重之差,即为总悬浮颗粒物的重量。

(2) 计算。

$$C = \frac{(W_2 - W_1) \times 1000}{V_0}$$

注:C 为总悬浮颗粒物的质量浓度(mg/m³)

W_1 为采样前滤膜重量(g)

W_2 为采样后滤膜重量(g)

V_0 为换算成标准大气压下的采样体积(m³)

标准状态下的采样体积换算:由于空气的体积随着温度、气压等气象因素的变化而变化,因此,须换算成标准状态下的空气体积,使其资料具有可比性。

$$V_0 = V_t \times \frac{T_0}{t} \times \frac{P}{P_0} = V_t \times \frac{273}{273 + t} \times \frac{P}{101.3\ (kPa)}$$

注:V_0 为换算成标准大气压下的采样体积(m³)

V_t 为实际采样体积(L 或 m³)

T_0 为标准状态下的绝对温度(273 K)

t 为采样时摄氏温度(℃)

P_0 为标准状态下的大气压(101.325 kPa)

P 为采样时的大气压(kPa)

(3) 注意事项。

①每张滤膜在使用前均需要光照检查,不能使用有针孔或有任何缺陷的滤膜采样。

②若需分析总悬浮颗粒物中 BaP 含量,滤膜在采样前应置于马福炉中 550℃烘烤 30 分钟,以去除有机杂质。若测定总悬浮颗粒物中重金属的含量,宜采用有机滤膜。

③在污染较重的地区采样或采样时间过长,滤膜上积尘太多会影响流量,故须及时更换滤膜并调节和保持流量。

④采样后用镊子小心取下滤膜,采样面对半折叠两次置于干燥器中。

⑤采样器在使用时应经常校准流量,采样前后流量校准误差应≤7%。

⑥要经常检查采样头是否漏气。当滤膜上颗粒物与四周白边之间的界限逐渐模糊时,则应更换面板密封垫。

⑦采样器的流量在排除电压不足等影响因素外,仍不能达到要求,此时应检查电机电刷是否磨损,若磨损则应及时更换。

第二节 大气中可吸入颗粒物（PM_{10}）的测定

一、实验目的和意义

通过实习掌握质量法测定大气中可吸入颗粒物的原理和操作方法。

二、实验方法和步骤

1. 原理

利用二段分离冲击式小流量采样器，在采样器规定的流量下采样，空气中颗粒物经惯性冲击分离，将空气动力学当量直径 <30 μm（$D_{50} = 10$ μm，几何标准差为 1.5 μm）的颗粒收集于已恒重的滤膜上。采样后，取下滤膜，称重，根据采样前后滤膜的质量差和采样体积来计算空气中可吸入颗粒物的浓度。

2. 仪器

（1）PM_{10} 采样器。

（2）气压计：最小分度值为 2 hPa。

（3）分析天平：感量为 0.1 mg。

（4）干燥器：内盛变色硅胶。

（5）滤膜：玻璃纤维滤膜，直径由所选用的采样器决定。

（6）镊子。

（7）滤膜贮存盒。

3. 方法

（1）采样。

将已恒重的滤膜（W_1），毛面向上，平置于采样夹中。按照所选择的采样器说明书操作，在采样器规定的流量下，采气 8～24 小时。同时记录采样时的气温和气压。采样后，取下滤膜，尘面向里对折，放于滤膜贮存盒中。放入干燥器中平衡 24 h，准确称量至恒重 W_2。采样前后滤膜质量之差，即为可吸入颗粒物的重量。

（2）计算。

$$C = \frac{(W_2 - W_1) \times 1000}{v_0}$$

注：C 为可吸入颗粒物的质量浓度（mg/m^3）

W_1 为采样前滤膜重量（g）

W_2 为采样后滤膜重量（g）

V_0 为换算成标准大气压下的采样体积（m^3）

（3）注意事项。

①采样期间流量应保持恒定。使用前应用皂膜流量计进行校准，误差应 <5%。

②采样前应认真清洁采样头的内外表面和分级喷嘴，安装时应防止漏气和压损滤膜。

③对采样滤膜的称量应进行质量控制。具体操作方法：在已平衡、称重的滤膜中，随

机抽取 4～5 张，每张反复平衡、称重 10 次以上，计算各张滤膜的质量均值，作为称量质量控制的"标准滤膜"。每次称量空白滤膜和采样后的滤膜时，必须同时称量两张"标准滤膜"。若用感量为 0.1 mg 的分析天平称量时，所称"标准滤膜"的质量与其均值之差应小于 0.45 mg，否则应重新平衡后再称量。

第三节 大气中细颗粒物（$PM_{2.5}$）的测定

一、实验目的和意义

通过实习掌握质量法测定大气中细颗粒物的原理和操作方法。

二、实验方法和步骤

1. 原理

通过具有一定切割特性的采样器，按恒定速度抽取一定体积的空气，使空气中细颗粒物被阻留在已恒重的滤膜上。采样后，取下滤膜，称重，根据采样前后滤膜的重量差和采样体积，计算空气中细颗粒物的浓度。

2. 仪器

（1）中流量采样器：流量范围为 60～125 L/min。

（2）$PM_{2.5}$ 切割器：切割粒径 D_{50} = 2.5 ± 0.2 μm，几何标准差为 1.2 ± 0.1 μm。

（3）分析天平：感量为 0.1 mg。

（4）干燥器：内盛变色硅胶。

（5）滤膜：超细玻璃纤维滤膜，直径由所选用的采样器决定。

（6）恒温恒湿箱：箱内空气温度在 15～30℃ 范围内连续可调，控温精度为 ±1℃；相对湿度控制在 50% ± 5%。

（7）镊子。

（8）滤膜贮存袋。

3. 方法

（1）采样。

将已恒重的滤膜（W_1），毛面向上，放于洁净采样夹内的滤网上。将滤膜牢固压紧至不漏气，开始采样。同时记录采样时的气温和气压。采样后，取下滤膜，尘面向里两次对折，放于滤膜贮存袋中。放入恒温恒湿箱中平衡 24 小时，称量至恒重 W_2。采样前后滤膜质量之差，即为细颗粒物的重量。

（2）计算。

$$C = \frac{(W_2 - W_1) \times 1000}{V_0}$$

注：C 为细颗粒物的质量浓度（mg/m³）

W_1 为采样前滤膜重量（g）

W_2 为采样后滤膜重量（g）

V_0 为换算成标准大气压下的采样体积（m^3）

（3）注意事项。

①采样器每次使用前须进行流量校准。

②检查滤膜：使用前将滤膜进行透光检查，确认无针孔或其他任何缺陷。滤膜称量时要消除静电的影响。

③检查采样头是否漏气：当滤膜放置正确，采样系统无漏气时，采样后滤膜上细颗粒物与四周白边之间界限应清晰，如出现界限模糊时，则应更换滤膜密封垫。

④采样前后，滤膜称量应使用同一台分析天平。

Experiment 15　Monitoring and Evaluation of Negative Ions in Air

Air negative oxygen ions (NAIs), which are formed by the combination of oxygen molecules and free electrons in the atmosphere, are colorless, odorless and also known as small particle negative ions. Negative oxygen ions can effectively reduce the concentration of particulate matter, especially $PM_{2.5}$ and PM_{10}, thus improving air quality, which are in the high concentration of the atmosphere such as forests, waterfalls and beaches, up to $0.5 \times 10^3 - 10 \times 10^3$ ions/cm^3. There are obvious daily, monthly and annual changes of negative oxygen ions, which are related to meteorological factors such as air temperature, humidity and precipitation, also related to forest vegetation and environmental conditions.

Small negative ions (or light negative ions) in the air have a promoting effect on human health, while high positive ions have a negative effect on human health. A high concentration of light negative ions indicates good air quality, while a high concentration of heavy ions or positive ions indicates heavy air pollution. It is of great significance to carry out air negative ion monitoring for disease convalescence, health promotion, meeting people's needs of ecological environment understanding, and making up for the deficiency of current environmental monitoring index system in China.

Ⅰ. Objectives

To master the use of air ion monitoring instrument and its monitoring technology and master the design key points of air ion monitoring scheme and the evaluation method of air ion through practice.

Ⅱ. Experiment Procedures

1. Selection of monitoring equipment

In order to comprehensively analyze the relationship between air ions and air quality, instruments capable of simultaneously monitoring air positive ions, negative ions, large ions and small ions should be selected. Generally, the instrument with high degree of automation can measure positive and negative ion concentration, recording environmental temperature and humidity at the same time, and automatically store digital records. Such as COM3800, 350U series air ion analyzer, NKMH103 series which made in Japan, DLY and ITC-201A produced by Southeast Electronic Research Institute in Zhangzhou, Fujian. Domestic instruments should comply with *The General Specification for Air Ion Measuring Instruments* (GB/T 18809-2002).

The high temperature and humidity environment may cause the instability of most of the brand instruments, so the instrument should be avoided in the high temperature and humidity environment as far as possible. The air negative ion monitoring should be carried out in sunny weather with little wind.

2. The design of the monitoring programme

At present our country has not specifical air ion monitoring specification. This experiment with reference to the Japanese *The Ion Density in the Air Act* (JIS-B9 929: 2006), *The Environmental Air Quality Monitoring Specification* (2007) (Trial), *Technical Specification for Ambient Air Quality Monitoring Points Layout* (HJ664-2013), *Manual Monitoring of environmental Air Quality Specification* (HJ 194-2017), *The Technical Specification for Soil Environmental Monitoring* (HJ/T 166-2004).

The determination area of air ions can be divided according to the difference of functional area or ecological environment: campus, residential area, street, lake, beach, park or green space, forest, suburb or countryside, etc.

(1) Selection of sampling area and point layout: sampling grid is set according to the detection purpose or the geomorphology, ecological balance and area of each area. In the relatively empty area, a sampling grid is set with the side length of 100-500 m, and the measurement point is in the center of each grid. When sampling in a large range, 5-10 sampling points are set when sampling less than 10 mu, 10-40 mu set with 10-15 sampling points, and 15-20 sampling points are set when sampling over 40 mu.

(2) Point distribution method: since the negative ions are greatly affected by air pollution, geomorphology and ecological environment, it is suggested to combine the sampling point distribution method of the air monitoring program and the soil monitoring program. The following methods can be used for layout: functional area, diagonal area(regular area), grid area(medium area), quincunx-shaped area(small and uniform area), serpentine area(large and uneven area), and fan-shaped (area with air pollution). The above methods of sampling and distribution can be used alone or in combination. The purpose is to reflect the distribution characteristics of negative ions representatively and provide reliable samples for monitoring.

(3) Design of monitoring time: it can be detected in the day (6:00-22:00) and night (22:00-6:00). The existence life of air negative ions is very short, generally only 1-2min. Therefore, when manual monitoring is conducted, the monitoring time should last at least 4-5d, which can cover different weather. Measure for at least 45 min each time and record more than 100 instantaneous data, or use an air negative ion online monitor to automatically record data.

(4) The use of the instrument: ① The placement of the instrument: The test height is 1.2 – 1.5 m, which is located at the same height with the temperature, humidity, wind speed and light. Under the condition of wind, the entrance direction of the instrument should be kept perpendicular to the wind direction as far as possible to minimize the interference of wind to the measurement results. For manual intermittent sampling, the height of the sampling port from the ground should be about 1.5 m. No strong reflection objects and shelters within 10 m. For automatic monitoring, the height of the sampling port or the monitoring beam from the ground should be within 3 – 15 m, and the distance of the sampling port of the monitoring instrument from the surface of the building walls, roofs and other supports should be more than 1 m. The instrument should be placed at a distance from the personnel. ② The operation of the instrument: Read the operation manual carefully in advance, and install the instrument correctly according to the manual. Verify that the ion density meter needs to be grounded before testing begins and that the enclosure of the meter must be free from any electrostatic effects. ③ Indoor measurement, the instrument must avoid close to plastic products and textiles and clothing which are made of synthetic fiber. If the air is not circulating, there may be a large gap in the value of ions. Moderate use of electric fans and other appliances, so that indoor air can flow, contribute to the uniform distribution of indoor air ions. ④ Data reading: Each grid should be measured at least 3 times at the same time interval. The measured amount is a time interval (usually seconds) at which at least 100 pieces of data are recorded. ⑤ Record the weather conditions and weather parameters (such as temperature, humidity, weather, ozone content, etc.), and record the environmental conditions of the detection point.

3. Calculation

The initial measurement of a few minutes, the measurement data is not stable, data processing should be removed. The instantaneous, daily, monthly, seasonal and annual concentrations of air ions can be evaluated for a single monitored area. According to the characteristics of detection points, the following methods were selected to conduct comprehensive air ion evaluation, respectively.

4. Evaluation

(1) Single-stage coefficient: the ratio of positive and negative ions in the air are called the unipolar coefficient. The unipolar coefficient of light ions are expressed as $n^+/n^- = q$, while that of heavy ions are expressed as $N^+/N^- = q$. The number of ions in the air and the unipolar coefficient can vary with various conditions. The unipolar coefficient is less than or equal to 1, to give a person comfort. If it is more than 50, the air is dirty.

(2) Abe air quality evaluation coefficient: According to the Abe coefficient, air quality is divided into 5 grades (Table 15 – 1). The Abe air ion evaluation coefficient (CI) model takes the urban residents of living area as the research object, and has better evaluation results for the negative ion status of urban residential areas.

$$CI = n^-/1000q$$

Note: n^- is the air negative ion concentration.

q is a single-stage coefficient.

Table 15 – 1 Air quality classification standard

Level	A	B	C	D	E
cleanliness	The most cleaning	General cleaning	Medium cleaning	Permissible value	The critical value
CI	>1.0	1.0 – 0.7	0.69 – 0.50	0.49 – 0.30	0.29

(3) Air negative ions coefficient: the scholar thinks, single stage-coefficient and abe air quality evaluation coefficient are not suitable for evaluating forest air negative ions, the single-stage coefficient values range is larger caused by the large number of negative ions in the forest, the dispersive results, bring some trouble to the data processing, thus put forward the coefficient of air negative ions, the formula is as follows:

$p = n^- / (n^+ + n^-)$

The negative ion coefficient is positively correlated with the air negative ion health care function and air cleanliness. When the air negative ion coefficient is greater than 0.5, the air cleanliness is high and beneficial to human body. The higher the negative ion coefficient is, the higher the air cleanliness is and the stronger the health care function of air negative ion is.

(4) Forest air ion evaluation Index (FCI): according to the characteristics of forest air ion and combined with the needs of people's tourism, FCI evaluation method was proposed (Table 15 – 2).

$FCI = n^- / 1000 \times P$

Note: P is the air negative ion coefficient.

1000 is the lowest negative ion concentration for human biological effect.

Table 15 – 2 Forest air ion classification standard and evaluation index classification standard

Level	I	II	III	IV	V
$n^- / (ion/cm^3)$	3000	2000	1500	1000	400
$n^+ / (ion/cm^3)$	300	500	700	900	1200
p	0.80	0.70	0.60	0.50	0.40
FCI	2.4	1.4	0.9	0.5	0.16

It is also possible to simply divide the air negative ion concentration level in the forest environment into 6 grades. >3000 is particularly fresh, 2000 – 3000 is very refreshing, 1500 – 2000 is relatively fresh, 1000 – 1500 is in general, 400 – 1000 is not fresh, <400 is particularly unrefreshing.

5. Notes

(1) Tests must be repeated many times or last for a certain period of time under stable environmental conditions in order to get more accurate test results.

(2) Pay attention to the applicable scope of the instrument, including temperature, relative humidity, wind speed and weather.

(3) Appropriate evaluation methods should be selected and the significance of measurement data should be correctly understood. At present, there is no unanimously recognized technical standard for the detection method of negative ion concentration at home and abroad. Therefore, it is a good idea to confirm the comparability of the test instruments and methods in advance.

实验十五　大气中负氧离子的监测与评价

大气负氧离子（negative air ions，NAIs）是指大气中的氧分子与自由电子结合而形成的带负电荷的氧气离子，无色无味，又称为小粒径负离子。负氧离子可有效降低颗粒物的浓度，尤其是 $PM_{2.5}$ 和 PM_{10}，从而改善空气质量，其在森林、瀑布、海滩等大气中含量较高，可达 $0.5 \times 10^3 \sim 10 \times 10^3$ ions/cm³。负氧离子存在较明显的日、月和年际变化，与气温、气湿、降水量等气象因素、森林植被、环境状况存在一定关联。

大气中小的负离子（或轻负离子）对人体的健康有促进作用，而正离子含量高时对人体健康有不利作用；轻负离子浓度高表明空气质量较好，而重离子或正离子含量高则表明空气污染较重。开展大气负离子监测，对人群疾病疗养、健康促进、满足人们对生态环境认识的需要、弥补我国当前环境监测指标体系不足具有重要意义。

一、实验目的

通过实习掌握大气离子监测仪器的使用及其监测技术，掌握大气离子监测方案设计要点及大气离子的评价方法。

二、实验方法和步骤

1. 监测设备的选择

为综合分析大气离子与大气质量的关系，应选择能够同时监测空气正离子、负离子、大离子、小离子的仪器。一般选择自动化程度较高的可测量正、负离子浓度，同时记录环境温度和湿度，自动储存数字记录的仪器。如日本产的 COM3800、350U 系空气离子测定器、NKMH103 系列、福建漳州东南电子研究所生产的 DLY、ITC-201A 等；国产的仪器应符合中国《空气离子测量仪通用规范》（GB/T 18809—2002）。

高温高湿环境可能造成大部分品牌仪器工作的不稳定性，应尽量避免仪器在高温高湿环境下工作，空气负离子监测应选择在晴朗少风的天气进行。

2. 监测方案的设计

目前我国尚未有专门针对空气离子监测的规范，本实验参照日本《空气中离子密度测定法》(JIS—B9 929：2006)、《环境空气质量监测规范》(2007)(试行)、《环境空气质量监测点位布设技术规范》(HJ664—2013)、《环境空气质量手工监测技术规范》(HJ 194—2017)、《土壤环境监测技术规范》(HJ/T 166—2004)。

大气离子的测定区域可根据功能区或生态环境差异划分：校园、居民区、街道、湖泊、海滩、公园或绿地、森林、郊区或农村等。

(1) 采样区域的选择及点位布设：根据检测目的或每个区域的地貌、生态的均衡性及面积设置采样网格。较为空旷的区域以100～500m为边长设采样网格，测量点在每个网格中心。较大范围采样时小于10亩5～10个采样点；10～40亩设10～15个采样点；大于40亩设15～20个采样点。

(2) 布点方法：由于负离子受大气污染、地貌和生态环境影响较大，因此建议结合大气监测方案的采样布点及土壤监测方案的布点方法进行。布点可参照以下方法：功能区布点、对角线布点（面积规则的地块）、网格布点（中等面积）、梅花形布点（面积较小，比较均匀的地块）、蛇形布点（面积较大，不太均匀）、扇形布点（有大气污染的区域）。以上几种采样布点方法，可以单独使用，也可以综合使用，目的就是要求有代表性地反映负离子的分布特征，为监测提供可靠的样品。

(3) 监测时间的设计：可在白天（6：00～22：00）和黑夜（22：00～6：00）检测，大气负离子的存在寿命极其短暂，一般只有1～2分钟，因此手工监测时，监测时间应该至少持续4～5天，可涵盖不同的天气。每次至少测量45分钟，并记录大于100个瞬时数据，或者用大气负离子在线监测仪，自动记录数据。

(4) 仪器的使用：①仪器的安放：测试高度为人口呼吸高度1.2～1.5m，与温度、湿度、风速、光照位于同一高度，在有风的条件下，应尽量保持仪器入口方向与风向垂直，最大限度地减少风对测量结果的干扰。对于手工间断采样，其采样口离地面的高度应在约1.5m；10m内无强烈反射物体和遮蔽物。对于自动监测，其采样口或监测光束离地面的高度应在3～15m范围内，监测仪器的采样口离建筑物墙壁、屋顶等支撑物表面的距离应大于1m；仪器放置点与人员应保持一定距离。②仪器的操作：事先仔细阅读使用说明书，正确按说明书进行安装操作。在检测开始前确认离子密度测量器需要接地，仪器的外壳必须不受到任何静电的影响。③室内测量时，仪器必须避免接近塑料制品和合成纤维制成的纺织品与衣物。空气若不流通，各处离子数值可能会有较大的差距。适度使用电风扇等器具，让室内的空气能够流动，有助于室内空气离子分布均匀。④数据的读取：每一网格至少测量3次，时间间隔相同。测量的量是一定时间间隔（通常为秒），至少记录100个数据。⑤同时记录天气状况及天气参数（如温度、湿度、天气、臭氧含量等），记录检测点环境状况。

3. 计算

初始测量的数分钟，测量数据不稳定，数据处理时应剔出。针对监测的单个区域，可评价大气离子的瞬时、日、月、季、年均浓度值。根据检测点特征，选择以下方法，分别进行综合大气离子评价。

4. 评价

(1) 单极系数：大气中正、负离子的比例称为单极系数。轻离子的单极系数以$n^+/n^- = q$

表示,重离子的单极系数以 $N^+/N^- = q$ 表示。空气中离子的数量和单极系数可因各种条件而发生变化。单极系数小于或等于1,才给人以舒适感;若大于50,表明空气较为污浊。

(2) 安培大气质量评价系数:根据安培系数的高低,将空气质量分为5个等级(表15-1)。安培空气离子评价系数(CI)模型以城市居民生活区为研究对象,其对城市居民区负离子状况评价结果较好。

$CI = n^-/1000q$

注:n^- 为空气负离子浓度。

q 为单极系数。

表15-1 大气质量分级标准

等级	A	B	C	D	E
清洁度	最清洁	一般清洁	中等清洁	容许值	临界值
CI	>1.0	1.0～0.7	0.69～0.50	0.49～0.30	0.29

(3) 负离子系数:有学者认为,单极系数和安培大气质量评价系数不太适合评价森林空气负离子,因为森林中较大的负离子数量造成单极系数取值范围较大,结果分散,给数据处理带来一定的麻烦,因此提出空气负离子系数,公式如下:

$p = n^-/(n^+ + n^-)$

负离子系数大小与大气负离子保健功能和空气清洁度大小呈正相关。当负离子系数大于0.5时,空气清洁度高,对人体有益。负离子系数越大,大气清洁度越高,大气负离子的保健功能越强。

(4) 森林空气离子评价指数(FCI):根据森林环境空气离子的特性,结合人们旅游的需要,提出 FCI 评价方法(表15-2)。

$FCI = n^-/1000 \times P$

注:P 为空气负离子系数。

1000 为人体生物学效应最低负离子浓度。

表15-2 森林大气离子分级标准及评价指数分级标准

等级	Ⅰ	Ⅱ	Ⅲ	Ⅳ	Ⅴ
$n^-/$(个/cm³)	3000	2000	1500	1000	400
$n^+/$(个/cm³)	300	500	700	900	1200
p	0.80	0.70	0.60	0.50	0.40
FCI	2.4	1.4	0.9	0.5	0.16

也可简单地将森林环境中大气负离子的浓度水平分为6个等级:>3000 为特别清新;2000～3000 为非常清新;1500～2000 较为清新;1000～1500 一般;400～1000 不清新;

<400 特别不清新。

5. 注意事项

（1）必须在稳定的环境条件下进行重复多次或者持续一定时间的测试，这样才能获得比较准确的检测结果。

（2）注意选用仪器的适用范围，包括温度、相对湿度、风速及天气。

（3）要选用适宜的评价方法并正确理解测量数据的意义，关于负离子浓度的检测方法，目前在国内外尚未有一致公认的技术标准。因此进行比较时最好能事先确认所使用的测试仪器、方法及其可比性。

Experiment 16　Determination of Biochemical Oxygen Demand in Water

Domestic sewage and industrial waste water contain a large number of organic pollutants, the decomposition of these organic pollutants need to consume a large amount of dissolved oxygen, resulting in the imbalance of oxygen in the water, the decline of dissolved oxygen content makes water quality worse, leading to the death of fish and other aquatic organisms.

It is difficult to determine the composition of organic matter in water because of its complex composition. In practice, the oxygen consumption by the decomposition of organic matter in water under certain conditions is usually used to indirectly reflect the content of organic matter in water, such as biochemical oxygen demand.

Biochemical Oxygen Demand (BOD) refers to the amount of dissolved oxygen consumed by aerobic microorganisms (mainly aerobic and facultative anaerobic bacteria) in the process of oxidative decomposition of organic matters in water.

In practical work, the reduced amount of dissolved oxygen (mg/L) in 1 L water after culture at 20℃ ±1℃ for 5 d is often expressed as BOD at 20℃ for 5 d, denoted as BOD_5^{20}, which is an indirect indicator of the degree of water pollution by organic matter.

The water sample of BOD was tested by dilution and inoculation method. During the collection, it should be filled and sealed in a brown glass bottle, the sample quantity should be no less than 1000 mL, and transported and stored in the dark at 0℃～4℃. Test and analysis are usually performed within 6 h. In case of long distance transport, storage time should not exceed 24 h in any case.

Ⅰ. Objectives

To master the principle and method of determination of dissolved oxygen by iodimetry; Familiar with the environmental hygiene significance of BOD_5^{20}.

II. Experimental methods and procedures

1. Principle

Two samples of original water or properly diluted water were taken, one was tested for dissolved oxygen at that time, the other was cultured at 20℃ for 5 d, and then the dissolved oxygen content was determined. The difference of the dissolved oxygen content between the two samples was BOD_5^{20}.

The determination of dissolved oxygen commonly used iodine quantity method, its principle is: add manganese sulfate solution and alkaline potassium iodide solution to water sample, produce manganese hydroxide flesh color precipitation, manganese hydroxide is very unstable, quickly oxidized by water dissolved oxygen into manganese acid or manganese manganese acid. Then add concentrated sulfuric acid to make high manganese react with potassium iodide to seperate out iodine. Taking starch as indicator, the dissolved oxygen was calculated by titrating the precipitated iodine with sodium thiosulfate standard solution.

$$MnSO_4 + 2NaOH \rightarrow Mn(OH)_2 \downarrow + Na_2SO_4$$
$$2Mn(OH)_2 + O_2 \rightarrow 2H_2MnO_3 \downarrow$$
$$H_2MnO_3 + Mn(OH)_2 \rightarrow MnMnO_3 + 2H_2O$$
$$MnMnO_3 + 3H_2SO_4 + 2KI \rightarrow 2MnSO_2 + I_2 + 3H_2O + K_2SO_4$$
$$I_2 + 2Na_2S_2O_3 \rightarrow 2NaI + Na_2S_4O_6$$

2. Instruments

(1) 250 mL dissolved oxygen bottle.

(2) 250 mL iodine measuring bottle.

(3) 250 mL triangulated bottle.

(4) 100 mL spherical straw, 10 mL straight straw, etc.

(5) Acid and base burette.

(6) Thermostat: 20℃ ±1℃.

(7) 20 L glass bottle.

(8) Aeration device: multi-channel air pump or other aeration device; Aeration may bring organic matter, oxidant and metal, and lead to air pollution. If there is pollution, the air should be filtered and cleaned.

3. Reagents

(1) Manganese sulfate solution: weigh 480 g AR $MnSO_4 \cdot 4H_2O$ (400 g $MnSO_4 \cdot 2H_2O$ or $MnCl_2 \cdot 2H_2O$), dissolve in distilled water, and dilute to 1000 mL after filtration.

(2) Alkaline potassium iodide solution: weigh 500 g AR sodium hydroxide and dissolve in 300 – 400 mL water; Weigh 150 g AR potassium iodide (or 135 g sodium iodide) dissolved in 200 mL distilled water. The above two solutions are combined, diluted to 1000 mL with distilled water, mixed well, and stood for 24 h to make sodium carbonate sink. Pour out the upper clarifying solution in a brown bottle with a rubber plug. After dilution and acidification, the

solution should not be blue against starch.

(3) Starch solution (5 g/L).

(4) AR concentrated sulfuric acid with a specific gravity of 1.84.

(5) Sodium thiosulfate standard solution (0.0250 mol/L).

① Preparation of concentrated solution and standard concentration: 25 g sodium thiosulfate ($Na_2S_2O_3 \cdot 5H_2O$) was weighed and dissolved in 1 L of distilled water, and 0.4 g sodium hydroxide was added to prevent decomposition. The concentration of this solution was about 0.1 mol/L. Store in a brown bottle and calibrate after a week.

Calibration method: weigh two parts of analyzed potassium iodate dried at 105 ℃ for 2h, each about 0.15 g, and put them into 250 mL iodine measuring bottle respectively. Add 100 mL distilled water to each bottle and heat to dissolve potassium iodate. Then add 3 g potassium iodide and 10 mL glacial acetic acid, and leave them in the dark for 5 min. Titrate the solution with sodium thiosulfate to be calibrated until it turns pale yellow. Add 5 g/L starch solution 1 mL to continue titrating until the blue faded, and record the dosage. The molarity of sodium thiosulfate solution can be calculated as follows:

$$Na_2S_2O_3 \ (mol/L) = \frac{m \ (KIO_3) \times 1000}{Na_2S_2O_3 \ (mL) \times 35.669}$$

m is the mass of potassium iodate

35.669 is the molar mass of potassium iodate, that is, the 1/6 amount of KIO_3

Finally, the result is expressed as the average of two parts.

② Dilution: The above demarcated sodium thiosulfate solution is diluted to 0.0250 mol/L with boiled and cooled distilled water.

(6) Inoculation water: take domestic sewage which is not polluted by industrial waste water, river water or lake water containing urban sewage, or effluent from sewage treatment plants, and place it at 20℃ for 24 – 36 h, and use the supernatant.

(7) Dilute water: Add a certain amount of distilled water or river water into a 20 L glass bottle, control the water temperature at 20℃ ± 1℃, and add 1 mL of each of the following salt solution to each liter of water as the nutrient for microorganisms.

① Magnesium sulfate solution: 22.5 g magnesium sulfate ($MgSO_4 \cdot 7H_2O$) is weighed and dissolved in 1 L distilled water.

② Calcium chloride solution: 27.5 g calcium chloride ($CaCl_2$) is weighed and dissolved in 1 L distilled water.

③ Ferric chloride solution: 0.25 g ferric chloride ($FeCl_3 \cdot 6H_2O$) is weighed and dissolved in 1 L distilled water.

④ Phosphate buffer solution: 8.5 g potassium dihydrogen phosphate (KH_2PO_4), 21.75 g potassium dihydrogen phospate (K_2HPO_4), 33.4 g disodium hydrogen phosphate ($NaHPO_4 \cdot 7H_2O$) and 1.7 g ammonium chloride (NH_4Cl) are dissolved in 1 L distilled water with a pH of 7.2.

After adding the nutrient solution, the distilled water was aerated for 2 d. During aeration, a medicinal charcoal device can be installed in the intake circuit to filter the incoming air. In order to stabilize the dissolved oxygen, it should be capped and left standing after aeration. The BOD for 5 d of diluted water should be less than 0.2 mg/L. Pollution on should be prevented during aeration, especially from introducing organic matter, metals, oxides or reducing substances. The mass concentration of oxygen in the diluted water shall not be supersaturated. It shall be left open for 1 h before use and shall be used within 24 h.

(8) Oxalic acid standard solution (0.0100 mol/L): 0.6304 g oxalic acid ($H_2C_2O_4 \cdot 2H_2O$) was dissolved in 100 mL distilled water at a concentration of 0.1000 mol/L. Then dilute it with distilled water for 10 times, which is 0.0100 mol/L.

(9) Potassium permanganate solution (0.1 mol/L): 3.16 g potassium permanganate was weighed, dissolved in 1.2 L distilled water, boiled for 10 – 15 min, and let stand for 7 – 10 d (its concentration was about 0.1 mol/L). For immediate use, 0.0100 mol/L oxalic acid was calibrated and diluted to 0.0100 mol/L.

(10) 1 : 3 sulfuric acid solution: Slowly add 1 part of concentrated sulfuric acid with a specific gravity of 1.84 to 3 parts (volume) distilled water.

4. Methods

(1) Diluted water sample.

For clean surface water, the dissolved oxygen content before and after 5 d can be directly measured without dilution. Water samples with heavy pollution should be diluted in different degrees according to the degree of pollution.

① Dilution ratio estimation: For the ideal diluted water sample, after culture at 20℃ for 5 d, it is more appropriate to reduce the dissolved oxygen by 40% – 60% or have at least 1 mg/L of remaining dissolved oxygen. Dilution ratios can be determined by the determination of total organic carbon (TOC), permanganate index (I_{Mn}), or chemical oxygen demand (COD_{Cr}) of the water sample. If chemical oxygen demand (COD_{Cr}) is used to estimate the appropriate dilution factor, assuming that the oxygen consumption is 10 mg/L, the sewage water sample can be diluted 5, 10, 15 times. Contaminated surface water samples are diluted 3, 5, 9 times. Individual special water sample can be diluted by a multiple.

② Method of water sample dilution: After the dilution ratio is determined, the sample of a certain volume is siphoned into the 1 L measuring cylinder of the dilution container with partial diluted water, diluted water is added or diluted water is inoculated to the scale, and the mixture is gently mixed to avoid residual bubbles. Siphoning the diluted water sample into two numbered oxygen bottles (one for the day of measurement and one for BOD_5^{20}); Tapping the bottle wall to remove bubbles that may cling to the wall, and finally tighten the cork. This is the first dilution ratio sample to be determined. The sample with different dilution ratio can be obtained by continuous dilution.

(2) Blank water sample.

Taking another two numbered dissolved oxygen bottles, fill them with diluted water with siphon and plug the bottle stopper, set as blank.

(3) Determination of water sample.

Take 1 bottle from each dilution factor and blank and determine the dissolved oxygen content on the same day. The other bottles were sealed with distilled water to prevent air from entering the bottle, and incubated at 20℃ ±1℃ for 5 d before taking out for BOD_5^{20} measurement.

Method of determination of dissolved oxygen in water by iodimetry: absorb 2 mL of manganese sulfate or manganese chloride solution into the dissolved oxygen bottle containing water sample, and insert the reagent below the water surface. Add 2 mL alkaline potassium iodide solution according to the above method, tighten the cork, and mix the bottle upside down for several times. At this time, there will be brown-yellow precipitation. Let it stand for 1 minute, and then turn the bottle upside down for several times to fully mix the precipitation. Then add 2 mL concentrated sulfuric acid, tighten the cork, mix it upside down and leave it for 5 minutes to dissolve the precipitate completely. 100 mL of the above solution was absorbed by a 100 mL spherical straw and placed in a 250 mL iodine measuring bottle. Immediately, 0.0250 mol/L sodium thiosulfate standard solution was used to titrate the solution to a yellowish color, 1 mL starch solution (5 g/L) was added, the end point was to continue titrating until the blue faded, and the dosage of sodium thiosulfate solution V was recorded.

(4) Calculation.

$$\text{Dissolved Oxygen }(O_2, \text{mg/L}) = \frac{v \times 0.0250 \times 8 \times 1000}{100}$$

$$BOD_5^{20}(O_2, \text{mg/L}) = \frac{(A_1 - A_2) - (B_1 - B_2) \times f_1}{f_2}$$

A_1 is the dissolved oxygen immediately after dilution of the water sample.

A_2 is the dissolved oxygen cultured at the end of 5 d.

B_1 is dissolved oxygen in diluted water.

B_2 is dissolved oxygen cultured in diluted water at the end of 5 d.

f_1 is the proportion of diluted water in a water sample.

f_2 is the proportion of the sample in the water sample.

(5) Notes.

① In the determination of dissolved oxygen, the reagent should be inserted below the liquid level and added slowly by the pipette, so as to avoid the error caused by bringing oxygen in the air into the water sample. Bubbles should be avoided during sampling and operation.

② When free acids and alkalis are contained in the water, it will inhibit microbial growth and should be neutralized first.

③ Excessive toxic substances in the water will inhibit the growth of microorganisms, which need to be diluted with diluted water; meanwhile, the inoculate water should be added to diluted water in advance to import microorganisms.

④ When a small amount of free chlorine is in the water, generally place it for 1 – 2 h and the free chlorine can disappear.

实验十六 水中生化需氧量的测定

生活污水和工业废水中含有大量的有机污染物，分解这些有机污染物需要消耗大量的溶解氧，造成水体中氧的不平衡，溶解氧含量下降使得水质恶化，导致鱼类及其他水生生物死亡。

水体中有机物的成分较复杂，难以一一测定其成分。实际工作中，通常采用水中有机物在一定条件下被分解所消耗的氧来间接反映水体中有机物的含量，如生化需氧量。

生化需氧量（biochemical oxygen demand，BOD）是指水中有机物在需氧微生物（主要是需氧及兼性厌氧细菌）的作用下，进行氧化分解过程中所消耗水中溶解氧的量。

实际工作中，常以20℃±1℃培养5天后，1 L水中溶解氧减少的量（mg/L）来表示，称为五日20℃生化需氧量，记为BOD_5^{20}，是一种间接表示有机物污染水体程度的指标。

采用稀释接种法检测生化需氧量的水样，采集时应注意充满并密封于棕色玻璃瓶中，样品量不小于1000 mL，于0～4℃暗处运输和保存。通常须于6小时内进行检测分析。如需进行长距离运输，在任何情况下，储存时间都不应超过24小时。

一、实验目的

通过实习掌握碘量法测定溶解氧的原理和方法；熟悉BOD_5^{20}的环境卫生学意义。

二、实验方法和步骤

1. 原理

取原水样或已适当稀释后的水样两份，一份测定当时的溶解氧量，另一份放入20℃恒温箱内培养5天，再测定溶解氧含量，前后两者溶解氧含量的差值即为BOD_5^{20}。

溶解氧的测定常用碘量法，其原理为：向水样中加入硫酸锰溶液和碱性碘化钾溶液，生成氢氧化锰肉色沉淀，氢氧化锰极不稳定，迅速被水中溶解氧氧化为锰酸或锰酸锰。然后加入浓硫酸，使高价锰与碘化钾反应析出碘。以淀粉作为指示剂，用硫代硫酸钠标准溶液滴定析出的碘，计算出溶解氧量。

$MnSO_4 + 2NaOH \rightarrow Mn(OH)_2 \downarrow + Na_2SO_4$

$2Mn(OH)_2 + O_2 \rightarrow 2H_2MnO_3 \downarrow$（肉色沉淀）

$H_2MnO_3 + Mn(OH)_2 \rightarrow MnMnO_3 + 2H_2O$

$MnMnO_3 + 3H_2SO_4 + 2KI \rightarrow 2MnSO_4 + I_2 + 3H_2O + K_2SO_4$

$I_2 + 2Na_2S_2O_3 \rightarrow 2NaI + Na_2S_4O_6$

2. 仪器

（1）250 mL 溶解氧瓶。

（2）250 mL 碘量瓶。

（3）250 mL 三角瓶。

（4）100 mL 球形吸管和10 mL 直形吸管等。

（5）酸式和碱式滴定管。

（6）恒温箱，20℃±1℃。

（7）20 L 大玻璃瓶。

（8）曝气装置：多通道空气泵或其他曝气装置；曝气可能带来有机物、氧化剂和金属，导致空气污染，如有污染，空气应过滤清洗。

3. **试剂**

（1）硫酸锰溶液：称取 480 g 分析纯 $MnSO_4 \cdot 4H_2O$（也可用 400 g $MnSO_4 \cdot 2H_2O$ 或 $MnCl_2 \cdot 2H_2O$），溶于蒸馏水中，过滤后稀释至 1000 mL。

（2）碱性碘化钾溶液：称取 500 g 分析纯氢氧化钠，溶于 300～400 mL 水中；称取 150 g 分析纯碘化钾（或 135 g 碘化钠）溶于 200 mL 蒸馏水中；将上述两种溶液合并，加蒸馏水稀释至 1000 mL，搅匀，静置 24 小时，使碘化钠下沉；倾出上层澄清液，盛于带橡皮塞的棕色瓶中。此液在稀释和酸化后，遇淀粉不应呈蓝色。

（3）淀粉溶液（5g/L）。

（4）分析纯浓硫酸，比重 1.84。

（5）硫代硫酸钠标准溶液（0.0250 mol/L）。

①配制浓溶液及标定浓度：称取 25 g 硫代硫酸钠（$Na_2S_2O_3 \cdot 5H_2O$），溶于 1 L 蒸馏水中，加入 0.4 g 氢氧化钠以防分解，此溶液浓度大约为 0.1 mol/L。储存于棕色瓶中，放置一周后进行标定。

标定方法：称取经 105℃ 干燥 2 小时的分析纯碘酸钾 2 份，每份约 0.15 g，分别放入 250 mL 的碘量瓶中；于每瓶中各加入 100 mL 蒸馏水，加热使碘酸钾溶解；再各加碘化钾 3 g 和冰醋酸 10 mL，置于暗处 5 分钟，用待标定的硫代硫酸钠滴定至溶液呈淡黄色时，加入 5 g/L 淀粉溶液 1 mL 继续滴定至蓝色刚褪去即为终点，记录用量；硫代硫酸钠溶液的摩尔浓度可按下式计算：

$$Na_2S_3O_3 (mg/L) = \frac{m(KIO_3) \times 1000}{硫代硫酸钠用量(mL) \times 35.669}$$

注：m 为碘酸钾的质量。

35.669 为碘酸钾的摩尔质量，即 KIO_3 1/6 的量。

最后用两份的平均值表示结果。

②稀释：将上述标定过的硫代硫酸钠溶液用煮沸冷却后的蒸馏水稀释成 0.0250 mol/L。

（6）接种水：取未受工业废水污染的生活污水，或含有城镇污水的河水或湖水，或污水处理厂的出水，于 20℃ 放置 24～36 小时，用上层清液。

（7）稀释水：在 20 L 大玻璃瓶中加入一定量的蒸馏水或河水，控制水温在 20℃±1℃，每升水中加入下列盐类溶液各 1 mL，作为微生物的营养料。

①硫酸镁溶液：称取 22.5 g 硫酸镁（$MgSO_4 \cdot 7H_2O$）溶于 1 L 蒸馏水中。

②氯化钙溶液：称取 27.5 g 氯化钙（$CaCl_2$）溶于 1 L 蒸馏水中。

③氯化铁溶液：称取 0.25 g 氯化铁（$FeCl_3 \cdot 6H_2O$）溶于 1 L 蒸馏水中。

④磷酸盐缓冲溶液：称取 8.5 g 磷酸二氢钾（KH_2PO_4），21.75 g 磷酸氢二钾

(K_2HPO_4), 33.4 g 磷酸氢二钠 ($NaHPO_4 \cdot 7H_2O$) 和 1.7 g 氯化铵 (NH_4Cl) 溶于 1 L 蒸馏水中, 此溶液 pH 值为 7.2。

加入上述营养液后, 蒸馏水曝气 2 天。曝气时可在进气路中安装一个药用炭装置, 用于过滤导入的空气。为使溶解氧稳定, 曝气后应加盖静置。稀释水的五日生化需氧量应在 0.2 mg/L 以下。在曝气的过程中应防止污染, 尤其是防止带入有机物、金属、氧化物或还原物。稀释水中氧的质量浓度不能过饱和, 使用前须开口放置 1 小时, 且应在 24 小时内使用。

(8) 草酸标准溶液 (0.0100 mol/L): 称取 0.6304 g 草酸 ($H_2C_2O_4 \cdot 2H_2O$) 溶于 100 mL 蒸馏水中, 其浓度为 0.1000 mol/L。再用蒸馏水稀释 10 倍, 即为 0.0100 mol/L。

(9) 高锰酸钾溶液 (0.1 mol/L): 称取 3.16 g 高锰酸钾, 溶于 1.2 L 蒸馏水中, 煮沸 10~15 分钟, 静置 7~10 天 (其浓度约为 0.1 mol/L)。临用时用 0.0100 mol/L 草酸标定, 稀释成 0.0100 mol/L。

(10) 1 : 3 硫酸溶液: 向 3 份 (容积) 蒸馏水中徐徐加入比重为 1.84 的浓硫酸 1 份。

4. 方法

(1) 稀释水样。

较清洁的地表水, 水样无须稀释, 直接测定其五天前后的溶解氧含量即可。污染较重的水样应根据污染轻重给予不同程度的稀释。

①估算稀释倍数: 理想的稀释后的水样, 在 20℃ 培养 5 天后, 溶解氧减少 40%~60% 或剩余溶解氧至少有 1 mg/L 较为合适。稀释倍数可根据水样的总有机碳 (TOC)、高锰酸盐指数 (I_{Mn}) 或者化学需氧量 (COD_{Cr}) 的测定值来确定。如用 COD_{Cr} 估计合适的稀释倍数, 假设耗氧量为 10 mg/L 时, 污水水样可稀释 5、10、15 倍。受污染的地面水水样稀释 3、5、9 倍。个别特殊的水样可多稀释一个倍数。

②稀释水样的方法: 确定稀释倍数后, 将一定体积的试样用虹吸管加入已加部分稀释水的稀释容器 1 L 量筒中, 加稀释水或接种稀释水至刻度, 轻轻混合避免残留气泡。用虹吸管将已稀释的水样加入两个已编号的溶解氧瓶内 (一个用于测当天溶解氧, 一个用于测 BOD_5^{20}); 轻击瓶壁, 以驱除可能附在瓶壁上的气泡, 最后塞紧瓶塞。此为第一稀释倍数样品, 待测定。可连续稀释, 即可得到不同稀释倍数的样品。

(2) 空白水样。

另取已编号的 2 个溶解氧瓶, 用虹吸管装入稀释水, 塞紧瓶塞, 作为空白。

(3) 水样的测定。

从每个稀释倍数和空白中各取 1 瓶, 分别测定当天溶解氧含量。其他各瓶用蒸馏水封口防止空气进入瓶内, 放入 20℃±1℃ 恒温箱中培养 5 天后取出测 BOD_5^{20}。

碘量法测定水中溶解氧的方法: 吸取 2 mL 硫酸锰或氯化锰溶液于装有水样的溶解氧瓶内, 加试剂时应插到水面下。按上法加 2 mL 碱性碘化钾溶液, 盖紧瓶塞, 将瓶颠倒混匀数次, 此时有棕黄色沉淀形成, 放置 1 分钟, 再将瓶颠倒数次, 使沉淀充分混匀。然后加入 2 mL 浓硫酸, 盖紧瓶塞, 颠倒混匀, 放置 5 分钟, 使沉淀完全溶解。用 100 mL 球形吸管吸取 100 mL 上述溶液置于 250 mL 碘量瓶中, 立即用 0.0250 mol/L 硫代硫酸钠标准溶液滴定至溶液呈淡黄色, 加入 5 g/L 淀粉溶液 1 mL, 继续滴定至蓝色刚褪去即为终点,记录硫代硫酸钠溶液用量 V。

（4）计算。

溶解氧（O_2，mg/L）$= \dfrac{v \times 0.0250 \times 8 \times 1000}{100}$

五日生化需氧量（O_2，mg/L）$= \dfrac{(A_1 - A_2) - (B_1 - B_2) \times f_1}{f_2}$

注：A_1 为水样经稀释后即时的溶解氧

A_2 为培养五日末的溶解氧

B_1 为稀释水的即时溶解氧

B_2 为稀释水培养五日末的溶解氧

f_1 为水样中稀释水所占的比例

f_2 为水样中样品所占的比例

（5）注意事项。

①测定溶解氧时，试剂的加入应将移液管插入液面以下，慢慢加入，以免将空气中的氧带入水样中而引起误差。采样和操作过程中应避免水中产生气泡。

②水中含游离酸和碱时，会抑制微生物生长，应先中和。

③水中含过量有毒物质时，会抑制微生物生长，须用稀释水稀释；同时所用稀释水事先应加接种水，以引入微生物。

④水中有少量游离氯时，一般放置 1~2 小时，游离氯即可消失。

Experiment 17 Determination of Available Chlorine in Bleaching Powder and the Amount of Residual Chlorine in Water

Part 1 Determination of available chlorine in bleaching powder

Chlorine containing disinfectants are some compounds with comparatively complex components, the chemical components are roughly: $3Ca(OCl)Cl \cdot Ca(OH)_2 \cdot nH_2O$, and the active component $Ca(OCl)Cl$ has sterilization and oxidation. Commercial bleaching powder contains 25% – 35% available chlorine, and commercial high test bleaching powder contains 60% – 70% available chlorine.

Available chlorine is used to represent the effective component of bleaching powder. It refers to the amount of chlorine generated after bleaching powder interacts with hydrochloric acid. It is expressed as a percentage. Available chlorine actually means the strength of oxidation reaction of chlorine-containing compounds in water.

The available chlorine in bleaching powder is generally determined by iodimetry.

Ⅰ. Objectives

To master the principle and method of determination of effective chlorine content in bleaching powder through practice.

II. Experimental methods and procedures

1. Principle

The available chlorine in bleaching powder reacts with potassium iodide in acidic solution to release a considerable amount of iodine, and then titrate with sodium thiosulfate standard solution. According to the dosage of sodium thiosulfate standard solution, the available chlorine in bleaching powder is calculated.

$2KI + 2CH_3COOH \rightarrow 2CH_3COOK + 2HI$

$2HI + Ca(OCl)Cl \rightarrow CaCl_2 + H_2O + I_2$

$I_2 + 2Na_2S_2O_4 \rightarrow 2NaI + Na_2S_4O_6$

2. Instruments

(1) The mortar.

(2) 250 mL iodine measuring bottle.

(3) 150 mL beaker.

3. Reagents

(1) Sodium thiosulfate standard solution (0.0500 mol/L).

(2) Starch solution (5 g/L).

(3) The potassium iodide.

(4) The glacial acetic acid.

4. Methods

(1) Weigh 0.71 g samples, which were grated powder in mortar, then add to the 150 mL beaker.

(2) Add about 5 mL of distilled water in the beaker, stir the powder into a paste with glass rod, coupled with distilled water to make it into a suspension. Pour it into the 100 mL volumetric flask. Rinse the beaker with distilled water for three times, dump all the washing fluid into the flask, add distilled water to the scale. Continuously oscillate the volumetric flask to mix it evenly.

(3) Dissolve about 0.75 g potassium iodide (10% KI solution, 7.5 mL) and 80 mL distilled water in the 250 mL iodine flask, then add 2 mL glacial acetic acid.

(4) Remove 25 mL sample suspension with straw from the flask, placed it in the 250 mL triangular flask, it immediately turn brown, after oscillation, put it aside for 5 mins.

(5) Add 0.0500 mol/L sodium thiosulfate standard solution with burette, continuously oscillate the iodine flask, till it turn light yellow, then add 1 mL starch solution, continue titration until the blue just fade, record the total dosage.

(6) Calculation.

$$\text{Available chlorine } (Cl_2, \%) = \frac{v \times 0.050 \times 70.91/2000 \times 100/25 \times 100}{0.71} = V$$

V: 0.0500 mol/L sodium thiosulfate standard solution dosage (mL).

Therefore, the milliliter of sodium thiosulfate standard solution (0.0500 mol/L) used in titration, directly represents the percentage of available chlorine in the bleaching powder.

Part 2 Determination of the amount of residual chlorine in water

Residual chlorine refers to the chlorine left in the water after the water is chlorinated and disinfected for a certain time. Its function is to ensure continuous sterilization and also to prevent any re-contamination of the water. There are three forms of residual chlorine:

(1) Total residual chlorine: HOCl、OCl$^-$、NH$_2$Cl、NHCl$_2$.

(2) Free residual chlorine: HOCl、OCl$^-$.

(3) Combined residual chlorine: NH$_2$Cl、NHCl$_2$、other chloramines.

The Hygienic Standard for Drinking Water of China (GB 5749 – 2006) stipulates that the free residual chlorine of centralized feed water shall not be less than 0.3 mg/L, the combined residual chlorine shall not be less than 0.5 mg/L, and the terminal water of the pipe network shall not be less than 0.05 mg/L.

Chlorination is the amount of chlorine added to a water sample.

The amount of required chlorine = Chlorine content-Residual chlorine.

The colorimetric method is generally used for the determination of residual chlorine in water.

Ⅰ. Objectives

To master the collection and preservation methods of water samples and the principle and method of determination of residual chlorine in drinking water. Understand the sanitary standard of residual chlorine in drinking water.

Ⅱ. Experimental methods and procedures

1. Principle

In an acidic solution with pH < 2, residual chlorine reacts with 3, 3, 5, 5-tetramethylbenzidine (C$_{16}$H$_{20}$N$_2$, hereinafter referred to as tetramethylbenzidine for short) to produce a yellow quinone compound, which is quantitated by visual colorimetry. The method can be used to prepare permanent residual chlorine standard color series with potassium dichromate solution.

2. Instruments

(1) Constant temperature water bath box.

(2) 50 mL colorimetric tube.

3. Reagents

(1) Potassium iodide-hydrochloric acid buffer (pH = 2.2): 3.7 g potassium chloride dried at 100℃ – 110℃ to constant weight was weighed, dissolved in pure water, 0.56 mL hydrochloric acid (ρ_{20} = 1.19 g/mL) was added, and diluted to 1000 mL with pure water.

(2) Hydrochloric acid solution (1 : 4)

(3) Tetramethylbenzidine solution (0.3 g/L): Weigh 0.03 g tetramethylbenzidine, add it in batches with 100 mL hydrochloric acid solution [C(HCl) = 0.1 mol/L] and stir to dissolve it in practice (heat and dissolve it if necessary). Mix well.

(4) Potassium dichromate-potassium chromate solution: 0.1550 g of potassium dichromate ($K_2Cr_2O_7$) and 0.4650 g of potassium dichromate (K_2CrO_4) which both dried at 120℃ to constant weight were weighed and dissolved in the buffer solution of potassium chloride-hydrochloric acid and diluted to 1000 mL. The color generated by this solution is equivalent to the color generated by the reaction of 1 mg/L residual chlorine with tetramethylbenzidine.

4. Methods

(1) Permanent residual chlorine standard colorimetric tubes are prepared as the following table.

Take 14 color comparison tubes, add potassium dichromate-potassium chromate solution into the 50 mL tube respectively, dilute with potassium chloride-hydrochloric acid buffer solution to the scale of 50 mL, it can be kept in the cold dark and used for 6 m.

Table 17-1 The preparation of 0.005-1.0mg/L permanent residual chlorine standard colorimetric solution

Residual chlorine/ (mg/L)	Potassium dichromate-potassium chromate solution /mL	Residual chlorine/ (mg/L)	Potassium dichromate-potassium chromate solution/mL
0.005	0.25	0.40	20.00
0.01	0.50	0.50	25.00
0.03	1.50	0.60	30.00
0.05	2.50	0.70	35.00
0.10	5.00	0.80	40.00
0.20	10.00	0.90	45.00
0.30	15.00	10.00	50.00

Note: If the residual chlorine of the water sample is greater than 1 mL/L, the concentration of potassium dichromate-potassium chromate solution can be increased by 10 times, and the standard color equivalent to 10 mg/L residual chlorine, which can be prepared into a permanent standard color series of 1.0-10 mL/L residual chlorine.

(2) Colorimetric.

Add 2.5 mL tetramethylbenzidine solution in a 50 mL colorimetric tube, then add clarify water sample in it, determine immediately after mixing, and get the colormetric result of free residual chlorine, then lay it still for 10 mins, and get the colormetric result of total residual chlorine.

(3) Calculation.

Chlorine content (Cl_2, mg/L) $= \dfrac{V_1 \times 1 \times 100}{V}$

The amount of required chlorine (Cl_2, mg/L) = Chlorine content (Cl_2, mg/L) − Residual chlorine (Cl_2, mg/L).

V_1：1.0 g/L standard solution dosage (mL).

V：the volume of water sample (mL).

1：1 g/L effective chlorine standard solution concentration is 1 mg/mL.

(4) Notes.

①The water sample of pH > 7 can be adjusted with hydrochloric acid solution to pH = 4 before determination.

②When Fe^- > 0.12 mg/L in water sample, 1 − 2 drops of Na_2EDTA solution can be added to each 50 mL water sample to eliminate interference.

③When the water temperature is less than 20℃, the sample can be heated to 25℃ − 30℃ to speed up the reaction.

④During the test, if the color is light blue, it indicates that the acidity of the color solution is obviously low, we can add more 1 mL reagent, then the normal color will appear. If the reagent turns orange, indicating a high residual chlorine content, the standard series of 1 − 10 mg/L residual chlorine can be used with an additional 1 mL reagent.

 实验十七　漂白粉中有效氯含量、水中余氯量的测定

第一节　漂白粉中有效氯含量的测定

含氯消毒剂是一些成分较复杂的化合物，化学成分大致为$3Ca(OCl)Cl \cdot Ca(OH)_2 \cdot nH_2O$，其有效成分$Ca(OCl)Cl$具有杀菌和氧化作用。商品漂白粉含25%～35%有效氯，商品漂粉精含60%～70%有效氯。

有效氯用来表示漂白粉的有效成分，指的是漂白粉与盐酸作用后所生成的氯量，用百分数表示。有效氯实际意义是表示含氯化合物在水中所起氧化反应的强度。

漂白粉中有效氯的测定，一般可采用碘量法。

一、实验目的

通过实习掌握测定漂白粉中有效氯含量的原理和方法。

二、实验方法和步骤

1. 原理

漂白粉中有效氯在酸性溶液中与碘化钾反应而释放出相当量的碘，再以硫代硫酸钠标

准溶液来滴定，根据硫代硫酸钠标准溶液的用量计算出漂白粉中有效氯的含量。

$2KI + 2CH_3COOH \rightarrow 2CH_3COOK + 2HI$

$2HI + Ca(OCl)Cl \rightarrow CaCl_2 + H_2O + I_2$

$I_2 + 2Na_2S_2O_4 \rightarrow 2NaI + Na_2S_4O_6$

2. 仪器

(1) 研钵。

(2) 250 mL 碘量瓶。

(3) 150 mL 烧杯。

3. 试剂

(1) 硫代硫酸钠标准溶液（0.0500 mol/L）。

(2) 淀粉溶液（5 g/L）。

(3) 碘化钾。

(4) 冰乙酸。

4. 方法

(1) 将具有代表性的样品用研钵研碎后，称取 0.71 g，放入 150 mL 烧杯内。

(2) 加 5 mL 左右蒸馏水于烧杯内，用玻璃棒搅拌成糊状。再加蒸馏水使其成悬浮液，倾入 100 mL 容量瓶内，用蒸馏水反复冲洗烧杯 3 次，将洗液全部倾入容量瓶，加蒸馏水至刻度。不断振荡容量瓶使其混合均匀。

(3) 向 250 mL 碘量瓶内加 0.75 g（10% 的 KI 溶液，7.5 mL）左右碘化钾和 80 mL 蒸馏水，使其溶解，再加入 2 mL 冰乙酸。

(4) 用吸管自容量瓶内取出样品悬浮液 25 mL，移入 250 mL 三角瓶内。此时立刻呈棕色，振荡混匀后，静置 5 分钟。

(5) 用滴定管加入 0.0500 mol/L 硫代硫酸钠标准溶液，不断振荡碘量瓶，直至变成淡黄色。然后加入 1 mL 淀粉溶液，继续滴定至蓝色刚褪去为终点，记录用量。

(6) 计算：

$$\text{有效氯}(Cl_2, \%) = \frac{v \times 0.050 \times 70.91/2000 \times 100/25 \times 100}{0.71} = V$$

式中，V: 0.0500 mol/L 硫代硫酸钠标准溶液用量（mL）。

因此，滴定时用去的 0.0500 mol/L 硫代硫酸钠标准溶液的毫升数，即直接代表该种漂白粉所含有效氯的百分数。

第二节　水中余氯量的测定

余氯是指水经加氯消毒，接触一定时间后，余留在水中的氯。其作用是保证持续杀菌，也可防止水受到任何再污染。余氯有三种形式：

(1) 总余氯：$HOCl$、OCl^-、NH_2Cl、$NHCl_2$。

(2) 游离性余氯：$HOCl$、OCl^-。

(3) 化合性余氯：NH_2Cl、$NHCl_2$、其他氯胺类化合物。

我国《生活饮用水卫生标准》（GB 5749—2006）中规定集中式给水出厂水的游离性余氯不低于 0.3 mg/L，化合性余氯不低于 0.5 mg/L，管网末梢水余氯不得低于 0.05 mg/L。

加氯量是指加入水样中的氯量。

需氯量 = 加氯量 - 余氯量。

水中余氯量的测定，一般可采用比色法。

一、实验目的

通过实习掌握水样的采集和保存方法，掌握测定生活饮用水中余氯的原理和方法；熟悉生活饮用水中余氯的卫生标准。

二、实验方法和步骤

1. 原理

在 pH < 2 的酸性溶液中，余氯与 3, 3, 5, 5-四甲基联苯胺（$C_{16}H_{20}N_2$，以下简称四甲基联苯胺）反应，生成黄色的醌式化合物，用目视比色法定量。该方法可用重铬酸钾溶液配制永久性余氯标准色列。

2. 仪器

（1）恒温水浴箱。

（2）50 mL 具塞比色管。

3. 试剂

（1）碘化钾-盐酸缓冲液（pH = 2.2）：称取 3.7 g 经 100℃~110℃ 干燥至恒重的氯化钾，用纯水溶解，再加 0.56 mL 盐酸（ρ_{20} = 1.19 g/mL），并用纯水稀释至 1000 mL。

（2）盐酸溶液（1:4）。

（3）四甲基联苯胺溶液（0.3 g/L）：称取 0.03 g 四甲基联苯胺，用 100 mL 盐酸溶液 [C（HCl）= 0.1 mol/L] 分批加入并搅拌使实际溶解（必要时可加温助溶），混匀，此溶液为无色透明，储存于棕色瓶中，在常温下可使用 6 个月。

（4）重铬酸钾-铬酸钾溶液：称取 0.1550 g 经 120℃ 干燥至恒重的重铬酸钾（$K_2Cr_2O_7$）及 0.4650 g 经 120℃ 干燥至恒重的铬酸钾（K_2CrO_4），溶解于氯化钾-盐酸缓冲溶液，并稀释至 1000 mL。此溶液生成的颜色相当于 1 mg/L 余氯与四甲基联苯胺反应生成的颜色。

4. 方法

（1）永久性余氯标准比色管（0.005~1.0 mg/L）的配制。

按下表所列用量分别吸取重铬酸钾-铬酸钾溶液注入 50 mL 具塞比色管中，用氯化钾-盐酸缓冲液稀释至 50 mL 刻度，在冷暗处保存可使用 6 个月（见表 17-1）。

表17-1　0.005～1.0 mg/L 永久性余氯标准比色溶液的配制

余氯/（mg/L）	重铬酸钾-铬酸钾溶液/mL	余氯/（mg/L）	重铬酸钾-铬酸钾溶液/mL
0.005	0.25	0.40	20.00
0.01	0.50	0.50	25.00
0.03	1.50	0.60	30.00
0.05	2.50	0.70	35.00
0.10	5.00	0.80	40.00
0.20	10.00	0.90	45.00
0.30	15.00	1.00	50.00

注：若水样余氯大于1ml/L时，可将重铬酸钾-铬酸钾溶液的浓度提高10倍，配成相当于10 mg/L 余氯的标准色，配制成1.0～10 mL/L的永久性余氯标准色列。

（2）比色。

于50 mL具塞比色管中，先加入2.5 mL四甲基联苯胺溶液，加入澄清水样至50 mL刻度，混合后立即比色，所得结果为游离性余氯；放置10分钟，比色所得结果为总余氯，总余氯减去游离性余氯即为化合性余氯。

（3）计算。

$$加氯量（Cl_2，mg/L）= \frac{V_1 \times 1 \times 100}{V}$$

需氯量（Cl_2，mg/L）= 加氯量（Cl_2，mg/L）- 余氯量（Cl_2，mg/L）

式中，V_1：1.0g/L 标准溶液用量（mL）

V：水样体积（mL）

1：1 g/L 有效氯标准溶液浓度是1 mg/mL

（4）注意事项。

①pH>7的水样可先用盐酸溶液调节至pH=4再行测定。

②水样中Fe^->0.12 mg/L时，可在每50 mL水样中加1～2滴Na_2EDTA溶液，以消除干扰。

③水温<20℃时，可先温热水样到25℃～30℃，以加快反应速度。

④测试时，如显浅蓝色，表明显色液酸度偏低，可多加1 mL试剂，则可出现正常颜色。如加试剂后显橘色，表明余氯含量偏高，可改用余氯1～10 mg/L的标准系列，并多加1 mL试剂。

Chapter Three Practical for Environmental Health
第三章 环境卫生学实验及案例

Experiment 18 Cases Study of the Relationship Between Environmental Pollution and Human Health

Part 1 Case study of air pollution

In recent years, with the rapid development of global economy and the continuous advancement of urbanization, the natural ecological environment has been damaged to different degrees. Air pollution can be divided into three categories: outdoor air pollution, indoor air pollution and air pollution caused by working factors. Fuel combustion, motor vehicle exhaust, dust from construction site and natural disasters are the main factors causing air pollution.

Ⅰ. Objectives

By discussing two classic cases of air pollution, this case will guide students to think about the relationship between human beings and the environment, and grasp the source of air pollution and its impact on human health.

Ⅱ. Cases and Questions

1. Case 1 Coal-burning smog events

From 5 to 9 December 1952, many parts of Britain were covered in thick fog and the atmosphere was in a temperature inversion. In London, the situation was the most serious. The temperature was between -3℃ and 4℃. There was no wind and the fog does not disperse, which lasts for 4～5 d. The concentration of pollutants in the atmosphere continued to increase, with the concentration of soot up to 4.46 mg/m^3, which was 10 times compared with the normal level. The concentration of SO_2 was up to 3.8 mg/m^3, which was 6 times compared with the normal level. At first, the animals had difficulty breathing, tongue trouble, and were sick and even died. Meanwhile, thousands of people had developed chest tightness, coughing, sore throats, vomiting, and the death toll of the disease had soared. During the week of December 7 to 13, the death toll soared, reaching to 4703. A following week, 3138 people died, followed by 8000 more in the next two months. A reanalysis of the data at the time suggested that the death toll was 12000.

Since 2013, the central and eastern regions of China have experienced severe haze weather on a large scale, which had a significant impact on urban atmospheric environment, public health, traffic safety and agricultural production. At the same time, as most of the severe haze weather is often difficult to dissipate once formed, such persistent haze weather is particularly serious to the urban environment, and is likely to bring strong social negative impact.

2. Case 2 Photochemical smog events

Los Angeles in the United States has experienced the photochemical smog event, successively in 1943, 1946, 1954, 1955, especially in 1955, the event lasted more than a week, the temperature was as high as 37.8℃, leading to the epidemic of asthma and bronchitis, 65 years old and above people's mortality increased, the average daily death of people was 70 to 317. Later investigation found that the soot is formed by NO_X and volatile organic compounds in the atmosphere under the ultraviolet rays of sunlight, and these two kinds of pollutants mainly come from automobile exhaust. At that time, Los Angeles had 3.5 million cars, consuming about 16 million liters of gas a day. Due to the low efficiency of automobile carburetors, more than 1000 tons of volatile organic compounds were discharged into the atmosphere every day.

Photochemical smog has also occurred in Lanzhou, Chengdu, Shanghai and Beijing in China.

3. Questions

(1) What are the main pollution sources of soot and photochemical smog events?

(2) What meteorological factors are respectively responsible for soot and photochemical smog events?

(3) What are the impacts of the two smog events on population health?

(4) What's the difference between Beijing's smog and these two typical smog events?

(5) What experiences and lessons should we draw from the air pollution incidents?

4. Notes

(1) The collection, presentation and discussion of relevant materials need the participation of teachers and students, which can be presented in forms of PPT and display board.

(2) Conduct discussion on the case and pay attention to form a relaxed interactive atmosphere.

(3) The practice process should reflect the principle of student-centered, teacher-led and problem-based.

Part 2 Case study of environmental pollution-related diseases

Environmental pollution is an important exogenous cause of disease that seriously threatens human health. Various environmental pollution factors, under certain intensity and time, can cause different degrees of damage to the human body, causing acute, chronic and long-term health effects on the exposed population, and in serious cases can lead to the occurrence of public hazards.

Any environmental pollution factor that can pollute the environment and worsen the environmental quality, and directly or indirectly make people sick, is collectively referred to as environmental-related pathogenic factor, so the disease caused among exposed people is called environmental-related disease.

Ⅰ. Objectives

Through the internship, students will master the harm of environmental pollution-related diseases, understand the relationship between people and the environment, and enhance students' awareness of participating in environmental protection.

Chapter Three Practical for Environmental Health
第三章 环境卫生学实验及案例

II. Cases and Questions

1. Case 1   Chronic cadmium poisoning

In May 2009, a 44-year-old villager from Shuangqiao village, Liuyang City, Hunan Province, died suddenly. The tests by authorities in Hunan Province showed excessive levels of cadmium in his body. A month later, another 61-year-old villager was hospitalized for respiratory symptoms and died shortly after, with urine cadmium more than four times compared with the recommended value. According to the investigation, there was a chemical enterprise in this area, which mainly produced powdered zinc sulfate and granular zinc sulfate. In April 2004, the company built a production line for indium refining without approval. Soon after that, a large number of trees around the enterprise withered and died, and some villagers suffered from systemic weakness, dizziness, chest tightness, joint pain and other symptoms. Relevant departments sampled and tested the soil, well water and surface irrigation water in the surrounding environment of the enterprise. The results showed that the cadmium content of most soil samples within 500 meters around the factory exceeded the standard, and some soil samples within 500 – 1200 m around the factory slightly exceeded the standard. According to the investigation, the waste residue, waste water, dust, surface runoff, transportation and stockpiling of raw materials, as well as the use of waste packaging materials and press cloth by some villagers were the main causes of soil cadmium pollution in this area, leading to the occurrence of chronic cadmium poisoning among people in this area. Subsequently, a comprehensive physical examination and epidemiological investigation were carried out on the population in the contaminated area, positive treatment was given to the patients, and certain compensation was made to the victims. The person responsible was transferred to the judiciary.

2. Case 2   Chronic methylmercury poisoning

In 1971, a national survey on the water quality of four major rivers found that the Songhua River was seriously polluted by mercury. The investigation confirmed that the source of pollution was the discharge of mercury-containing industrial waste from Jilin Chemical Plant into the river water, and a large amount of methylmercury was accumulated in the river fish, which became an significant way for the residents along the river who liked to eat river fish to absorb methylmercury. The epidemiological survey on the health status of the residents along the polluted river showed that a large number of people were polluted by methylmercury, and the intake of methylmercury in more than half of the residents in the seriously polluted areas exceeded the estimated limit recommended by WHO. Many people had accumulated mercury in their bodies, and 100 percent of the mercury in the hair of the fishermen tested along the river exceeded the safe limit. Some people had reached the harmful level, with clinical signs such as narrow visual field and peripheral hypoesthesia associated with methylmercury poisoning. After the environmental treatment, the mercury accumulation in the organisms in the water area is gradually reduced, and the harm caused by mercury pollution is effectively controlled. At present, the mercury pollution of Songhua

River is limited in scope, the exposed population is fixed, the incidence of the affected population is low, the patients have mild symptoms, the course of the disease is stable, and it is effectively monitored and treated.

3. Questions

(1) Analyze the causes of chronic cadmium poisoning and chronic methylmercury poisoning.

(2) What are the clinical manifestations and diagnostic basis of chronic cadmium poisoning and chronic methylmercury poisoning respectively?

(3) Analyze the role of food chain in biological amplification.

(4) Is there a global legal basis for the determination of public hazards?

(5) How to understand the relationship between people and the environment.

4. Notes

(1) The collection, presentation and discussion of relevant materials need the participation of teachers and students, which can be presented in forms of PPT and display board.

(2) Conduct discussion on the case and pay attention to form a relaxed interactive atmosphere.

(3) The practice process should reflect the principle of student-centered, teacher-led and problem-based.

实验十八　环境污染与人群健康的案例分析

第一节　大气污染案例分析

近年来，随着全球经济的快速发展和城市化进程的不断推进，自然生态环境遭到不同程度的破坏。大气污染分为室外空气污染、室内空气污染及工作因素造成的空气污染三大类。燃料的燃烧、机动车尾气、建筑处扬尘、自然灾害等是造成大气污染的主要因素。

一、目的

本案例通过针对两个经典的大气污染案例讨论，引导学生思考人类与环境之间的关系，掌握大气污染的来源及对人类健康的影响。

二、案例与问题

1. 案例一　煤烟型烟雾事件

1952年12月5日至9日，英国很多地区被浓雾覆盖，大气呈逆温状态。其中伦敦的情况最有严重，气温位于-3℃～4℃间，无风，浓雾不散，持续4～5天不变。大气中的污染物浓度不断增加，烟尘浓度最高达4.46 mg/m³，是平时的10倍。SO_2浓度最高达3.8 mg/m³，是平时的6倍。最开始，牲畜出现了呼吸困难、舌头吐露，患病甚至死亡的现象。与此同时，数千市民出现胸闷、咳嗽、咽痛、呕吐等症状，因该病死亡的人数骤增。12

月 7 日至 13 日这一周，死亡人数猛增，达到 4703 人。之后的第二周，死亡人数达 3138 人，在此后的两个月内，陆续有 8000 人死亡。对当时的数据进行重新分析后发现，这次事件造成的超额死亡人数达 12000 人。

自 2013 年以来，我国中东部地区曾大范围出现过严重的雾霾天气，对城市大气环境、群众健康、交通安全、农业生产等带来的影响十分显著。同时，由于大部分严重的雾霾天气一旦形成往往很难消散，此类持续性雾霾天气对城市环境的危害尤其严重，并容易带来较强的社会负面影响。

2. 案例二　光化学型烟雾事件

美国洛杉矶先后于 1943、1946、1954、1955 年发生光化学型烟雾事件，尤其是在 1955 年持续一周多的事件期间，气温高达 37.8℃，导致哮喘、支气管炎的流行，65 岁及以上人群的死亡率增高，平均每日死亡 70～317 人。后来调查发现煤烟是由大气中 NO_x 和挥发性有机物在日光紫外线的照射下形成的，而这两类污染物主要来源于汽车尾气。当时洛杉矶有 350 万辆汽车，每天消耗约 1600 万升汽油。因汽车汽化器的汽化效率低，每天仅挥发性有机物就有 1000 多吨排入大气。

光化学型烟雾在我国的兰州、成都、上海、北京等地也都有发生过。

3. 问题

（1）煤烟型烟雾事件和光化学型烟雾事件的主要污染来源分别是什么？
（2）煤烟型烟雾事件和光化学型烟雾事件分别受哪些气象因素的影响？
（3）两起烟雾事件对人群健康的影响有哪些？
（4）北京雾霾与两起典型的烟雾事件之间有什么区别？
（5）从大气污染事件中，我们应该吸取什么经验和教训？

4. 注意事项

（1）相关资料的收集、展示和讨论需要师生共同参与，可以 PPT、展板等形式展示。
（2）围绕案例进行讨论，注意形成轻松的互动氛围。
（3）实习过程应体现以学生为主体、以教师为主导、以问题为中心的原则。

第二节　环境污染性疾病案例分析

环境污染是严重威胁人类健康的重要外源性病因。各种环境污染因素在一定强度和时间作用下可对人体造成不同程度的损伤，在受暴露人群中引发急性、慢性、远期健康影响，严重时可导致公害病的发生。

凡能污染环境，使环境质量恶化，而直接或间接使人患病的环境污染因素，统称为环境污染性致病因素（environmental pollution-related pathogenic factor），因此在暴露人群中引发的疾病称为环境污染性疾病（environmental pollution-related disease）。

一、目的

通过实习，使学生掌握环境污染性疾病的危害，理解人与环境之间的关系，同时提高学生参与环境保护的意识。

二、案例与问题

1. 案例一　慢性镉中毒

2009年5月,湖南浏阳市双桥村一名44岁的村民突然死亡,经湖南省相关机构检测,死者体内镉严重超标。一个月后,另一名61岁的村民因呼吸系统病症入院治疗,不久后不治身亡,检测其尿镉超出参考值4倍多。经调查,该地区有一家化工企业,主要生产粉状硫酸锌和颗粒状硫酸锌。2004年4月,这家企业未经审批擅自建设一条冶炼生产线。此后不久,厂区周围树林大片枯死,部分村民相继出现全身无力、头晕、胸闷、关节疼痛等症状。相关部门对该企业周边环境的土壤、井水、地表灌溉水进行采样检测,结果表明,厂区周边500米范围内大部分土壤样品镉含量超标,厂区周边500～1200米范围内部分土壤样品镉含量轻度超标。调查认为,该化工企业的废渣、废水、粉尘、地表径流、原料产品运输与堆存,以及部分村民使用废旧包装材料和压滤布等,是造成这一区域土壤镉污染的主要原因,引发了该地区人群出现慢性镉中毒患者。随之对污染区的人群进行了全面的身体检查和流行病学调查,对患者进行了积极治疗,并对受害者进行了一定的补偿。相关责任人被移送司法机关。

2. 案例二　慢性甲基汞中毒

1971年,全国四大主要江河水质调查发现松花江受汞污染严重。经调查证实,污染源为吉林化工厂含汞工业废物排入江水造成污染,江鱼体内富集大量甲基汞,成为喜食江鱼的沿江居民甲基汞摄入的重要途径。对污染江段沿江居民健康状况的流行病学调查结果表明,大量人群受到甲基汞污染,污染严重地区半数以上居民甲基汞摄入量超过世界卫生组织推荐的测算限量;许多人体内有汞蓄积,沿江受检渔民(头)发汞100%超过安全界限值;一部分人已达到危害的程度,出现视野狭窄、末梢感觉减退等与甲基汞中毒有关的临床体征。经过环境治理后,该水域生物体内汞蓄积逐渐减少,汞污染造成的危害得到有效的控制。目前松花江汞污染范围得到限制,暴露人群固定,受影响人群发病率低,病人病征轻微,病程稳定,得到有效监控和治疗。

3. 问题

（1）分析引起慢性镉中毒和慢性甲基汞中毒的原因。
（2）慢性镉中毒和慢性甲基汞中毒的临床表现和诊断依据分别是什么?
（3）分析食物链在生物放大中的作用。
（4）公害病的判定在全球是否具有法律依据?
（5）如何理解人与环境之间的关系。

4. 注意事项

（1）相关资料的收集、展示和讨论需要师生共同参与,可以PPT、展板等形式展示。
（2）围绕案例进行讨论,注意形成轻松的互动氛围。
（3）实习过程应体现以学生为主体、以教师为主导、以问题为中心的原则。

Chapter Three Practical for Environmental Health
第三章 环境卫生学实验及案例

Experiment 19　Investigation on the Effects of Environmental Arsenic Pollution on the Health of Population

Ⅰ. Objectives

In environmental health work, the methods of environmental epidemiology and environmental toxicology are mainly used to explore and evaluate the relationship between environmental exposure and population health and its influencing factors. Through the analysis of environmental pollution background data, master one of the basic research methods of environmental epidemiology: the investigation and analysis of dose-response (effect) relationship, in order to evaluate the impact of environmental factors on population health.

Ⅱ. Content and Methods

First read the following survey and analysis materials, then follow the guidelines for class assignments and discussion.

Case Description: A city is a small south-to-north blind canyon basin, with a population of about 120000. There is a tin smelter in the northwest of the city, 2 residential regions and about 13 residential point areas in the leeward side. The plant mainly produces refined tin, and the main pollutants are arsenic, lead and fluorine. About 9.5 tons of arsenic have been discharged into the environment every year, and arsenic discharge accounts for 19% of the input volume. If the polluted area is 3 km^2, the environmental arsenic load is about 3.18 tons/ (km^2 · year). According to the local health department, the city has had several acute and sub-acute arsenic poisoning incidents, which seriously affected the production and life of the city's residents.

In order to investigate the impact of arsenic pollution on the health of residents in the city, the researchers conducted the following work: ①Survey or the enviromental arsenic exposive status; ②Survey on the health status of residents; ③Investigation on the relationship between environmental arsenic exposure dose and health effects of residents.

Selection of investigation sites: The researcher took two residential regions (13 residential point areas in total), A and B, downwind side of the pollution source (tin smelter), as the polluted area, and the residents in the polluted area as the investigation objects. The residents of an agricultural area 30 km east of the city were taken as the control group. The economy, culture and living habits of this area were similar to the polluted area, but there was no agricultural or industrial arsenic pollution.

Question 1: In order to understand the impact of environmental arsenic pollution on the health of the residents in this city, what aspects should this study begin to work on?

Question 2: Please draw a schematic diagram of the selection of survey points according to the case data.

1. Investigation of environmental arsenic exposure

(1) Investigation results of the current situation of arsenic pollution in the environment: Air, indoor air, source water, groundwater and soil in the polluted area and control area were collected and the arsenic content was determined respectively. The results are shown in Table 19-1.

Table 19-1　Arsenic content in atmosphere, indoor air, water and soil in a polluted area and control area of a city

Plot	Atmosphere/ ($\mu g/m^3$)			Indoor air/ ($\mu g/m^3$)		
	Average daily concentration range	Average daily overshoot rate/%	Annual average concentration	Kitchen	Bedroom	
				Autumn	Autumn	Winter
Polluted area A	0.1 – 6.8	30.0	2.3	3.0	2.7	1.2
Polluted area B	0.0 – 8.0	20.0	1.2	2.0	1.0	0.9
Control area	0.0 – 1.0	0.0	0.2	0.0	0.0	0.0

Plot	Source water/ (mg/L)		Underground water/ (mg/L)		Soil/ ($\mu g/g$)	
	Maximum value	Mean value	Maximum value	Mean value	Plough layer	Deep layer
Polluted area A	50.53	21.33	0.003	0.002	221.4	80.70
Polluted area B	52.37	25.40	0.003	0.002	238.0	95.19
Control area	0.07	0.03	0.005	0.002	26.4	85.43

Question 3: Is there significant environmental arsenic pollution in the city? If so, what might be the route of its pollution?

Question 4: There is no significant difference in arsenic content in groundwater and deep soil between the polluted area and the control area. What is the possible reason?

(2) Residents arsenic intake survey results: five settlements in different distance from pollutants and control areas, random 10 homes as arsenic intake survey results, with a home survey for five days in a unit, on a daily basis to investigate the average of all kinds of food, water and air intake, at the same time to collect all kinds of food, water and air samples, such as measure its arsenic content respectively, different approaches to calculate each standard average arsenic intake every day. The results are shown in Table 19-2.

Table 19-2 Intake of arsenic by different routes in the survey area [μg/(d·standard people)]

Plot	The total intake	Food Intake	Food Rate of contribution/%	Water Intake	Water Rate of contribution/%	Air Intake	Air Rate of contribution/%
Polluted area A							
a	526.9**	492.8**		10.0		24.1**	
b	672.3**	612.3**		45.7**		14.3**	
c	359.5*	346.0		6.3		7.2**	
Polluted area B							
a	285.3	259.8		13.9**		11.6**	
b	392.6*	371.9		11.5*		9.2**	
Control area	262.7	258.4		4.3		0.0	

Note: * Compared with the control area, $P < 0.05$; ** compared with the control area, $P < 0.01$.

Question 5: Calculate the contribution rate of arsenic intake from different ways to total arsenic intake, and explain the types and characteristics of environmental pollution in this city.

(3) Investigation of population arsenic exposure: The researchers investigated the average levels of arsenic in hair and urine of residents in the polluted area and the control area, and the results were shown in Table 19-3.

Table 19-3 Determination values of arsenic in hair and arsenic in urine of residents in the investigation area

Plot	Hair arsenic/(μg/g)			Urine arsenic/(mg/L)		
	The number of survey	Scope	Median	The number of survey	Scope	Median
Polluted area A	850	0.00–160.35	13.40**	804	0.07–1.65	0.12**
Polluted area B	346	1.18–113.59	7.76**	586	0.01–0.60	0.13**
Control area	351	0.00–18.00	0.98	348	0.00–0.27	0.05

Note: ** compared with control area, $P < 0.01$.

Question 6: What do the results in Table 19-3 tell us Is it appropriate to use the median evaluation? Please accordingly explain the results in Table 19-3.

Question 7: Table 19-4 shows the arsenic hypernormalcy of 321 smokers and 875 non-smokers in the polluted area. What problems do the analysis results show?

Table 19-4 Influence of smoking on hair arsenic content of residents in polluted areas

Exposure index	The number of survey	The number of hair arsenic excess	Hair arsenic abnormal rate/%	P
Smokers	321	212	66.04	$u = 1.23$
Non-smokers	875	544	62.17	$P > 0.05$
Total	1196	756	63.21	

Note: The normal value of hair arsenic in this city is (0.69 ± 0.12) μg/g.

2. A survey of the health effects of the population

(1) The results of retrospective investigation on the causes of death of residents from 1982 to 1986 are shown in Table 19-5.

Table 19-5 Mortality rates and tumor mortality rates in the survey area (1982–1986)

Plot	The number of population	Mortality rate/‰				Specific rate of tumor death/ (1/100000)			
		The number of deaths	Crude mortality	Expected deaths	Age-adjusted mortality rate	The number of deaths	Crude mortality	Expected deaths	Age-adjusted mortality rate
Polluted area A	9120	37	4.06	40		11	120.61	7	
Polluted area B	97379	558	5.73	559		52	53.40	110	
Control area	15841	91	5.74	85		5	31.56	5	

Question 8. Calculate the age-adjusted mortality rate and age-adjusted mortality rate of tumors death in two polluted areas and control areas. What implications do the results provide for further research?

(2) The survey results of neonatal malformations from 1983 to 1987 are shown in Table 19-6 and Table 19-7.

Table 19-6 Neonatal malformation rate of residents in the survey area (1983–1987)

Plot	Number of newborn	Number of deformity	Deformity rate/‰	P
Polluted area A	1461	21	14.37	>0.05
Polluted area B	151	2	13.25	>0.05
Control area	208	1	4.81	

Table 19-7 Relationship between arsenic exposure history of puerpera and incidence of neonatal deformity in polluted areas (1983-1987)

Arsenic exposure history	number of survey	Number of deformity	Deformity rate/‰
Yes	92	2	21.74
No	1520	21	13.83

Question 9: According to the results in Table 19-6 and Table 19-7, there is no significant difference in the rate of neonatal malformation between the polluted area and the control area. Please explain the possible reasons. What should we do next?

(3) Sister chromatid exchange (SCE) and micronucleus assay results of maternal and neonatal peripheral blood lymphocytes, are shown in Table 19-8.

Table 19-8 Maternal and neonatal SCE and micronucleus rates in the survey area

Plot	Puerpera		Newborn	
	SCE	Micronucleus rate/‰	SCE	Micronucleus rate/‰
Polluted area A	9.47*	1.57	9.01**	1.46
Polluted area B	8.93	1.77**	9.45**	1.49
Control area	7.23	1.45	5.27	1.32

Note: * Compared with the control area, $P<0.05$; ** compared with control area, $P<0.01$.

Question 10: According to the results in Table 19-8, what is the significance of SCE and micronucleus in judging the effects of environmental pollution on population health? Is there anything wrong with the results of this table?

(4) Investigation results on the prevalence of chronic arsenic poisoning in the polluted areas: The researchers investigated 4848 residents with no history of occupational arsenic exposure in the polluted areas and found 440 patients with chronic arsenic poisoning. The main clinical features of the patients were slow onset and mild symptoms, including dizziness (52.27%), joint pain (47.68%), abdominal distension (17.05%) and abdominal pain (15.91%), etc. The main signs were skin lesions, including hyperkeratosis (85.99%), pigmentation spots (37.50%), decolorization spots (32.95%) and nasal mucosal hyperemia (16.36%), etc. Age-adjusted prevalence rates of chronic arsenic poisoning in polluted area A and polluted area B were 8.73% and 10.74% respectively. The minimum age of the patients was 12 years old, and the minimum living time in the contaminated area was 10 years.

At present, there is no unified diagnostic criteria for chronic arsenic poisoning, and the diagnostic criteria stipulated in this survey are: ① Living in arsenic-polluted areas for more than

10 years; ② Arsenic in hair or urine exceeds the upper limit of local normal value; ③ At the same time accompanied by one of the following signs: non-exposed skin has obvious hypopigmentation spots or pigmentation spots, skin has hyperkeratosis, nasal mucosa has scars, nasal septum perforation, skin cancer and lung cancer.

3. Exposure-effect relationship

Exposure-effect relationship is one of the basic research methods to elucidate the influence of environmental factors on population health. There are many methods to classify exposure level gradient. Based on the reality, the researchers took the residential area and its land ownership relationship as the unit to divide the exposure level and the effect level. Arsenic content in soil, arsenic intake per capita and average arsenic exposure level of population were taken as environmental and biological exposure inderes the age-adjusted prevalence rate of chronic arsenic poisoning in residents was used as health effect index and regression analysis was conducted. The results are shown in Table 19 - 9.

Table 19 - 9 Analysis data of exposure-effect relationship

Survey plot of contaminated area	Distance from source/ km	Arsenic in soil/ ($\mu g/g$)	Arsenic intake/ [μg/(d · standard people)]	Average hair arsenic level/ ($\mu g/g$)	Age-adjusted prevalence of chronic arsenic poisoning/%
a	1.75	503.8	526.9	7.76	17.35
b	1.25	960.2	672.3	9.09	13.81
c	1.75	822.7		12.80	13.67
d	1.25	72.1		5.00	3.68
e	2.50	591.6	359.5	5.74	4.62
f	4.40	104.4		4.08	5.01
g	2.50	146.4		3.56	9.56
h	3.50	115.7	285.3	3.00	2.55
i	3.25	79.7		2.17	4.02
j	5.50	32.9		2.75	10.20
k	4.75	123.0		4.00	6.17
l	8.00	178.6	392.6	4.50	4.40
m	0.75	221.4		13.40	12.00

Question 11: According to the data in Table 19 - 9, calculate the regression equation of the relationship between the age-adjusted prevalence rate of chronic arsenic poisoning and the distance from the pollution source, and the reference value of the edge of the pollution area form the downwind side of the pollution source.

Question 12: According to the data in Table 19 – 9, calculate the regression equation of the relationship between arsenic content in soil and the age-adjusted prevalence rate of chronic arsenic poisoning among residents, and the reference limit value of total arsenic content in soil.

Question 13: According to the data in Table 19 – 9, calculate the regression equations of the relationship between arsenic intake, average hair arsenic level and age-adjusted prevalence rate of chronic arsenic poisoning respectively, and analyse the results.

Question 14. What do you think of the epidemiological investigation of the impact of environmental pollution on population health? Please draw up an outline of an epidemiological investigation of the effects of environmental arsenic pollution on population health and analyse what other deficiencies exist in the materials provided in this case.

 实验十九　环境砷污染对居民健康影响的调查研究

一、目的

在环境卫生工作中，主要采用环境流行病学和环境毒理学的方法探讨和评价环境暴露与人群健康之间的关系及其影响因素。通过对环境污染背景资料的分析，掌握环境流行病学基本研究方法之一——剂量－反应（效应）关系的调查与分析，以评价环境因素对人群健康的影响。

二、实习内容与方法

首先阅读下述调查和分析资料，然后按照指导提纲进行课堂作业和讨论。

案例简介：某市为一南北向盲状峡谷小盆地，常年风向频率以南风为主，人口约12万。市区西北侧有一锡冶炼厂，下风侧有2个居民区，约13个居民点。该厂以生产精锡为主，主要污染物有砷、铅和氟等。该厂每年排入环境中的砷约9.5吨，砷排出量占投入量19%，如以污染面积3 km² 计算，环境中砷负荷约 3.18 t/(km²·y)。根据当地卫生部门资料介绍，该市曾数次发生急性、亚急性人畜砷中毒事件，严重影响了该市居民的生产、生活。

为了调查该市环境砷污染对居民健康的影响，研究者开展了以下工作：① 环境砷暴露状况的调查；② 居民健康状况的调查；③ 环境砷暴露剂量与居民健康效应关系的调查。

调查点的选择：研究者将污染源（锡冶炼厂）下风侧 A、B 两个居民区（共13个居民点）作为污染区，污染区内的居民作为调查对象。以该市以东 30 km 的一农业区居民作为对照，该区经济、文化、生活习惯与污染区相近，但无农业及工业性砷污染存在。

问题1：为了解该市环境砷污染对居民健康的影响，本研究应从哪些方面着手开展工作？

问题2：请根据案例资料绘制出调查点选择的示意图。

1. 环境砷暴露状况的调查

(1) 环境中砷污染现状的调查结果：采集污染区和对照区大气、室内空气、水源水、地下水和土壤，分别测定其中砷的含量，结果见表 19-1。

表 19-1　某市污染区和对照区大气、室内空气、水和土壤中砷的含量

调查区	大气/($\mu g/m^3$)			室内空气/($\mu g/m^3$)		
	日均浓度范围	日均超标率（%）	年均浓度	厨房	卧室	
				秋	秋	冬
污染区 A	0.1～6.8	30.0	2.3	3.0	2.7	1.2
污染区 B	0.0～8.0	20.0	1.2	2.0	1.0	0.9
对照区	0.0～1.0	0.0	0.2	0.0	0.0	0.0

调查区	水源水/(mg/L)		地下水/(mg/L)		土壤/($\mu g/g$)	
	最大值	平均值	最大值	平均值	耕作层	深层
污染区 A	50.53	21.33	0.003	0.002	221.4	80.70
污染区 B	52.37	25.40	0.003	0.002	238.0	95.19
对照区	0.07	0.03	0.005	0.002	26.4	85.43

问题 3：请问该市是否存在明显的环境砷污染？若有，其污染的途径可能是什么？

问题 4：污染区和对照区的地下水、深层土壤中砷含量无明显差异，可能的原因是什么？

(2) 居民砷摄入量的调查结果：在距污染物不同距离的 5 个居民点和对照区，随机抽取 10 户作为砷摄入量的调查结果，以户为单位逐日连续调查 5 天，调查其各种食物、水及空气的平均摄入量，同时采集各种食物、水及空气等样品，分别测定其砷的含量，计算不同途径每个标准人每天平均砷摄入量。结果见表 19-2。

表 19-2　调查区居民砷不同途径摄入量 [$\mu g/$(d·标准人)]

调查点	总摄入量	食物		饮水		空气	
		摄入量	贡献率/%	摄入量	贡献率/%	摄入量	贡献率/%
污染区 A							
a	526.9**	492.8**		10.0		24.1**	
b	672.3**	612.3**		45.7**		14.3**	
c	359.5*	346.0		6.3		7.2**	
污染区 B							

续表 19-2

调查点	总摄入量	食物		饮水		空气	
		摄入量	贡献率/%	摄入量	贡献率/%	摄入量	贡献率/%
a	285.3	259.8		13.9**		11.6**	
b	392.6*	371.9		11.5*		9.2**	
对照区	262.7	258.4		4.3		0.0	

注：* 与对照区比较，$P<0.05$；** 与对照区比较，$P<0.01$。

问题 5：计算居民不同途径砷摄入量对总砷摄入量的贡献率，说明该市环境污染的类型和特点。

（3）人群砷暴露水平的调查：研究者调查了污染区和对照区居民的发砷、尿砷平均水平，结果见表 19-3。

表 19-3　调查区居民发砷、尿砷测定值

调查点	发砷/（μg/g）			尿砷/（mg/L）		
	调查人数	范围	中位数	调查人数	范围	中位数
污染区 A	850	0.00～160.35	13.40**	804	0.07～1.65	0.12**
污染区 B	346	1.18～113.59	7.76**	586	0.01～0.60	0.13**
对照区	351	0.00～18.00	0.98	348	0.00～0.27	0.05

注：** 与对照区比较，$P<0.01$。

问题 6：表 19-3 的结果说明了什么问题？采用中位数评判是否合适？请对表 19-3 的结果做出相应的解释。

问题 7：表 19-4 为污染区 321 名吸烟者和 875 名非吸烟者的发砷超常率，该分析结果说明了什么问题？

表 19-4　污染区居民吸烟对发砷含量的影响

暴露指标	调查人数	发砷超常人数	发砷超常率/%	P
吸烟	321	212	66.04	$u=1.23$
不吸烟	875	544	62.17	$P>0.05$
合计	1196	756	63.21	

注：该市发砷正常值为 $(0.69±0.12)$ μg/g。

2. 居民健康效应的调查

（1）1982—1986 年居民死亡原因的回顾性调查结果见表 19-5。

表 19-5 调查区居民死亡率和肿瘤死亡专率（1982—1986 年）

调查区	人口数	死亡率/‰				肿瘤死亡专率/（1/10 万）			
		死亡数	粗死亡率	期望死亡数	年龄调整死亡率	死亡数	粗死亡率	期望死亡数	年龄调整死亡率
污染区 A	9120	37	4.06	40		11	120.61	7	
污染区 B	97379	558	5.73	559		52	53.40	110	
对照区	15841	91	5.74	85		5	31.56	5	

问题 8：计算两个污染区和对照区的年龄调整死亡率和肿瘤年龄调整死亡率，其结果为进一步研究提供了什么启示？

（2）1983—1987 年新生儿畸形调查结果见表 19-6、表 19-7。

表 19-6 调查区居民新生儿畸形率（1983—1987 年）

调查区	新生儿数	畸形数	畸形率/‰	P
污染区 A	1461	21	14.37	>0.05
污染区 B	151	2	13.25	>0.05
对照区	208	1	4.81	

表 19-7 污染区产妇砷接触史与畸形儿发生率的关系（1983—1987 年）

砷接触史	调查人数	畸形数	畸形率/‰
有	92	2	21.74
无	1520	21	13.83

问题 9：表 19-6、表 19-7 的结果显示新生儿畸形率在污染区与对照区无显著性差异，其可能的原因是什么？下一步工作应该如何开展？

（3）产妇和新生儿外周血淋巴细胞姐妹染色单体交换（SCE）和微核测定结果见表 19-8。

表 19-8 调查区产妇及新生儿 SCE 及微核率

调查区	产妇		新生儿	
	SCE	微核率/‰	SCE	微核率/‰
污染区 A	9.47*	1.57	9.01**	1.46
污染区 B	8.93	1.77**	9.45**	1.49
对照区	7.23	1.45	5.27	1.32

注：* 与对照区比较，$P<0.05$；** 与对照区比较，$P<0.01$。

问题10：根据表19-8的结果，SCE、微核在判断环境污染对人群健康效应方面有何意义？该表结果有无不当之处？

（4）污染区慢性砷中毒患病情况的调查结果：研究者共调查了污染区无职业砷接触史居民4848人，发现慢性砷中毒患者440人。临床特点多为起病缓、症状轻，患者主要症状有头晕（52.27%）、关节痛（47.68%）、腹胀（17.05%）、腹痛（15.91%）等。主要体征为皮肤病变，有皮肤角化过度（85.99%）、色素沉着斑（37.50%）、脱色斑（32.95%）、鼻黏膜充血（16.36%）等。污染区A和污染区B慢性砷中毒年龄调整患病率分别为8.73%和10.74%。患者最小年龄为12岁，污染区居住年限最短为10年。

目前，慢性砷中毒尚无统一的诊断标准，此次调查中规定的诊断标准为：① 生活在砷污染区10年以上。② 发砷或尿砷含量超过本地正常值上限。③ 同时伴有下列体征之一者：非暴露部位皮肤有明显的色素减退斑或沉着斑，皮肤有角化过度，鼻黏膜有瘢痕、鼻中隔穿孔、皮肤癌及肺癌。

3. 暴露-效应关系

暴露-效应关系是阐明环境因素对人群健康状况影响的基本研究方法之一。暴露水平梯度划分方法很多，研究者从实际出发，以居民点及其土地归属关系作为划分暴露水平及效应水平的单元，以土壤中砷含量、居民人均砷摄入量和人群发砷平均水平为环境及生物学暴露指标，以居民慢性砷中毒年龄调整患病率为健康效应指标。最后，进行回归分析。结果见表19-9。

表19-9 暴露-效应关系分析资料

污染区调查点	距污染源距离/km	土壤中砷/(μg/g)	砷摄入量/[μg/(d·标准人)]	发砷平均水平/(μg/g)	慢性砷中毒年龄调整患病率/%
a	1.75	503.8	526.9	7.76	17.35
b	1.25	960.2	672.3	9.09	13.81
c	1.75	822.7		12.80	13.67
d	1.25	72.1		5.00	3.68
e	2.50	591.6	359.5	5.74	4.62
f	4.40	104.4		4.08	5.01
g	2.50	146.4		3.56	9.56
h	3.50	115.7	285.3	3.00	2.55
i	3.25	79.7		2.17	4.02
j	5.50	32.9		2.75	10.20
k	4.75	123.0		4.00	6.17
l	8.00	178.6	392.6	4.50	4.40
m	0.75	221.4		13.40	12.00

问题11：根据表19-9中的资料，求出慢性砷中毒年龄调整患病率和距污染源距离之间关系的回归方程，并找出污染源下风侧污染区边缘的参考值。

问题12：根据表19-9中的资料，求出土壤砷含量与居民慢性砷中毒年龄调整患病率关系的回归方程，并计算土壤总砷含量的参考界限值。

问题13：根据表19-9中的资料，分别求出砷摄入量、发砷平均水平与慢性砷中毒年龄调整患病率之间关系的回归方程，并分析其结果。

问题14：你对环境污染对人群健康影响的流行病学调查有什么体会？请拟订一个关于环境砷污染对人群健康影响的流行病学调查研究提纲，同时分析本实习中所提供的材料还存在哪些缺陷。

（肖　莎）

Chapter Four | Practice for Occupational Hygiene

第四章 | 职业卫生学实验及案例

Chapter Four Practice for Occupational Hygiene
第四章 职业卫生学实验及案例

 Experiment 20 Determination of δ-amino-γ-ketovalic Acid (δ-ALA) in Urine

Lead is an important occupational harmful factor of heavy metals. The data from the incidence of occupational diseases in recent years shows that chronic occupational lead poisoning accounts for a high proportion of chronic occupational poisoning. When lead poisoning occurs, the content of δ-amino-γ-ketovalic acid (δ-ALA) in urine increases, so the determination of δ-ALA content in urine is helpful to the diagnosis of lead poisoning.

Ⅰ. Objective

To understand the significance of the urine δ-ALA detection and master the detection method of urine δ-ALA.

Ⅱ. Principle

The principle of experiment (Ethyl acetate extraction, Para-dimethylaminobenzaldehyde colorimetry) is: when the pH is 4.6 and the temperature is 100℃, δ-ALA condensed in urine with ethyl acetoacetate produce pyrrole compounds. The compounds are extracted with ethyl acetate and could react with chromogenic agent (Para-dimethylaminobenzaldehyde) to form red compound. Then colorimetric quantification is carried out according to absorbance.

Ⅲ. Materials

1. Instruments

The following instruments will be used in this experiment:

Spectrophotometer, urinometer, boiling water bath, electric furnace, centrifuge (1500 ~ 2000 r/min), 20 pieces of 10 mL colorimetric tube, 1 piece of 2 mL pipettes, 4 pieces of 10 mL straw, 1 piece of 5 mL straw, and 2 pieces of 2 mL straws, 10 pieces of 10 mL centrifuge tube.

2. Reagents

(1) Ethyl acetoacetate, ethyl acetate.

(2) Preparation of reagents.

① Acetate Buffer (pH = 4.6): add 57 mL glacial acetic acid and 82 g anhydrous sodium acetate to 700 mL distilled water. After dissolution, add water to 1000 mL.

② Chromogenic agent: add 1 g Para-dimethylaminobenzaldehyde, 30 mL glacial acetic acid, 5 mL perchloric acid (70%) and 5 mL distilled water in sequence into a 50 mL graduated cylinder. After dissolution, dilute to 50 mL with glacial acetic acid, then blend and store in refrigerator.

③ ALA standard solution.

Storage solution: accurately weigh 12.8 mg δ-amino acetylacetate (δ-ALA · HCl), and add into a 100 mL capacity bottle, then dilute to 100 mL with distilled water. Then 1 mL the liquid contains 100 g δ-ALA. Storage solution can be kept effective in refrigerator for two months.

Application liquid: take the storage solution 10 mL into 100 mL capacity bottle and dilute to 100 mL. Then, 1 mL the liquid contains 10 μg δ-ALA.

IV. Experiment Procedures

1. Drawing of standard curves

Take 6 pieces of 10 mL colorimetric tube, prepare the standard color column according to Table 20 – 1.

Table 20 – 1 Volume and content of ALA standard curve

Reagents	ALA standard tubes number					
	0	1	2	3	4	5
ALA Standard application liquid/mL	0.0	0.1	0.3	0.5	0.7	1.0
Distilled water/mL	2.0	1.9	1.7	1.5	1.3	1.0
ALA content /μg	0	1	3	5	7	10

(1) Add 2 mL acetic acid buffer solution and 0.4 mL ethyl acetoacetate into 0~6 tubes, mix well, then take a water bath heating for 10 min in boiling water, take out and cool down to room temperature.

(2) Add 4 mL ethyl acetate into each tube, shake the tubes well for 1 min, centrifuge for 5 mins, then take out and wait to stratification.

(3) Add 2 mL ethyl acetate extract solution into another 6 pieces of 10 mL colorimetric tubes, add 2 mL chromogenic agent into each tube, cover tubes and shake well, be static for 10 mins.

(4) Measure the absorbance with spectrophotometry (wavelength 554 nm), using zero tube as reference. Draw the standard curve according to the relationship between ALA concentration and absorbance.

2. Determination of urine sample

(1) Add 1 mL urine sample with a specific gravity of 1.010 to 1.035 into two 10 mL colorimetric tubes respectively, add 1 mL distilled water and 2 mL acetic acid buffer solution in each tube, then shake well. One of them is the sample tube, the other is the blank tube of urine sample. Add 0.4 mL ethyl acetoacetate solution the sample tube, add 0.4 mL acetic acid buffer solution to the blank tube of urine sample, mix well, heat in boiling water bath for 10 mins, take out and cool down to room temperature.

(2) The following steps are carried out according to step 2 – 4 of drawing of standard curves mentioned above, do the colorimetric quantification by spectrophotometry, and use ethanol acetate

as reference.

3. Calculation

The absorbance of processed compound substance: sample tube absorbance minus the blank tube absorbance of urine sample. Then check the standard curve with the processed compound substance absorbance to obtain the ALA content (μg) of urine sample.

$$ALA \; (\mu g/mL) = \frac{M}{V} \times \frac{1.020 - 1000}{K - 1000} \qquad (\text{Formula } 20-1)$$

ALA: the ALA concentration in urine sample (μg/mL);

M: ALA content in the sample tube (μg);

V: the volume of urine (mL) in the experiment, $V = 1$ mL;

K: Specific gravity of the sample urine, it is measured by urinometer.

4. Points for attention

(1) Ethyl acetate and ethyl acetoacetate should be recent reagents. And the chromogenic agent should be freshly prepared.

(2) After adding chromogenic agent and being static for 10 mins, colorimetric determination should be completed within half an hour.

(3) Urine samples are easy to rot. If the urine rots, it can be able to increase pH, and affect the results of the determination. If it is not measured in time, urine samples should be stored in the refrigerator.

(4) If the specific gravity of urine sample is within normal range, the measured results can be calculated according to the following formula in the experiment, the volume of urine is 1 mL, so the concentration of ALA in the urine sample is M (μg/mL):

Urine ALA (μg/mL) = sample tube ALA content (μg) (Formula 20-2)

(5) Other substances that can react with chromogenic agents are not extracted by ethyl acetate, so they do not interfere with the determination.

(6) The linear range of method is 0-5 μg/0.5 mL. The lower limit of urine sample determination is 0.3 mg/L.

实验二十 尿中δ-氨基-γ-酮戊酸（δ-ALA）的测定

铅是重要的重金属类职业性有害因素，近几年的职业病发病数据显示，慢性职业性铅中毒在慢性职业中毒中所占比例较高，是慢性职业中毒的主要组成部分。在发生铅中毒时，工人尿中δ-氨基-γ-酮戊酸（δ-ALA）的含量增高，故测定尿中δ-ALA的含量，有助于铅中毒的诊断。

一、实验目的

本实验使学生了解尿δ-ALA检测的意义，掌握δ-ALA检测方法。

二、实验原理

乙酸乙酯萃取，对-二甲氨基苯甲醛比色法检测尿液中 δ-ALA 的含量实验原理：在 pH 为 4.6 及温度为 100℃ 的条件下，尿中 δ-ALA 与乙酰乙酸乙酯缩合生成吡咯化合物。此化合物用乙酸乙酯提取，并与显色剂（对-二甲氨基苯甲醛）作用生成红色化合物。根据颜色深浅进行比色定量。

三、实验材料

1. 仪器设备

本次实验用到的实验仪器设备如下：分光光度计；尿比重测定仪；沸水浴锅；电炉；离心机（1500～2000 r/min）；20 支 10 mL 具塞比色管；1 支 2 mL 移液管；4 支 10 mL 吸管、1 支 5 mL 吸管、2 支 2 mL 吸管；10 支 10 mL 离心管。

2. 主要试剂及配制

（1）乙酰乙酸乙酯、乙酸乙酯。

（2）试剂配制。

①醋酸盐缓冲液（pH = 4.6）：于 700 mL 水中加入 57 mL 冰乙酸，82 g 无水醋酸钠，溶解后加水至 1000 mL。

②显色剂：于 50 mL 量筒中依次加入 30 mL 冰乙酸、1 g 对-二甲氨基苯甲醛、5 mL 高氯酸（70%）、5 mL 水。溶解后，用冰乙酸稀释至 50 mL，混匀，贮于冰箱中保存。

③ALA 标准溶液。

贮备液：准确称取 δ-氨基乙酰丙酸盐（δ-ALA·HCl）12.8 mg 于 100 mL 容量瓶中，用水溶解并稀释至刻度，此时 1 mL 稀释液 δ-ALA 含量为 100 g。贮存冰箱中可保存两个月。

应用液：取贮备液 10 mL 于 100 mL 容量瓶中并稀释至刻度，此液 1 mL 相当于 10 μg δ-ALA。

四、实验方法和步骤

1. 标准曲线的绘制

取 6 支 10 mL 具塞比色管，按下表配制标准体系。

表 20-1 ALA 标准曲线加样体积和含量

试剂	ALA 标准试管编号					
	0	1	2	3	4	5
ALA 标准应用液/mL	0.0	0.1	0.3	0.5	0.7	1.0
蒸馏水/mL	2.0	1.9	1.7	1.5	1.3	1.0
ALA 含量/μg	0	1	3	5	7	10

(1) 各管中加入 2 mL 乙酸缓冲液、0.4 mL 乙酰乙酸乙酯，混匀，沸水浴加热 10 分钟，取出冷却至室温。

(2) 各管中加入 4 mL 乙酸乙酯，加塞振摇 1 分钟，离心 5 分钟，取出静置分层。

(3) 取乙酸乙酯提取液 2 mL 于另外 6 支 10 mL 具塞比色管中，各加入 2 mL 显色剂，加塞振摇，静置 10 分钟。

(4) 用分光光度法（波长 554 nm），以零号管作为参照管，测其吸光度。根据 ALA 浓度与吸光度的关系绘制标准曲线。

2. 尿比重测定

(1) 分别取 1 mL 尿比重在 1.010～1.035 的尿样于两支 10 mL 具塞比色管内，各加蒸馏水 1 mL，乙酸缓冲液 2 mL，混匀。其中一管作为样品管，另一管为尿样空白管。向样品管中加入 0.4 mL 乙酰乙酸乙酯，向尿样空白管中加入 0.4 mL 乙酸缓冲液，充分混匀，同时置沸水浴中加热 10 分钟，取出冷却至室温。

(2) 以下步骤按标准曲线绘制的第 2 步至第 4 步进行，以乙酸乙醇作为参照管，用分光光度法进行比色定量。

3. 计算

实验所需吸光度为：样品管吸光度减去尿样空白管吸光度，将处理后的吸光度值代入标准曲线，查得样品管中 ALA 含量（μg）。

$$ALA\ (\mu g/mL) = \frac{M}{V} \times \frac{1.020 - 1000}{K - 1000} \qquad (公式 20 - 1)$$

ALA：尿样中 ALA 浓度（μg/mL）；

M：检测尿样中 ALA 的含量（μg）；

V：实验中所用尿样体积（mL）；

K：检测尿样的尿比重。

4. 注意事项

(1) 乙酸乙酯、乙酰乙酸乙酯最好为近期产品，显色剂宜新鲜配制。

(2) 加入显色剂后，静置 10 分钟，应在半小时内完成比色。

(3) 尿样易腐败，可导致 pH 增高，影响测定结果。如不能及时测定，应将尿样保存在冰箱中。

(4) 如尿样比重在正常范围内，测得结果可按公式 20 - 2 计算（本实验中尿样 ALA 单位是 μg，体积单位是 mL，ALA 的浓度单位是 μg/mL，而 μg/mL = mg/L），当体积为 1 mL 时：

$$尿中 ALA\ (mg/L) = 样品管中 ALA 含量\ (\mu g) \qquad (公式 20 - 2)$$

(5) 其他能与显色剂反应的物质，不被乙酸乙酯萃取，故不干扰测定。

(6) 方法的线性检测范围为 0～5 μg/0.5 mL，尿样检测下限为 0.3 mg/L。

Experiment 21 Determination of Cholinesterase Activity in Whole Blood by Spectrophotometry—by Ferric Trichloride Method

Ⅰ. Objectives

The aim of this experiment is to be familiar with determination of cholinesterase (ChE) activity in whole blood by spectrophotometry. Students are expected to reach the following requirements:

(1) To understand the mechanism of organophosphorus pesticide poisoning.

(2) To master the significance of ChE activity determination in whole blood.

(3) To master the principle and method of ChE activity determination in whole blood.

Ⅱ. Principle

Acetylcholine (ACh) can be hydrolyzed into choline and acetic acid by ChE in the blood. When the reaction terminates, the remnant ACh in the blood will react with alkaline hydroxylamine and produce acetyl-hydroxylamine, which will react with ferric trichloride and produce reddish brown hydroxamic acid iron complexes in the acidic environment. The color depth is directly proportional to the amount of acetylcholine remnant, which means the deeper the color solution, the more amount of acetylcholine remnant. Therefore, the amount of remnant acetylcholine can be determined by spectrophotometer, and the cholinesterase activity can be calculated by the amount of hydrolyzed acetylcholine, which can be calculated by formula.

Ⅲ. Materials

1. Instruments

The following instruments will be used in this experiment:

spectrophotometer, colorimetric tubes, constant temperature water bath, hemoglobin straw (20 μL scale), scale straw, glass tubes, and funnels.

2. Reagents

Reagents should be analytically pure, the water should be distilled water or deionized water.

(1) Phosphate buffer solution (Pbs, pH = 7.40).

(2) Alkaline hydroxylamine solution (Ahs).

(3) Hydrochloric acid solution (Has, 1 : 2).

(4) 10% Ferric chloride solution (Fcs).

(5) Acetylcholine chloride standard solution (Acs, 7μmol/mL).

3. Sampling and preservation

Firstly, add 0.98 mL phosphate buffer solution into the colorimetric tube. Secondly, assimilate participant' blood 20 μL with hemoglobin straw, poured into the same colorimetric tube,

Chapter Four Practice for Occupational Hygiene
第四章 职业卫生学实验及案例

and detected immediately.

If not determined immediately, take 0.5 mL blood into the glass tube, which includes heparin anticoagulant, and mix. The blood samples need to be transported in low-temperature or ice environment. It can be stored for a week in a 4 ℃ refrigerator.

Ⅳ. Experiment Procedures

1. Procedures

Table 21 – 1 shows the experiment procedures step by step. The blank tube is used as the reference sample. The absorbance values are determined by spectrophotometer at the wavelength of 520 nm, and the ChE activity is calculated by Formula 21 – 1 and Formula 21 – 2.

Table 21 – 1 The experiment reagents and procedures (mL)

Steps	Reagents	Test tubes			
		Sample tube (A)	Control tube (B)	Standard tube (C)	Blank tube
Step 1	Phosphate buffer solution	0.98	0.98	1	1
Step 2	Blood	0.02	0.02	–	–
Step 3	To preheat the tubes in 37℃ water for 5 mins				
Step 4	Acetylcholine chloride standard solution	1	–	1	–
Step 5	Distilled Water	–	1	–	1
Step 6	To place the tubes in 37℃ water for 30 mins				
Step 7	Alkaline hydroxylamine solution	4	4	4	4
Step 8	To take the tubes out of warm water and shake them for 2 mins				
Step 9	Hydrochloric acid solution	2	2	2	2
Step 10	To shake the tubes for 2 mins				
Step 11	Ferric chloride solution	2	2	2	2
Step 12	To shake the tubes and filter the liquid				

Note: " – " means that no reagent is added.

2. Calculation

(1) Calculate the absolute value of blood ChE activity according to the following formula.

$$Xs = \frac{C + B - A}{C} \times 7 \qquad \text{(Formula 21 – 1)}$$

Xs: Hydrolysis of acetylcholine concentration, μmol (0.02 mL, 37 ℃, 30 mins);

A: The absorbance value of sample tube (A);

B: The absorbance value of control tube (B);

C: The absorbance value of standard tube (C);

(2) The relative value of blood ChE activity (%).

$$X_{SR} = \frac{Xs}{M} \times 100 \qquad \text{(Formula 21-2)}$$

X_{SR}: The relative value of blood ChE activity (%);

Xs: Hydrolysis of acetylcholine concentration, μmol (0.02 mL, 37 ℃, 30 mins);

M: The normal reference values;

The normal reference values (a region in China): male 3.22 ± 0.336 μmol; female 3.19 ± 0.398 μmol.

3. Evaluation

According to the evaluation criteria of pesticide poisoning in Table 21-2, the pesticide poisoning degree of the tested objects was evaluated.

Table 21-2 Criteria for judging the degree of pesticide poisoning based on ChE activity

Poisoning classification	ChE activity
Normal	≥70%
Mild poisoning	50% - 70%
Moderate poisoning	30% - 50%
Severe poisoning	<30%

4. Points for attention

(1) Prepare test tubes and add phosphate buffer before blood collection.

(2) Strictly disinfect before the blood collection, place the used cotton balls and needle in a medical garbage bag, and take disinfection disposal finally.

(3) Accurately control the water bath temperature and setting time.

(4) Complete the colorimetry after adding ferric chloride within 20 mins.

实验二十一　全血胆碱酯酶的测定——三氯化铁比色法

一、实验目的

血液胆碱酯酶是有机磷农药中毒的重要诊断指标，是中毒治疗后的效果观察指标，亦是接触有机磷农药人员健康状况的动态观察指标。测定有机磷农药接触者血液胆碱酯酶活性，有助于有机磷农药中毒的诊断和治疗效果的评价。

(1) 加深对有机磷农药中毒机制的认识。

(2) 掌握全血 ChE 活性测定的意义。

(3) 掌握全血 ChE 活性测定原理、方法。

二、实验原理

血液内的乙酰胆碱可以被胆碱酯酶水解为胆碱和乙酸,若胆碱酯酶活性被抑制,则无法水解乙酰胆碱,乙酰胆碱被蓄积在血液中,剩余的乙酰胆碱可以与碱性羟胺反应生成乙酰羟胺,乙酰羟胺在酸性条件下与三氯化铁反应生成棕红色的络合物羟肟酸铁。棕红色越深,表示反应产物羟肟酸铁越多,在三氯化铁充足的条件下,提示乙酰羟胺越多。以此类推,说明血液中乙酰胆碱剩余越多,进而说明胆碱酯酶活动越低。

三、实验材料

1. 实验试剂

磷酸盐缓冲液(pH=7.40),碱性羟胺溶液,1:2盐酸溶液,10%三氯化铁溶液,乙酰胆碱标准应用液(1 mL 含 7 μmol)。

2. 实验仪器

分光光度计,比色管,恒温水浴箱,血红蛋白吸管(20 μL 刻度),刻度吸管,试管,漏斗。

3. 采样和保存

第一步,取 0.98mL 磷酸盐缓冲液注入比色管中;第二步,用血红蛋白吸管采集末梢循环静脉血 20μL 注入盛有磷酸盐缓冲液的比色管中,立即进行测定。

四、实验过程

1. 实验步骤

用三氯化铁比色法,依据表 21-1 所列的全血胆碱酯酶活性检测实验试剂和操作步骤,依次加入下列试剂后测量吸光度。吸光度测定波长为 520 nm,以空白管作为调零管。最后将吸光度结果代入公式 21-1 和公式 21-2,计算检测对象胆碱酯酶的绝对活性值和相对活性值。

表 21-1 胆碱酯酶活性的实验试剂和操作步骤

单位:mL

步骤	试剂	试管编号			
		样品管(A)	对照管(B)	标准管(C)	空白管
第1步	磷酸盐缓冲液	0.98	0.98	1	1
第2步	静脉血(肝素抗凝)	0.02	0.02	—	—
第3步	置37℃水浴中预热5分钟				
第4步	乙酰胆碱标准应用液	1	—	1	—
第5步	蒸馏水	—	1	—	1
第6步	置37℃水浴中反应30分钟,准时取出				

续表 21-2

步骤	试剂	试管编号			
		样品管（A）	对照管（B）	标准管（C）	空白管
第 7 步	碱性羟胺溶液	4	4	4	4
第 8 步	充分振摇 2 分钟				
第 9 步	1+2 盐酸溶液	2	2	2	2
第 10 步	充分振摇 2 分钟				
第 11 步	三氯化铁溶液	2	2	2	2
第 12 步	充分振摇，用滤纸过滤				

注："—"表示不需要加对应的试剂。

2．计算

（1）按以下公式计算血液胆碱酯酶活性绝对值。

$$Xs = \frac{C+B-A}{C} \times 7 \qquad \text{（公式 21-1）}$$

Xs：水解乙酰胆碱的浓度，μmol（0.02 mL，37℃，30 分钟）；

A：样品管（A）的吸光度值；

B：对照管（B）的吸光度值；

C：标准管（C）的吸光度值。

（2）胆碱酯酶活性相对值（%）。

$$X_{SR} = \frac{X_S}{M} \times 100 \qquad \text{（公式 21-2）}$$

X_{SR}：胆碱酯酶活性相对值（%）；

X_S：水解乙酰胆碱的浓度，μmol（0.02 mL，37℃，30 分钟）；

M：健康人胆碱酯酶活性绝对值；

健康人胆碱酯酶活性绝对值（中国某地区）：男：3.22 ±0.336 μmol；女：3.19 ± 0.398 μmol。

3．评价

依据表 21-2 中的农药中毒评估标准，评估本实验检测对象的农药中毒情况。

表 21-2 依据胆碱酯酶活性判断农药中毒程度的标准

中毒级别	胆碱酯酶活性
未中毒	≥70%
轻度中毒	50%～70%
中度中毒	30%～50%
重度中毒	<30%

4. 注意事项

（1）采血前先准备好试管，加入磷酸盐缓冲液。

（2）采血时严格消毒，用过的棉球、刺针集中放置。

（3）准确控制水浴温度和放置时间。

（4）加三氯化铁显色后，在 20 分钟内比色。

Experiment 22　Determination of Total Dust Concentration and Dispersion

Productive dust is the main pathogenesis of pneumoconiosis, so monitoring productive dust is an important measure to prevent pneumoconiosis. Dust concentration refers to the quality or quantity of dust in per unit volume air. In the hygienic standard in China, the maximum allowable concentration of dust is represented by mass concentration, for expressing as mg/m^3. Dust dispersion refers to the distribution of dust particles of different sizes in per unit volume air. It includes quantitative dispersion and quality dispersion, and the current hygienic standard in China adopts quantitative dispersion. In this experiment, the contents include two parts: one is determination of total productive dust concentration, the other is determination of dust dispersion.

Part 1　Determination of total productive dust concentration —Filter membrane quality method

Ⅰ. Objective

To learn and master the measurement method of productive total dust concentration.

Ⅱ. Principle

A certain volume of dust-containing air is extracted and the dust is left on the filter membrane that is weighed before sampling. The mass (mg/m^3) of dust in unit volume air is obtained by the increment of the filter membrane after sampling.

Ⅲ. Materials

Instruments: The following instruments or materials will be used in this experiment.

Dust sampler (use explosion-proof sampler in explosion-proof workplace), perchloroethylene fiber filter membrane, filter clamp, sample box, tweezers, analytical balance, stopwatch, dryer (discoloration silica).

Ⅳ. Experiment Procedures

1. Filter membrane preparation

Remove the lining paper on both sides of the filter membrane with tweezers and weigh the filter membrane on the analytical balance. The number and quality are recorded on lining paper. Open the filter clamp, lay the wool surface of the 40 mm diameter filter membrane upward on the conical ring, tighten the fixed ring, make sure the filter membrane has no fold or crack, and put it into the sample box.

2. Sampling

(1) Sampling points: The sampler is placed within the range of workers' daily activities, and the height from the floor is the breathing zone of workers and dust distribution is relatively uniform. When there is influence of the wind flow, the downwind side or the return side of the working place should be chosen, and the moving dust point should be located in the representative places of the worker's activities, or set up on the mobile equipment.

(2) First, a filter membrane holder with a filter membrane (no need to weigh the filter membrane) can be clamped into the sampling head, start the sampler and adjust to the required flow, then the filter membrane is replaced by the weighed filter membrane, and make the filter membrane surface facing the dust-containing airflow. When the dust sample can't avoid the mud and sand pollution, the dust surface can be sideways.

(3) Sampling flow rate: If the diameter of filter membrane is 40 mm, sampling flow rate is 15 – 40 L/min. If the filter membrane is funnel-shaped, the flow rate can be increased appropriately, but no more than 80 L/min.

(4) The sampling duration is determined according to the estimate values of dust concentration at the sampling point and the dust increment (40 mm filter membrane shall not be less than 1 mg, but not more than 10 mg. The dust increment of the funnel filter membrane with a diameter of 75 mm is not subject to this limit), and generally no less than 10 mins (when the dust concentration is higher than 10 mg/m^3, the volume of collecting air shall not be less than 0.2 m^3; when the dust concentration is below 2 mg/m^3, the volume of collecting air should be limited between 0.5 – 1 m^3). Record filter membrane number, sampling time, air flow rate and conditions of sampling point.

(5) After sampling, the filter membrane is removed from the filter clamp with tweezers, the filter membrane with dust-face is folded inward several times, then wrapped with liner paper, and stored in the sample box, or placed in the sample clamp, and brought back to the laboratory.

(6) The filter membrane that has been sampled is generally weighed without drying. When the relative humidity of the field air is more than 90% or there is water mist, the filter membrane should be placed in the dryer for 2 h and then weighed; 30 mins in the dryer later, weigh again. If the difference between two adjacent weights is less than 0.1 mg, take the minimum value.

3. Calculation

The dust concentration is calculated by the following formula:

$$C = \frac{m_2 - m_1}{Q \cdot t} \times 1000 \qquad \text{(Formula 22 – 1)}$$

C: Dust concentration, mg/m^3;

m_1: Filter membrane weight before sampling, mg;

m_2: Filter membrane weight after sampling, mg;

t: Sampling time, min;

Q: Air flow rate, L/min.

4. Notes

(1) It is the basic method to detect productive dust concentration in the current health standards in China. If other instruments or methods are used to detect dust mass concentrations, this method must be used as a benchmark.

(2) The surface of perchloroethylene fiber filter membrane is fine villous, not brittle, which has obvious static electricity and hydrophobicity. And the fiber filter membrane can firmly adsorb dust, but it doesn't bear high temperature and easily dissolves in organic solvents. The sampled filter membrane can be used as a material for the determination of dust dispersion or for the determination of free silica by alkali-melted molybdenum blue colorimetric method. If the environmental temperature of sampling site is above 55℃, the perchloroethylene fiber filter membrane should be changed to glass fiber filter membrane.

(3) When there is oil mist in the air of the sampling site, the sampled filter membrane should be washed by petroleum ether or aviation gasoline, and then dried before weighing.

Part 2　Determination of productive dust dispersion
　　　　—Filter membrane dissolving smear

Ⅰ. Objective

To learn and master the measurement method of productive dust dispersion.

Ⅱ. Principle

The sampled filter membrane is dissolved in organic solvent to form the suspension solution of dust particles, then make the smears and calculate the dispersion under microscope.

Ⅲ. Materials

1. Instruments

The following instruments or materials will be used in this experiment: small beaker or small test tube, small glass rod, glass dropper or straw, slide, biological microscope, eyepiece micrometer, and objective micrometer.

2. Reagents

Butyl acetate.

IV. Experiment Procedures

1. Procedures

(1) Put the sampled filter membrane into a small beaker or test tube, add 1 – 2 mL butyl acetate into the beaker or test tube with a straw or dropper, stir well with a glass rod to form uniform suspension dust solution. Then immediately absorb a drop of dust suspension solution on the slide with dropper, evenly coated. When the dust suspension solution on the slide volatilizes naturally into a transparent film, write the number, sampling place and date on the label of slide.

(2) The objective micrometer is a standard scale with a total length of 1 mm, which is divided into 100 equal scales, so each scale is 10 μm (Figure 22 – 1).

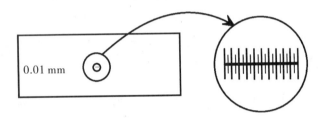

Figure 22 – 1   Objective micrometer

(3) Calibration of the eyepiece micrometer: Place the eyepiece micrometer to the eyepiece tube, and place the objective micrometer on the loading platform. Firstly, find the scale line of the objective micrometer under the low magnification, then move it to the center of the vision field. Secondly, change the objective micrometer to 400 – 600 times magnification, and adjust calibration screw to the scale line clear. Thirdly, move the platform, make a scale line of the objective micrometer coincide with a scale of the eyepiece micrometer, and then find out another coincidence scale. Count the number of the scale lines of objective and eyepiece micrometers respectively between the two coincidence scale lines (Figure 22 – 2).

Calculate the spacing of each scale of the eyepiece micrometer (μm):

$$\text{eyepiece micrometers per scale (μm)} = \frac{a}{b} \times 10 \text{ (μm)} \qquad \text{(Formula 22 – 2)}$$

a: The scale number of objective micrometer;
b: The scale number of eyepiece micrometer;
10: The spacing of objective micrometers per scale, μm.

If 45 scales of eyepiece micrometer are equivalent to 10 scales of objective micrometer, then one scale of eyepiece micrometer is equivalent to 2.2 μm as Figure 22 – 2 shows.

$$\frac{10}{45} \times 10 \text{ (μm)} = 2.2 \text{ (μm)} \qquad \text{(Formula 22 – 3)}$$

(4) Take off the objective micrometer, place the dust specimen on the platform. Firstly, find the dust particle with the low magnification, then measure the size of each dust particle with the

calibrated eyepiece micrometer under the high magnification (Figure 22 – 3). Move the dust particles enter to the scope of eyepiece microscale vision, and measure each dust particle's diameter (long diameter or short diameter). At least 200 dust particles were measured for each specimen. According to Table 22 – 1, record the number of dust particles by groups, and calculate the percentage.

Table 22 – 1 Measurement record of dust dispersion

Unit _____ Sampling locations _____ Sampling time _____ Filter membrane number _____

Content	Diameter/μm	<2	2 –	5 –	≥10	Total
Number of dust particles						
Percentage/%						100%

Gauger _____

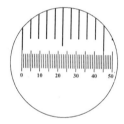
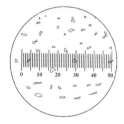

Figure 22 – 2 Calibration of eyepiece micrometers   Figure 22 – 3 Measurement of dust dispersion

2. Notes

(1) All the equipment must be cleaned before using to avoid dust contamination. The prepared smear specimen should be kept in a glass plate.

(2) When the dust particles of the smear specimen are too dense and affect the measurement, the dust suspension can be remade with appropriate amount of butyl acetate dilution.

(3) A calibrated eyepiece micrometer can be only applied at magnification of the eyepiece and objective lens which have been used for calibration.

(4) The parts of the smear specimens with more uniform dust distribution should be selected for measurement to reduce the error.

(5) This method does not apply to dust that can be dissolved in organic solvents and fibrous dust, the measurement method of such dust is natural deposition.

实验二十二 总粉尘浓度及分散度的测定

生产性粉尘是引起尘肺病的主要病因，因此对生产性粉尘的监测是防止尘肺病的重要措施。生产性粉尘浓度是指单位体积空气中所含粉尘的质量或数量，在我国卫生标准中，生产性粉尘最高容许浓度采用质量浓度，以 mg/m^3 表示。粉尘分散度是指空气中不同大小粉尘颗粒的分布程度，用百分构成比表示。有数量分散度和质量分散度两种，我国现行卫生标准采用数量分散度。因此本实验内容包含两部分：总生产性粉尘浓度的测定和生产性粉尘分散度的测定。

第一节 总生产性粉尘浓度的测定
——滤膜质量法

一、实验目的
使学生学习和掌握生产性总粉尘浓度的测定方法。

二、实验原理
用粉尘采样器将已称量重量的过氯乙烯纤维滤膜装在采样器上，打开采样器采取一定体积的含尘空气，采集完毕后，取下滤膜称重，滤膜采样前后的增量，则为粉尘重量，依次可求出单位体积空气中粉尘的质量（mg/m^3）。

三、实验材料
实验器材：粉尘采样器，过氯乙烯纤维滤膜，滤膜夹，样品盒，镊子，分析天平，秒表，内盛变色硅胶的干燥器。

四、实验过程
1. **滤膜准备**

用镊子取下滤膜两面的夹衬纸，将滤膜放在分析天平上称量，将编号和质量记录在衬纸上。打开采样器滤膜夹，将直径 40 mm 的滤膜毛面向上平铺于锥形环上，旋紧固定环，使滤膜无褶皱或裂隙，放入样品盒。

2. **采样**

（1）采样点：采样器置于接尘作业人员经常活动的范围内，多为粉尘分布较均匀的呼吸带位置。有风流影响时，一般应选择在作业地点下风侧或回风侧；在移动的扬尘点，应位于作业人员活动中有代表性的地点，或架设于移动设备上。

（2）先用一个装有滤膜（未称量滤膜即可）的滤膜夹装入采样头中旋紧，开动采样器调节至所需流量，然后将已称量滤膜换入采样头，使滤膜受尘面迎向含尘气流。当迎向含尘气流无法避免飞溅的泥浆、砂粒对样品污染时，受尘面可侧向。

（3）采样流量：用 40 mm 滤膜时为 15～40 L/min；用漏斗状滤膜时，可适当加大流量，但不得超过 80 L/min。

（4）根据采样点的粉尘浓度估计值及滤膜上所需粉尘增量（直径 40 mm 平面滤膜，不得少于 1 mg，但不得多于 10 mg。直径 75 mm 的漏斗状滤膜粉尘增量不受此限制）确定采样持续时间，但一般不得小于 10 分钟（当粉尘浓度高于 10 mg/m³ 时，采气量不得少于 0.2 m³；低于 2 mg/m³，采气量应为 0.5～1 m³）。记录滤膜编号、采样时间、气体流量和采样点生产工作情况。

（5）采样结束后，用镊子将滤膜从滤膜夹上取下，受尘面向内折叠几次，用衬纸包好，贮于样品盒中，或装入自备的样品夹中，带回实验室。

（6）已采样滤膜，一般情况下不需要做干燥处理，即可称量。如果采样时现场空气相对湿度在 90% 以上或有水雾，应将滤膜放在干燥器内 2 小时后称量，然后再放入干燥器中 30 分钟，再次称量。当相邻两次的称量结果之差小于 0.1 mg 时，取其最小值。

3. 计算结果

将本次实验数据代入公式 22-1，计算实验结果。

$$C = \frac{m_2 - m_1}{Q \cdot t} \times 1000 \qquad\qquad (公式\ 22-1)$$

C：粉尘浓度，mg/m³；

m_1：采样前滤膜质量，mg；

m_2：采样后滤膜质量，mg；

t：采样时间，min；

Q：采气流量，L/min。

4. 注意事项

（1）本方法为我国现行卫生标准采用的基本方法。如果使用其他仪器或方法测定粉尘质量浓度时，必须以本方法为基准。

（2）过氯乙烯纤维滤膜表面呈细绒毛状，不易脆裂，具有明显的静电性和憎水性，能牢固地吸附粉尘，但不耐高温，易溶于有机溶剂。已采样滤膜可留作测定粉尘分散度或作为碱熔钼蓝比色法测定游离二氧化硅的材料。在 55 ℃ 以上现场采样测定粉尘质量浓度时不宜应用，可改为玻璃纤维滤膜。

（3）采样现场空气中有油雾时，可用石油醚或航空汽油浸洗，晾干后再称量。

第二节　生产性粉尘分散度的测定
——滤膜溶解涂片法

一、实验目的

使学生学习和掌握生产性粉尘分散度的测定方法。

二、实验原理

采样后滤膜溶解于有机溶剂中,形成粉尘粒子的混悬液,制成涂片标本,在显微镜下测定。

三、实验材料

1. 实验耗材

本次实验用到的耗材如下:小烧杯或小试管、玻璃棒、玻璃滴管或吸管、载玻片、生物显微镜、目镜测微尺、物镜测微尺。

2. 试剂

乙酸丁酯。

四、实验方法和步骤

1. 操作步骤

(1) 将采有粉尘的过氯乙烯纤维滤膜放入小烧杯或试管中,用吸管或滴管加入 1~2 mL 醋酸丁酯,用玻璃棒充分搅拌,制成均匀的粉尘悬液,立即用滴管吸取一滴于载玻片上,均匀涂片,待自然挥发成透明膜,贴上标签,注明编号、采样地点、日期。

(2) 物镜测微尺是一标准尺度,其总长为 1 mm,分为 100 等分刻度,每一分度值为 0.01 mm,即 10 μm,见图 22-1。

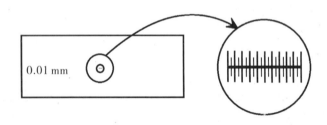

图 22-1 物镜测微尺

(3) 目镜测微尺的标定:将待标定的目镜测微尺放入目镜镜筒内,物镜测微尺置于载物台上,先在低倍镜下找到物镜测微尺的刻度线,移至视野中央。然后将物镜换成 400~600 倍,放大倍率,调至刻度线清晰,移动载物台;使物镜测微尺任一刻度线与目镜测微尺的任一刻度线相重合,然后找出两尺另外一条重合的刻度线,分别数出两条重合刻度线间物镜测微尺和目镜测微尺的刻度数,见图 22-2。

计算目镜测微尺每刻度的间距(μm):

$$目镜测微尺每刻度间距 = \frac{a}{b} \times 10 (\mu m) \qquad (公式 22-2)$$

公式中,a:物镜测微尺刻度数;

b:目镜测微尺刻度数;

10:物镜测微尺每格刻度距离,μm。

图 22-2 中，目镜测微尺的 45 个刻度相当于物镜测微尺的 10 个刻度，则目镜测微尺的 1 个刻度相当于 2.2 μm：

$$\frac{10}{45} \times 10 = 2.2 \ (\mu m) \qquad\qquad (公式 22-3)$$

（4）取下物镜测微尺，将粉尘涂片放在载物台上，先用低倍镜找到粉尘粒子，然后在标定目镜测微尺时所用的放大倍率下，用目镜测微尺测量每个粉尘粒子的大小，见图 22-3。移动涂片，使粉尘粒子依次进入目镜测微尺的范围，遇长径量长径，遇短径量短径，测量每个尘粒。每个标本至少测量 200 个尘粒。按表 22-1 分组记录，算出百分数。

表 22-1 粉尘分散度测量记录

单位_____ 采样地点_____ 采样时间_____ 滤膜编号_____

	粒径/μm	<2	2～	5～	≥10	总计
尘粒数/个						
百分数/%						100%

测量者_____

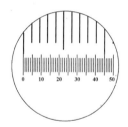 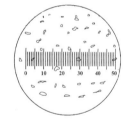

图 22-2 目镜测微尺的标定　　图 22-3 粉尘分散度的测量

2. 注意事项

（1）所用器材在用前必须擦洗干净，避免粉尘污染。已制好的涂片标本应放置玻璃平皿内保存。

（2）当发现涂片标本因尘粒过密而影响测量时，可再加适量醋酸丁酯稀释，重新制作涂片标本。

（3）已标定的目镜测微尺只能在标定时所用的目镜和物镜放大倍率下应用。

（4）应选择涂片标本中粉尘分布较均匀的部位进行测量，以减少误差。

（5）本法不适用于可溶于有机溶剂中的粉尘和纤维状粉尘，此类粉尘应用自然沉降法测量。

Experiment 23 Case Study of Occupational Diseases and Occupational Health

Part 1 Case study on pneumoconiosis

Ⅰ. Objectives

In China, occupational pneumoconiosis is the most common occupational disease, accounting for more than 80% of new occupational diseases every year. The prevention and treatment of pneumoconiosis is the focus of occupational disease prevention in China. In this experiment, learning objectives and requirements to students are as follows:

(1) To master the analysis method of occupational pneumoconiosis cases.

(2) To master the main exposure opportunities, clinical manifestations, preventive measures of pneumoconiosis.

(3) To be familiar with pneumoconiosis diagnosis and treatment principles.

(4) To understand the main contents of on-site occupational health investigation.

Ⅱ. Case study and analysis

Wang ×, male, 28 years old, worked in a wear-resistant material factory from August 2004 to October 2007, had worked more than 3 years as miscellaneous worker and crushing workers, exposed to a large amount of productive dust. Since August 2007, Wang had symptom of cough and chest tightness, and treated as cold, but had never been cured. Then Wang went to the hospital for examination. From the chest X-ray, doctor found shadows on both lungs, and several doctors of several hospitals suspected that was pneumoconiosis. However, the diagnosis of the local occupational disease prevention and control institute is "Zero phase of pneumoconiosis (medical observation) with pulmonary tuberculosis". Finally, Wang took the pathological diagnosis of lung tissue to prove that he did suffer from pneumoconiosis in June 2009. Wang was diagnosed with the third phase of silicosis, and received a total of 615000 RMB of compensation in September 2009.

[Questions]

(1) Why did Wang suffer from silicosis?

(2) What are the clinical manifestations of silicosis?

(3) What is the main diagnostic basis of silicosis?

(4) From this case, what are the problems in the prevention and control of occupational diseases in China?

Part 2 Case study on occupational lead poisoning

Ⅰ. Objectives

Occupational poisoning is a major category of occupational diseases, including acute occupational poisoning and chronic occupational poisoning. Chronic lead poisoning is the most common disease of chronic occupational poisoning, which is an important content for students to learn. Through this study, students reach the following requirements:

(1) To master the analysis methods of occupational poisoning cases.

(2) To master the main exposure opportunities, clinical manifestations and preventive measures of occupational lead poisoning.

(3) To be familiar with the principles of diagnosis and treatment of occupational lead poisoning.

(4) To understand the main contents of on-site occupational health survey.

Ⅱ. Case study and analysis

The patient, Li ×, male, 37 years old, had been suffering from insomnia, headache, dizziness, memory loss, general fatigue, joint pain and loss of appetite since 1986. In the past three years, the above symptoms had been aggravated, accompanied by frequent periumbilical and unfixed abdominal cramps, which can be relieved by pressing the abdomen by hand. He was hospitalized in 1992. Medical examination found that the conscious was normal, temperature was 37.2℃, pulse was 72 times/min, respiratory rate was 20 times/min, blood pressure was 120/70 mmHg, cardiopulmonary function is normal, liver and spleen was normal, abdomen was flat and soft. Periumbilical abdomen had slight pressing pain, but no rebound tenderness. The sense of pain touch in the extremities was normal, and did not draw forth pathological reflex. Blood and urine routine was normal, liver and cardiac function was normal, chest X-ray photos were normal.

[Questions 1]

(1) What else materials do you think should be added to the above information?

(2) If you are a doctor, when you encounter a patient with abdominal cramps, what diseases might you be thinking about?

(3) What poisons can cause abdominal cramps? Workers of which occupations might expose to these poisons?

Upon further inquiry of the patient's occupation history, it was found that the patient had been engaged in the casting of the printing plant since 1984, pouring molten lead water into the typehead; there was a large amount of lead vapor escaped into the air in the process. And the workers worked eight hours a day. According to this information, the patient may have chronic lead poisoning.

[Questions 2]

(4) What are the differences in clinical manifestations between acute and chronic lead poisoning?

(5) What other clinical tests should be done to confirm that the patient suffered from lead poisoning?

(6) What occupational health surveys should be conducted in the patient's workplace?

Through the investigation of the patient's workplace, it was found that the concentration of lead smoke in the air of the workplace was 0.4 – 0.8 mg/m^3. According to the patient's occupational exposure history and clinical manifestations, it was considered as occupational poisoning, and the patient was transferred to the occupational disease prevention hospital for further diagnosis and treatment. Examination on admission to hospital results showed that the concentration of lead in urine was 12.3 μmol/L, ALA concentration in urine was 80.4 μmol/L, and the concentration of free protoporphyrin in red blood cells was 3.6 μmol/L. The diagnosis was chronic lead poisoning.

[Questions 3]

(7) What are the antidotes for chronic lead poisoning? What should we pay attention to when taking medicine?

(8) In addition to detoxification treatment, what adjuvant treatment should be given?

An investigation team organized by the occupational disease prevention and control hospital went to the workshop of printing plant to investigate, and found that the process produced blue-gray smoke when workers poured the plate, and there was no detoxification cover in the workshop. Workers rarely used protective equipment such as protective clothing, masks, and gloves. According to a survey of other workers in the same workshop, most of them reported that they had symptoms, such as headache, dizziness, memory loss, limb weakness and muscle pain, while a few workers had abdominal pain. The occupational disease prevention and control hospital organized a physical examination for workers in the workshop. The results showed that 6 of the 8 workers had higher urine lead, and ALA in urine was higher than normal, and 3 of the 6 workers had numbness in their extremities.

[Questions 4]

(9) What occupational health problems did exist in the workplace? How can it be improved?

Part 3　Occupational health surveillance case analysis

Ⅰ. Objectives

Occupational health surveillance is a health monitoring method and process for prevention, which continuously monitors the health status of workers with various examinations according to their occupational exposure history, and finds early symptoms of health damage in time. Occupational health surveillance is an important guarantee for the fulfillment of the employer's obligations and the realization of the workers' rights. It is also the basis for the implementation of the occupational-disease-diagnosis appraisal system and the work-related injury protection system. The purpose of this case analysis is as follows:

(1) To master the basic contents of occupational health surveillance.

(2) To be familiar with occupational disease diagnosis procedures.

II. Case study and analysis

Liu × ×, male, 46 years old, lives in Liuzhuang, Ping-an Town, B County, A City. Liu had worked wollastonite grinding job for 5 years since June 2013 in the branch of refractory material factory in B County. However, the labor contract was not signed until March 10, 2018. In November 2018, Liu began to appear symptoms of cough, chest tightness, fatigue, and dyspnea, so he had an occupational health examination.

[Questions 1]

(1) What disease may Liu suffer from? And why?

(2) What is occupational health examination? What are the categories? Please describe the purpose and objects of various occupational health examinations.

(3) What is occupational health surveillance? What is the relationship between occupational health examination and occupational health surveillance?

(4) Where should workers go for occupational health examination? At present, how to obtain the qualification of occupational health examination institutions in China? What is the basis?

Liu had an occupational health examination at the C Occupational Disease Diagnosis Institution (hereinafter referred to as the "C Diagnostic Institution", it's with occupational health examination qualification) in B county on December 30 in 2018. The C Diagnostic Institution concluded that the diagnosis was suspected as occupational pneumoconiosis, and recommended a reexamination 3 months later. On March 30 in 2019, doctor according to the reexamination concluded that Liu was suspected to have occupational pneumoconiosis, and recommended Liu for an occupational disease diagnosis.

[Questions 2]

(5) What items should be examined in light of Liu's situation?

(6) What is the classification of occupational health examination reports?

(7) Was it appropriate that the C Diagnostic Institution handled the examination results of Liu? Why?

Then Liu applied for an occupational disease diagnosis in C Diagnostic Institution, and the C Diagnostic Institution informed Liu to provide the materials of occupational-disease-inductive contact history (hereinafter referred to as "occupational contact history"). But the factory didn't provide the materials in the beginning, and provided evaluation report of the workplace occupational-disease-inductive factors after urged by health administrative department of B county. The report showed that the concentration of wollastonite powder dust of grinders' workplace was

C_{TWA} = 20.5 mg/m^3, over the occupational exposure limit of China's workplace harmful factors (5.0 mg/m^3). Liu said that he needed to work five days a week, and ten hours a day. He contacted a lot of dust during the work, and the factory provided only 3 disposable masks a week.

[Questions 3]

(8) What materials should be provided by the employer when employees apply for occupational disease diagnosis?

(9) If the employer refuses to provide diagnostic information, what should we do?

(10) What is the occupational exposure limit? What are the contents of occupational exposure limits for chemical factors in workplace?

On October 10 in 2019, Liu went to the C Diagnostic Institution for occupational disease diagnosis, submitted his occupational contact history and the court's Civil Mediation document. C Diagnostic Institution organized a consultation of three occupational disease diagnosis doctors. According to the diagnostic criteria of occupational pneumoconiosis, Liu was diagnosed with stage II silicosis on January 16 in 2020, and the Occupational Disease Diagnosis Certificate was delivered to Liu and the employer. The employer disagreed with the diagnosis, and applied for an occupational disease appraisal application to the Health Commission of A city. The Health Commission accepted the application, and randomly selected five occupational disease appraisal experts from the province to verdict. According to the occupational disease diagnosis standard and full deliberation, the expert group concluded that Liu's disease was stage II silicosis after reviewing the identification information. Finally, the employer and Liu all accepted the conclusion.

[Questions 4]

(11) Please introduce the procedures of the occupational disease diagnosis.

(12) If the parties disagree with the conclusion of the occupational disease diagnosis, how should they do?

Part 4　Case analysis of occupational noise-induced deafness

I. Objective

To master the diagnostic method of occupational noise-induced deafness.

II. Case study and analysis

The patient, male, 47 years old, worked in material grinder section of a cement factory from August 2008 to August 2014. He worked for about 8 hours a day in three shifts. During the work, he was exposed to noise and dust, and wore earplugs intermittently. The patient felt hearing loss in both ears, accompanied by tinnitus for 5 years and aggravated for 1 year, without diagnosis and treatment. One year ago, the result of the occupational health examination gave the following warning: "The left ear had a slight hearing loss in speech sound frequency, while the right ear had a moderate hearing loss." The occupational health examination authority, according to the "suspected occupational noise-induced deafness", advised the patient to apply for an occupational disease diagnosis from a qualified agency for the diagnosis of occupational diseases.

[Questions]

(1) As an occupational diagnosis expert, what will you do if you receive that patient?

(2) If the diagnosis of occupational noise-induced deafness can't be excluded after completing the materials of occupational disease diagnosis, which tests will be performed to make the diagnosis and classification?

实验二十三 职业病与职业卫生案例分析

第一节 尘肺病案例分析

一、实习目的

在中国，职业性尘肺病是最主要的一种职业病，在每年新发职业病中占比均在80%以上，尘肺病是中国职业病防治的重点。通过本次学习，学生须达到以下要求：

(1) 掌握职业尘肺病案例的分析方法。

(2) 掌握尘肺病的主要接触机会、临床表现、预防措施。

(3) 熟悉尘肺病的诊断及处理原则。

(4) 了解现场职业卫生学调查的主要内容。

二、案例与分析

王某，男，28岁，2004年8月至2007年10月在某耐磨材料厂打工，做过杂工、破碎工，其间接触到大量粉尘。2007年8月开始咳嗽、胸闷，按照感冒治疗，久治未愈，到医院做胸片检查，发现双肺有阴影，多家医院的医生怀疑其为尘肺病。但当地职业病诊断机构诊断为"尘肺0期（医学观察）合并肺结核"。在多方求助无门后，王某于2009年6月选择了取肺组织进行病理学尘肺病诊断。王某最终被确诊为尘肺Ⅲ期，并于2009年9月获得各种赔偿共计61.5万元。

[问题讨论]

(1) 该工人为什么会患上尘肺病？

(2) 尘肺病的临床表现有哪些？

(3) 尘肺病的主要诊断依据是什么？

(4) 本案例反映出我国职业病防治工作中还存在哪些问题？

第二节 职业性铅中毒案例分析

一、实习目的

职业中毒是职业病中的一大类，包括急性职业中毒和慢性职业中毒，而慢性铅中毒则是慢性职业中毒的主要职业病，是学生学习的重要内容。通过本次学习，学生须达到以下要求：

(1) 掌握职业中毒案例的分析方法。
(2) 掌握职业性铅中毒的主要接触机会、临床表现、预防措施。
(3) 熟悉职业性铅中毒的诊断及处理原则。
(4) 了解现场职业卫生学调查的主要内容。

二、案例与分析

患者李×，男，37岁，自1986年以来经常失眠、头痛、头晕、记忆力减退、全身乏力、关节酸痛、食欲不振。近3年来，上述症状加重，并出现经常性的脐周、下腹部无固定点绞痛，用手按压腹部可使其缓解，于1992年住院治疗。体格检查发现：患者神志清楚，一般情况尚可，体温37.2℃，脉搏72次/分，呼吸20次/分，血压120/70 mmHg，心肺功能正常，肝脾不大，腹平软，脐周有轻微的压痛，无反跳痛，四肢痛触觉未见异常，未引出病理反射，血、尿常规正常，肝功能、心电图正常，胸部X线照片未见异常改变。

[问题讨论1]

(1) 上述资料中，你认为还应该补充哪些内容？
(2) 当遇到腹绞痛患者时，你会考虑可能是哪些疾病？
(3) 引起腹绞痛常见的毒物有哪些？哪些职业的工人可能会接触这些毒物？

进一步询问患者的职业史，发现该患者从1984年开始从事印刷厂的浇板工作，即把熔融的铅水浇进字模当中，在浇板时有大量的铅蒸气逸散到空气中。工人每天工作8小时。据此推断该患者可能是慢性铅中毒。

[问题讨论2]

(4) 急性和慢性铅中毒的临床表现有哪些不同？
(5) 要证实该患者是铅中毒，还应做哪些临床检验？
(6) 对患者的工作场所应进行哪些职业卫生学调查？

通过对该患者的工作场所进行调查，发现车间空气中铅烟浓度为 $0.4 \sim 0.8$ mg/m³，根据患者的职业接触史及其临床表现，认为是职业中毒，该患者被转至职业病防治院进行进一步诊治。入院时检查发现：尿铅浓度为 12.3 μmol/L，尿中 ALA 浓度为 80.4 μmol/L，血红细胞游离原卟啉浓度为 3.6 μmol/L，据此诊断为慢性铅中毒。

[问题讨论3]

(7) 慢性铅中毒常用的解毒剂有哪些？用药时应注意哪些问题？
(8) 除进行解毒治疗外，还应给予哪些辅助性治疗？

职业病防治院组织了一个调查组到该印刷厂的浇板车间进行调查，发现工人们在浇板时有蓝灰色的烟雾产生，车间内没有安装排毒罩。工人们也很少用防护服、口罩、手套等防护用品。调查同车间的其他工人，大多数工人都反映有头痛、头昏、记忆力减退、四肢无力、肌肉酸痛等症状，少数工人有腹痛的症状。职业病防治院组织该车间工人进行体检，结果 8 名工人中有 6 人的尿铅、尿 ALA 高于正常值，其中 3 人有肢端麻木。

［问题讨论 4］

（9）该工作场所中存在哪些职业卫生问题，应该怎样改进？

第三节　职业健康监护案例分析

一、实习目的

职业健康监护是以预防为目的，根据劳动者的职业接触史，通过各种检查连续性监测劳动者的健康状况，及时发现早期健康损害征象的一种健康监控方法和过程。职业健康监护是落实用人单位义务、实现劳动者权利的重要保障，是实施职业病诊断鉴定制度和工伤保障制度的基础。该案例的实习目的如下：

（1）掌握职业健康监护的基本内容。

（2）掌握职业病诊断程序。

二、案例与分析

刘××，男，46 岁，家住 A 市 B 县平安乡刘庄。刘××自 2013 年 6 月起在 B 县耐火材料厂原料分厂粉磨岗位从事硅灰石的粉磨工作 5 年，但直到 2018 年 3 月 10 日才签订劳务合同。2018 年 11 月，刘××开始出现咳嗽、咳痰、胸闷、乏力、呼吸困难症状，因此进行了职业健康检查。

［问题讨论 1］

（1）刘××所患疾病可能是什么病，为什么？

（2）什么是职业健康检查？它分为哪几类？请介绍各类职业健康检查的目的和对象。

（3）什么是职业健康监护？职业健康检查和职业健康监护有什么关系？

（4）劳动者应到哪里去做职业健康检查？现阶段我国职业健康检查机构资质如何获得，有何依据？

刘××于 2018 年 12 月 30 日到 B 县 C 职业病诊断机构（以下简称为"C 诊断机构"，具有职业健康检查资质）进行职业健康检查。经检查，C 诊断机构得出检查结论为疑似职业性尘肺病，建议 3 个月后复查。2019 年 3 月 30 日复查结论为疑似职业性尘肺病，医生建议刘××进行职业病诊断。

［问题讨论 2］

（5）针对刘××的情况，应该检查哪些项目？

（6）职业健康体检报告分为哪几种？

（7）C 诊断机构对刘××检查结果的处理是否妥当，为什么？

刘××即向C诊断机构要求进行职业病诊断，C诊断机构告知刘××须用人单位提供其职业病危害接触史（以下简称"职业接触史"）等资料。但用人单位B县耐火材料厂一直不提供，经B县卫生行政部门督促后，B县耐火材料厂提供了工作场所职业病危害因素检测评价报告，检测结果为粉磨工硅灰石粉尘$C_{TWA}=20.5\ mg/m^3$，超过了我国工作场所有害因素职业接触限值（$5.0\ mg/m^3$）。据刘××描述，其每周工作5天，每天工作10小时，工作期间会接触大量粉尘，且单位每周只提供3个一次性防尘口罩。

[问题讨论3]

（8）申请职业病诊断时，用人单位应提供哪些资料？

（9）如果用人单位拒绝提供诊断相关资料，我们应该怎么办？

（10）什么是职业接触限值？工作场所化学因素的职业接触限值包括哪些？

2019年10月10日，刘××到C诊断机构进行职业病诊断，自述职业接触史并提供法院的《民事调解书》。C诊断机构组织了三名职业病诊断医师会诊，依据职业性尘肺病诊断标准，于2020年1月16日，诊断刘××为硅肺Ⅱ期，并向刘××和用人单位送达了《职业病诊断证明书》。用人单位B县耐火材料厂对诊断结果有异议，向A市卫健委提出职业病鉴定申请，A市卫健委受理后，从该省职业病诊断鉴定专家库中随机抽取5名专家组成职业病鉴定专家组。专家组对鉴定资料进行审阅，依照职业病诊断标准，经充分合议后，做出了"硅肺Ⅱ期"的鉴定结论，用人单位B县耐火材料厂和刘××均表示接受鉴定结论。

[问题讨论4]

（11）请说说职业病的诊断程序。

（12）如果当事人对职业病诊断机构做出的职业病诊断结论有异议，他们该怎么办？

第四节 职业性噪声聋案例分析

一、实习目的

使学生掌握职业性噪声聋的诊断方法。

二、案例与分析

患者，男，47岁，2008年8月至2014年8月在某水泥厂生料磨工段从事粉磨作业，每天工作约8小时，三班倒，工作中接触噪声及粉尘，间断性佩戴耳塞，自觉双耳听力下降伴耳鸣5年，加重1年，未诊治。1年前单位职业健康体检电测听提示："左耳语频段听力轻度下降，右耳语频段听力中度下降。"该职业健康检查机构按"疑似职业性噪声聋"建议患者到有职业病诊断资质的机构申请职业病诊断。

[问题讨论]

（1）作为职业病诊断医师，如果你接诊了该患者，将做何处理？

（2）如果在完善职业病诊断相关资料后仍不能排除职业性噪声聋的诊断，将进行哪些检测方可做出诊断与分级？

Chapter Four　Practice for Occupational Hygiene
第四章　职业卫生学实验及案例

 Experiment 24　The Measurement and Evaluation of Productive Noise

Ⅰ. Objectives

Productive noise has become one of the most important physical harmful factors that affects the workers' health, so the prevention and control of productive noise is very important to protect the health of occupational population. Through this experiment, students should be familiar with the usage of sound level meter, and master the measurement calculation and evaluation methods of productive noise.

Ⅱ. Materials

The following instruments will be used in this experiment: sound level meter (SL-5856), tape measure.

Ⅲ. Experiment Procedures

(1) To choose the measuring points.

The measuring points should be the workers frequently operate, and the normal height of the points should be as high as the man's ears (1.5 m height will be chosen in this experiment). The number of the measuring points depends on the distribution of the noise source. If the noise sources are abundant and dispersive, the workshop should be divided into several areas, and the difference of sound level within the same area should be less than 3 dB. There should not be any shelter around the measuring points, otherwise the measuring result will be affected and incorrect.

The simulation site: The distance between the worker's operating point and the noise source is assumed as 1 – 2 m in this experiment, therefore the measuring point will be 1 – 2 m in front of the noise source. At the same time, students will measure the sound level in the office next to the measuring site.

(2) To install the batteries, which will be appropriated for the power, and switch "ON" position to connect the power.

(3) To choose the measuring level at "fast" or "slow" button.

Note: The sound level meter should be set as "fast" when the noise is steady, and the result will be recorded as the mean value of readings within 5 s; while the sound level meter should be set as "slow" when the noise is unsteady, and the measurement time should be determined by the changes of noise.

—In this experiment, we choose "fast", students will measure the noise for three times, calculate and record the mean value.

(4) To record the results in the recording sheet.

199

The values displayed on the monitor are the measured values. Record the measured results in the recording sheet (Table 24 – 1).

Table 24 – 1 Recording sheet of noise measurement (dB)

Measuring point	NO. 1 value (V_1)	NO. 2 value (V_2)	NO. 3 value (V_3)	mean value (V_{mean})
workshop				
office				

(5) To press "HOLD" button gently when measuring the sound level. If the monitor displays "max", it means the maximum measuring value will be held. To press the "HOLD" button again and the HOLD function will be canceled. Now, the displayed value on the monitor means the instantaneous measuring value.

(6) To switch the power button to "OFF" when the measurement is completed.

(7) To evaluate the results.

Students will evaluate the intensity level of noise measured in the simulative workshop, the lounge and the office, then to determine if the noise levels are complied with the noise standard. Standard for evaluation: *The National Standard for Industrial Noise Control* (GB/T50087 – 2013). Details are in Table 24 – 2.

Table 24 – 2 The noise standards of industrial enterprises in various locations

Number	Category of measuring point	Standard of noise/dB
1	Productive workshop, workplaces (continuous noise for 8h/d)	85
2	Workshop duty room, observation room, rest room, laboratory	70
3	Office, laboratory, design room	70
4	Central Laboratory which belongs to the factory (including laboratory, test room and measuring room)	60
5	Infirmary, classroom, dormitory on duty	55

实验二十四　生产性噪声的测定与评价

一、实验目的

生产性噪声已成为影响职业人群健康的最主要的物理性有害因素，因此对生产性噪声的防控对保护职业人群健康至关重要，掌握对生产性噪声的测定和评价方法则有助于对生产性噪声的防控。

（1）掌握声级计的使用方法。

（2）掌握工厂内噪声的测量、计算及评价方法。

二、实验材料

电子声级计（sound level meter）（SL-5856），卷尺。

三、实验方法和步骤

（1）测量点的选择：测点应选在工人生产操作经常停留的地点，测点位置高度以人耳的高度为准。测点数目根据目的要求和噪声源分布情况确定。如果声源比较多且很分散，则应将现场划分为若干个小区，每一小区内各处声级的差别不应大于3 dB。测点附近避免有物体遮挡，以免影响噪声测量结果。

本次模拟现场：假设工人生产操作经常停留地点为距噪声源前方1~2米范围内，因此测量点为噪声源前方1~2米处。同时测量模拟现场隔壁休息室噪声强度。

（2）安装电池，将电源开关拨到"ON"位置，接通电源。

（3）将"快""慢"开关拨到合适的位置。测量稳态噪声应使用声级计"快档"，一次测量应取5秒内的平均读数；测量非稳态噪声应使用声级计"慢档"，并应根据噪声变化特性确定测量时间。

——本次实验选择"快"，取5秒内的平均读数；测量3次，取平均值。

（4）把结果记录在记录表上。

监视器上显示的值是测量值，将测量结果记录在记录表中（见表24-1）。

表24-1 模拟车间及办公室噪声测量结果记录

单位：dB

测量场所	第一次测量	第二次测量	第三次测量	平均值
工作车间				
办公室				

（5）在进行声级测量时，轻按"HOLD"键，显示器上出现"max"字符，表示保持测定期间内的最大值。若取消保持功能，只需要再按一下"HOLD"键即可，此时，显示器上的数字即为瞬时测量值。

（6）测量完毕，将电源开关拨到"OFF"，关掉电源。

（7）对结果进行评价。

对模拟车间、休息室和办公室现场测量的噪声强度值进行评价，判定所测现场噪声强度是否符合噪声标准。评价依据：《工业企业噪声控制设计规范》（GB/T50087—2013），见表24-2。

表 24-2　工业企业厂区内各类地点噪声标准

序号	地点类别	噪声限制值/dB
1	生产车间及作业场所（每天连续噪声 8 小时）	85
2	车间内值班室、观察室、休息室、实验室	70
3	车间所属办公室、实验室、设计室	70
4	厂部所属中心实验室（包括试验、化验、计量室）	60
5	医务室、教室、值班宿舍	55

Experiment 25　Determination of Meteorological Conditions

Ⅰ. Objectives

To understand the significance of meteorological condition measurement, to master the usage of commonly used meteorological condition measuring instruments, which can solve the practical problems encountered in the field of meteorological condition measurement and improve the work adaptability.

Ⅱ. Materials

The following instruments or materials will be used in this experiment: dry and wet bulb thermometer, hot-wire electric anemometer, and aneroid barometer.

Ⅲ. Experiment Procedures

1. Determination of air temperature and humidity

(1) Instrument: Dry and wet bulb thermometer.

(2) Procedures.

① Check whether the dry and wet bulb thermometer readings are consistent before use. Make sure the difference is less than 0.1℃.

② The wet bulb is fully wet wrapped in wetted gauze by adding distilled water with the rubber ball. Note: Do not turn the instrument upside down when adding water, and pay attention to prevent wet gauze clogging the casing.

③ The dry and wet bulb thermometer is suspended vertically at the measuring point for about 3 – 5 mins.

Record temperature readings of the dry bulb and wet bulb thermometer. The dry bulb temperature represents the air temperature.

The relative humidity is calculated from relative humidity table using the difference in readings of the two thermometers.

Chapter Four Practice for Occupational Hygiene

(3) Result.

The laboratory is seen as simulated workplace, and measure the temperature and humidity of the laboratory. Measure three times, record them in Table 25 – 1, and calculate the mean value.

Table 25 – 1 Wet-and-dry-bulb thermometer measurement record sheet

Records	NO. 1 value (V_1)	NO. 2 value (V_2)	NO. 3 value (V_3)	mean value (V_{mean})
Dry bulb (℃)				
Wet bulb (℃)				
Difference of the two thermometers (℃)				
Relative humidity (%)				

2. Determination of wind speed

(1) Instrument: hot-wire electric anemometer.

(2) Procedures.

① Switch calibration button to "off" position and calibrate to zero point.

② Insert plug in the socket and seal the probe. Then switch calibration button to "full scale" position and adjust "full scale" knob to make electric meter at zero point.

③ Switch calibration button to zero point, then control the electric meter at zero point using the coarse adjustment and fine adjustment. Reveal the probe and make the red dot face the wind. The reading once every 0.5 min and average the results of 3 times. The wind speed was obtained according to calibration curve.

(3) Result.

The laboratory is seen as simulated workplace, and measure the wind speed of the laboratory. Measure three times, record them in Table 25 – 2, and calculate the mean value.

Table 25 – 2 Wind speed measurement record sheet (m/s)

value NO. 1 (V_1)	NO. 2 value (V_2)	NO. 3 value (V_3)	mean value (V_{mean})

Note: wind velocity according to calibration curve.

3. Determination of air pressure

(1) Instrument: aneroid barometer.

The pressure of the atmosphere is measured by an aneroid barometer, which is an empty metal box (close to a vacuum in the box). Aneroid barometer is composed of induction, transmission and indexing, and could compresse or expand when the pressure changes through the spring sheet balance. As the aneroid barometer compresses or expands, the pressure value can be indicated directly by passing the extension motion to the pointer by amplification.

(2) Procedures.

①Calibration of instrument: Calibration of instrument: Calibrate the aneroid barometer to the location/altitude with a mercury barometer or the current barometer pressure from a local weather forecast. Turn the barometer's center knob so that the arrow rests directly above the indicator arrow (this is the current barometric pressure for your location). The empty box barometer is calibrated every 3 to 6 months.

② Measurement: Open the aneroid barometer cover, read the temperature firstly, accurate to 0.1℃, tap the box surface to overcome the mechanical friction in the aneroid barometer, wait for the needle swing static reading. When reading, the line of sight should be perpendicular to the scale line of the pointer. The value shown at the tip of the pointer is x 10 (mmHg).

(3) Result.

The laboratory is seen as simulated workplace, and measure the air pressure of the laboratory. Measure three times, record them in Table 25 – 3, and calculate the mean value.

Table 25 – 3 Air pressure measurement record sheet (mmHg)

NO. 1 value (V_1)	NO. 2 value (V_2)	NO. 3 value (V_3)	mean value (V_{mean})

实验二十五　气象条件的测定

一、实验目的

了解气象条件测定的意义，掌握常用测定气象条件仪器的使用方法，能解决气象条件测定现场所遇到的实际问题，提高工作应变能力。

二、实验材料

干球湿球温度计，热球式电风速计，气压盆。

三、实验方法和步骤

1. 气温和气湿的测定

(1) 实验仪器。

本次实验使用干湿球温度计同时测定气温和气湿。

（2）测定方法。

①使用前请检查干湿球温度计读数是否一致，确保温差小于 0.1℃。

②湿球温度计球用湿纱布包裹湿球，用橡皮球加入蒸馏水，使湿球充分湿润，加水时仪器不得倒置，并注意防止湿纱布堵塞套管。

③将干湿球温度计垂直悬挂在测量点处约 5min。

④记录干球温度计和湿球温度计的温度读数，干球温度表示空气温度。

⑤相对湿度需要根据两个温度计读数的差值从相对湿度表中计算出来。

（3）结果。

用实验室模拟工作场所，检测实验室的温度和湿度，测量三次并取平均值。结果记录在表 25 - 1 上。

表 25 - 1　工作场所温度湿度测量结果

结果	第一次测量值（V_1）	第二次测量值（V_2）	第三次测量值（V_3）	平均值（$V_{平均}$）
干球温度（℃）				
湿球温度（℃）				
干球 - 湿球温度差（℃）				
相对湿度（%）				

2. 风速测定

（1）实验仪器。

用热球式电风速计测量风速。

（2）使用方法。

①校正开关置于"关"的位置，按常规校正机械调零。

②将插杆插头插在插座上，使杆呈垂直位，螺塞压紧使探头密封。"校正开关"置于"满度"位置，慢慢调整"满度调节"旋钮，使电表指在零点位置。

③将"校正开关"置于"零位"的位置，慢慢调整"粗调""细调"两个旋钮，使电表指在零点位置。然后，轻轻拉动螺塞使测杆探头露出，将测头上的红点面对风向。测定时每 0.5 分钟读数 1 次，连续 3 次，取平均值。此时，可从电表上读数，再查阅校正曲线，得出被测风速。

（3）结果。

将实验室模拟工作场所，检测实验室的风速，测量三次并取平均值。结果记录在表 25 - 2 上。

表25-2 风速测量结果（m/s）

第一次测量值（V_1）	第二次测量值（V_2）	第三次测量值（V_3）	平均值（$V_{平均}$）

3. 气压测定（空盒气压表）

（1）实验仪器：空盒气压表。

大气压力是由无液气压表来测量，无液气压表也称空盒气压表，盒内接近真空，其有感应、传递和指标三部分组成。当气压变化时，气压表通过弹簧片调节平衡气压盒的压缩或膨胀，随着压缩或膨胀，通过传递放大，把伸张运动传给指针，就可以直接指示气压值。

（2）测定方法。

①仪器的校准：用水银气压表或当地天气预报提供的气压计，将无液气压表校准到所处的位置/高度。转动气压计的中心旋钮，使指针位于指示箭头的正上方（这是您所在位置的当前气压），无液气压表每隔3~6个月校准一次。

②现场测量：打开气压表盒盖后，先读温度，准确到0.1℃，轻敲盒面（克服空盒气压表内机械摩擦），待指针摆动静止后读数。读数时视线需垂直指针刻度线，读数指针尖端所示的数值×10（mmHg）。

（3）结果。

用实验室模拟工作场所，检测实验室的气压，测量三次并取平均值。结果记录在表25-3上。

表25-3 气压测量结果

单位：mmHg

第一次测量值（V_1）	第二次测量值（V_2）	第三次测量值（V_3）	平均值（$V_{平均}$）

（于德娥）

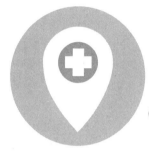

Chapter Five | Experiments and Cases of Nutrition and Food Hygiene

第五章 | 营养与食品卫生学实验及案例

Chapter Five Experiments and Cases of Nutrition and Food Hygiene
第五章 营养与食品卫生学实验及案例

Experiment 26 Determination of Reducing Sugar Content in Food

Ⅰ. Objectives

(1) To learn and master the principle and method of direct titration in the determination of reducing sugars in food.

(2) Understand the method of food sample pretreatment.

Ⅱ. Principle

After removing protein from food samples, titrating the calibrated alkaline copper tartrate solution (calibrate the alkaline copper tartrate solution with standard reducing sugar solution) with methylene blue as indicator under heating conditions, and calculating the reducing sugar content in sample according to the consumed volume of the sample.

Ⅲ. Materials

1. Samples

(1) Sprite.

(2) Coconut water.

2. Reagents

(1) Alkaline cupric tartrate solution A (ACTS A): weigh 15 g copper sulfate ($CuSO_4 \cdot 5H_2O$) and 0.05 g methylene blue, dissolve in water and dilute to 1000 mL.

(2) Alkaline copper tartrate solution B (ACTS B): weigh 50 g sodium potassium tartrate and 75 g sodium hydroxide, dissolve in water, then add 4 g potassium ferrocyanide, completely dissolve, dilute with water to 1000 mL, and store in rubber plug glass bottle.

(3) Glucose standard solution: accurately weigh 1.0000 g of pure glucose (98 ± 2 ℃ dry 2 hours), dissolve in water, then add 5 mL of hydrochloric acid, and dilute with water to 1000 mL, the solution is equivalent to 1.0 mg glucose per milliliter.

The reagents used in this method are all pure analytical reagents.

3. Instruments

(1) 2000 mL volumetric flask.

(2) 100 mL beaker.

(3) Funnel.

(4) Filter paper.

(5) Glass bar.

(6) 20 mL, 50 mL measuring cylinder.

(7) 25 mL acid burette.

(8) Adjustable furnace with asbestos sheet.

(9) 150 mL conical flask.

IV. Experiment Procedures

1. Sample treatment

(1) Sprite: Take about 50 mL sample and place it in a small beaker. After removing carbon dioxide by water bath, 25 mL samples were measured and moved into 2000 mL volumetric flask. And wash the measuring cylinder with water, wash the liquid into the volumetric bottle, and then add water to the scale and mix for backup.

(2) Coconut water: Cut open the coconut, attract and filter the coconut water, measure 40 mL filtrate, and move it into the 2000 mL volumetric bottle. And wash the measuring cylinder with water, wash the liquid into the volumetric bottle, and then add water to the scale and mix for backup.

Note: The final concentration of reducing sugar in the diluted sample should be close to that of the standard solution of glucose.

2. Calibrate alkaline copper tartrate solution

Attract 5.0 mL ACTS A and 5.0 mL ACTS B, put them into a 150 mL conical flask, add 10 mL water and 2 glass beads. Add about 9 mL standard solution of glucose from the burette and control it to boil in 2 minutes. Continue adding the standard solution of glucose at the rate of 1 drop every 2 seconds when it is hot until the blue of the solution just disappears as the end point. The total volume of the consumed standard solution of glucose was recorded, and the average value of the three experiments was taken to calculate the quality (mg) equivalent to glucose per 10 mL alkaline copper tartrate solution (5 mL of solution A and solution B).

3. Sample solution prediction

Attract 5.0 mL ACTS A and 5.0 mL ACTS B, put them into a 150 mL conical flask, add 10 mL water and 2 glass beads. Heat to boil within 2 minutes, add the sample solution from the burette while it is hot at a fast speed and then a slow speed (Note: Keep the solution boiling). When the solution becomes lighter, titrating at the rate of 1 drop every 2 seconds until the blue color fades, and record the consumed volume of the sample solution.

4. Determination of sample solution

Attract 5.0 mL ACTS A and 5.0 mL ACTS B, put them into a 150 mL conical flask, add 10 mL water and 2 glass beads. Add a sample solution of 1 mL less than the predicted volume from the burette, heat to boil within 2 minutes, continue adding the sample solution at the rate of 1 drop every 2 seconds when it is boiling until the blue of the solution just disappears as the end point. The total volume of the consumed sample solution was recorded, and the average value of the three experiments was calculated.

5. Calculation of results

The content of reducing sugar in the sample (in terms of some reducing sugar) is calculated by the following formula.

$$X = \frac{\frac{A}{V_2} \times \frac{2000}{V_0}}{1000}$$

X—The content of reducing sugar in the sample (in terms of some reducing sugar) (g/100 mL);

A—Alkaline copper tartrate solution (half A, half B) corresponds to the quality of some kind of reducing sugar (mg), $A = V_1 * 1 \text{mg/mL}$.

V_0—The consumption of sample (sprite or coconut water).

V_1—The average volume of consumed standard glucose dilution during determination.

V_2—The average volume of consumed sample dilution during determination.

6. Matters needing attention

(1) The preparation of reagents should follow the operating procedures. Pay attention to your safety.

(2) When titrating a boiling solution, be careful not to let the reagent splash into your eyes.

实验二十六　食品中还原糖含量的测定

一、实验目的

(1) 学习和掌握直接滴定法测定食品中还原糖的原理和方法。
(2) 了解食品样品预处理的方法。

二、实验原理

食品样品去除蛋白质后，在加热条件下以次甲基蓝做指示剂，滴定标定过的碱性酒石酸铜溶液（用还原糖标准溶液标定碱性酒石酸铜溶液），根据样品消耗的体积计算样品还原糖含量。

三、实验材料

1. 样品
(1) 雪碧。
(2) 椰子水。

2. 试剂
(1) 碱性酒石酸铜甲液：称取 15 g 硫酸铜（$CuSO_4 \cdot 5H_2O$）及 0.05 g 次甲基蓝，溶于水中并稀释至 1000 mL。
(2) 碱性酒石酸铜乙液：称取 50 g 酒石酸钾钠及 75 g 氢氧化钠，溶于水中，再加入 4 g 亚铁氰化钾，完全溶解后，用水稀释至 1000 mL，贮存于橡胶塞玻璃瓶内。

(3) 葡萄糖标准溶液：精确称取 1.0000 g 经过 98±2℃ 干燥 2 小时的纯葡萄糖，加水溶解后加入 5 mL 盐酸，并以水稀释至 1000 mL，此溶液每毫升相当于 1.0 mg 葡萄糖。

本方法中所用试剂均为分析纯试剂。

3. 仪器

(1) 2000 mL 容量瓶。
(2) 100 mL 烧杯。
(3) 漏斗。
(4) 滤纸。
(5) 玻璃棒。
(6) 20 mL、50 mL 量筒。
(7) 25 mL 酸式滴定管。
(8) 带石棉板的可调电炉。
(9) 150 mL 锥形瓶。

四、方法和步骤

1. 样品处理

(1) 雪碧：取约 50 mL 样品置于小烧杯中。水浴除去二氧化碳后量取 25 mL 样品移入 2000 mL 容量瓶中。并用水洗涤量筒，洗液并入容量瓶中，再加水至刻度线混匀后备用。

(2) 椰子水：砍开椰子，吸取椰子水过滤，量取滤液 40 mL，移入 2000 mL 容量瓶中。并用水洗涤量筒，洗液并入容量瓶中，再加水至刻度线混匀后备用。

注意：稀释的样品中的还原糖的最终浓度应接近于葡萄糖标准液的浓度。

2. 标定碱性酒石酸铜溶液

吸取 5.0 mL 碱性酒石酸铜甲液及 5.0 mL 乙液，置于 150 mL 锥形瓶中，加水 10 mL，加入玻璃珠 2 粒，从滴定管滴加约 9 mL 葡萄糖标准溶液，控制在 2 分钟内加热至沸腾，趁热以每 2 秒 1 滴的速度继续滴加葡萄糖标准溶液，直至溶液蓝色刚好褪去为终点，记录消耗的葡萄糖标准溶液总体积，同时平行操作 3 份，取其平均值，计算每 10 mL（甲、乙液各 5 mL）碱性酒石酸铜溶液相当于葡萄糖的质量（mg）。

3. 样品溶液预测

吸取 5.0 mL 碱性酒石酸铜甲液及 5.0 mL 乙液，置于 150 mL 锥形瓶中，加水 10 mL，加入玻璃珠 2 粒，控制在 2 分钟内加热至沸腾，趁热以先快后慢的速度，从滴定管中滴加样品溶液（注意：要保持溶液沸腾状态），待溶液颜色变浅时，以每 2 秒 1 滴的速度滴定，直至溶液蓝色褪去，记录样品溶液消耗体积。

4. 样品溶液测定

吸取 5.0 mL 碱性酒石酸铜甲液及 5.0 mL 乙液，置于 150 mL 锥形瓶中，加水 10 mL，加入玻璃珠 2 粒，从滴定管中滴加比预测体积少 1 mL 的样品溶液，控制在 2 分钟内加热至沸腾，然后趁沸腾继续以每 2 秒 1 滴的速度滴定至终点。记录消耗样品溶液的总体积，同法平行操作 3 份，得出平均消耗体积。

5. 结果计算

样品中还原糖的含量（以某种还原糖计）按下式公式计算。

$$X = \frac{\frac{A}{V_2} \times \frac{2000}{V_0}}{1000}$$

式中，X—样品中还原糖的含量（以某种还原糖计）（g/100 mL）；

A—碱性酒石酸铜（甲、乙液各半）相当于某种还原糖的质量（mg），$A = V_1 * 1\mathrm{mg/mL}$

V_0—样品（雪碧或椰子水）的消耗量。

V_1—测定时平均消耗标准葡萄糖稀释液的体积。

V_2—测定时平均消耗样品稀释液的体积。

6. 注意事项

（1）配制试剂时要遵守操作规程，注意安全。

（2）在溶液沸腾的状态下，滴定时要注意避免让试剂溅入眼睛。

Experiment 27　Determination of Vitamin C Content in Foods

Ⅰ. Objectives

(1) Learn and master the principle and method of determination of reduced ascorbic acid in food.

(2) To further understand the important role of ascorbic acid in food on body health.

Ⅱ. Principle

The ascorbic acid in fresh food mainly exists in the reduced form, so the determination of reduced ascorbic acid can roughly understand the level of ascorbic acid in food. The reduced ascorbic acid can reduce the dye 2, 6-dichlorophenol indophenol. The ascorbic acid solution was calibrated with the standard potassium iodate solution, and then the 2, 6-dichlorophenol indophenol dye solution was calibrated with the calibrated ascorbic acid solution, and then the ascorbic acid in the sample was titrated with the dye 2, 6-dichlorophenol indophenol. 2, 6-dichlorophenol indophenol is red in an acidic solution and fades after reduction. The measured solution in excess of 1 drop of dye will appear red, indicating the end point. With no impurity interference, the amount of the solution to be measured is proportional to the concentration of ascorbic acid.

Ⅲ. Materials

1. Samples
(1) Apple.
(2) Guava.

2. Reagents
(1) 1% oxalic acid.
(2) 2% oxalic acid.
(3) White clay.
(4) 0.0100 mol/L potassium iodate standard reserve solution: Precisely weigh 0.2140 g of dry potassium iodate (GR or AR grade), dissolve in distilled water in 100 mL volumetric flask and dilute to scale.
(5) 0.0010 mol/L potassium iodate standard application solution: Dilute 10 mL of potassium iodate standard reserve solution to 100 mL. The 1.0 mL solution is equivalent to 0.088 mg of ascorbic acid.
(6) 1% starch solution: Weigh 0.5 g of soluble starch, add 1 drop of water, stir into paste, pour into 50 mL boiling water, mix well, refrigerate for later using.
(7) 6% potassium iodate solution: Weigh 0.6 g of potassium iodate and dissolved in 10 mL distilled water (prepared before using).
(8) Ascorbic acid solution: Weigh 20 mg of pure ascorbic acid powder, dissolve with 1% oxalic acid in 100 mL volumetric bottle, dilute to scale, shake well, and store in cold storage.
(9) Sodium bicarbonate solution: Weigh 40.2 g sodium bicarbonate and dissolve in 200 mL boiling water.
(10) 2,6-dichlorophenol indophenol: Dissolve 50 mg of 2,6-dichlorophenol in the hot solution of sodium bicarbonate, cool it, put it in the refrigerator overnight, filter it into a 250 mL volumetric flask on the next day, dilute it with distilled water to scale, and shake well. Store in a brown bottle and refrigerate.

3. Instruments
(1) Tissue mower.
(2) Micro burette.
(3) Conical flask.
(4) 100 mL measuring cylinder with plug.

Ⅳ. Experiment Procedures

1. Calibration of 2,6-dichlorophenol indophenol solution
(1) Calibration of ascorbic acid standard solution: Attract 2 mL ascorbic acid solution into a conical flask, then add 5 mL 1% oxalic acid, 0.5 mL 6% potassium iodide solution, and 2 drops of 1% starch solution, then take 0.0010 mol/L potassium iodate standard liquid droplet to

determine to the end point as light blue.

Computing method: Ascorbic acid concentration (mg/mL) = consumed mL of 0.0010 mol/L potassium iodate solution ×0.088 ÷ consumed mL of ascorbic acid that was taken.

(2) Calibration of 2,6-dichlorophenol indophenol solution: Attract 5 mL of the calibrated ascorbic acid solution and 5 mL of 1% oxalic acid solution into a conical flask, and titrate the uncalibrated 2,6-dichlorophenol indophenol solution to a reddish color until the solution is fade-free within 15 s. The milligrams of ascorbic acid equivalent to 1 mL dye = ascorbic acid concentration (mg/mL) × milliliters of ascorbic acid solution ÷ milliliters of consumed dye in titration.

2. Sample determination

(1) Take 100 g sample, chop it slightly, then put it into the crusher, add 2% oxalic acid solution in equal amount to make homogenate.

(2) Weigh 10 g homogenate in a small beaker, carefully wash the sample into 100 mL measuring cylinder with 1% oxalic acid, dilute to scale, shake well and set.

(3) Filtrate the upper liquid. 5 mL of the filtrate was attracted into a conical flask, and the calibrated 2,6-dichlorophenol solution was titrated to a reddish color until the solution was fade-free within 15 s.

(4) Use distilled water as a blank titration. If the dye concentration is too high, it should be properly diluted.

3. Calculation of results

Reduced ascorbic acid (mg/100 g) $= \dfrac{(V_1 - V_2) \times T}{W}$

In the formula:

V_1: The amount of dye used in titration of the sample (mL);

V_2: The amount of dye used in the blank titration (mL);

W: The amount of sample contained in the sample diluent used for titration (g);

T: The milligrams of ascorbic acid equivalent to 1 mL dye.

4. Notice

(1) The operation process should be rapid, because the reduced ascorbic acid is easy to be oxidized, generally no more than 2 minutes.

(2) When raw food homogenate is shaken in the measuring cylinder, foam may be produced. A few drops of isopentyl alcohol can be added to remove the foam.

(3) If the sample is colored, pour 20 mL of the upper liquid of the sample into a conical flask, add a spoonful of white clay, shake it several times to make it fully decolorized, and then take the upper liquid for determination after static. At the same time, take a conical flask, add 20 mL 1% oxalic acid, add a spoonful of white clay, shake several times, as blank.

(4) The white clay with strong decolorization power and no adsorption of ascorbic acid should be selected. The recovery rate of each batch of new white clay should be determined.

(5) If the sample is not easy to be filtered, the supernatant can be selected for determination after centrifugation.

(6) There may be other impurities in the sample which can also reduce 2,6-dichlorophenol indophenol, but the reduced rate of it is slower than ascorbic acid, so the titration ends with the pink not fading with in 15 s.

实验二十七　食品中维生素C含量的测定

一、实验目的

（1）学习和掌握食品中还原型抗坏血酸测定的原理和方法。

（2）进一步了解食物中抗坏血酸对机体健康的重要作用。

二、实验原理

新鲜食品中的抗坏血酸主要以还原型的形式存在，因此测定还原型抗坏血酸可粗略了解该食品中抗坏血酸浓度的高低。还原型抗坏血酸可将染料2,6-二氯酚靛酚还原。用标准碘酸钾溶液标定抗坏血酸溶液，然后以标定的抗坏血酸溶液标定2,6-二氯酚靛酚染料溶液，再用此染料滴定样品中的抗坏血酸。2,6-二氯酚靛酚在酸性溶液中呈红色，被还原后红色褪去。当被测溶液过量1滴染料时即显红色，以示终点。在无杂质干扰时，被测溶液还原染料的量与其中所含抗坏血酸浓度成正比。

三、实验材料

1. 样品

（1）苹果。

（2）番石榴。

2. 试剂

（1）1%草酸。

（2）2%草酸。

（3）白陶土。

（4）0.0100 mol/L碘酸钾标准储备液：精密称取干燥的碘酸钾（GR或AR级）0.2140 g，用蒸馏水溶解于100 mL容量瓶中并定容至刻度。

（5）0.0010 mol/L碘酸钾标准应用液：取碘酸钾标准储备液10 mL稀释至100 mL。此液1.0 mL相当于抗坏血酸0.088 mg。

（6）1%淀粉溶液：称取可溶性淀粉0.5 g，加水1滴，搅拌成糊状以后倒入50 mL沸水中，混匀，冷藏待用。

（7）6%碘酸钾溶液：称取碘酸钾0.6 g溶解于10 mL蒸馏水中，临用前配制。

（8）抗坏血酸溶液：称取纯抗坏血酸粉末20 mg，用1%草酸溶解于100 mL容量瓶中并稀释至刻度，摇匀，冷藏保存。

（9）碳酸氢钠溶液：称取碳酸氢钠 40.2 g，溶解在 200 mL 沸水中。

（10）2,6-二氯酚靛酚：称取 2,6-二氯酚靛酚 50 mg 溶解在上述碳酸氢钠热溶液中，冷却后放冰箱中，过夜，次日过滤在 250 mL 容量瓶中，用蒸馏水稀释至刻度，摇匀。贮于棕色瓶中，冷藏保存。

3. 仪器

（1）组织捣碎机。

（2）微量滴定管。

（3）锥形烧瓶。

（4）100 mL 具塞量筒。

四、方法和步骤

1. 2,6-氯酚靛酚溶液的标定

（1）抗坏血酸标准溶液的标定：吸取抗坏血酸溶液 2 mL 于锥形瓶中，再加入 1% 草酸 5 mL，6% 碘化钾溶液 0.5 mL，1% 淀粉溶液 2 滴，再以 0.0010 mol/L 碘酸钾标准液滴定至终点为淡蓝色。计算方法：抗坏血酸浓度（mg/mL）= 消耗 0.0010 mol/L 碘酸钾溶液毫升数 × 0.088 ÷ 所取抗坏血酸毫升数。

（2）2,6-二氯酚靛酚溶液的标定：吸取已标定过的抗坏血酸溶液 5 mL 及 1% 草酸溶液 5 mL 于锥形瓶中，以待标定的 2,6-二氯酚靛酚溶液滴定至溶液呈淡红色，在 15 秒内不褪色为止。1 mL 染料相当于抗坏血酸的毫克数 = 抗坏血酸浓度（mg/mL）× 抗坏血酸溶液的毫升数 ÷ 滴定消耗染料的毫升数。

2. 样品测定

（1）取样品 100 g 稍加切碎后置捣碎机中，加入等量的 2% 草酸溶液，制成匀浆。

（2）称取 10 g 匀浆于小烧杯中，小心地以 1% 草酸将样品洗入 100 mL 量筒内，稀释至刻度，摇匀，静置。

（3）取上层液过滤。吸取滤液 5 mL 于锥形瓶中，以标定过的 2,6-二氯酚靛酚溶液滴定至溶液呈淡红色，15 秒内不褪色为止。

（4）用蒸馏水作空白滴定，如染料浓度过高，应适当稀释。

3. 结果计算

$$还原型抗坏血酸（mg/100\ g） = \frac{(V_1 - V_2) \times T}{W}$$

式中，V_1：样品滴定时所用的染料量（mL）；

V_2：空白滴定时所用的染料量（mL）；

W：滴定时所用样品稀释液中含样品的量（g）；

T：1 mL 染料相当于抗坏血酸毫克数。

4. 注意事项

（1）操作过程要迅速，因还原型抗坏血酸易被氧化，一般不超过 2 分钟。

（2）生食物匀浆在量筒内振摇可能会产生泡沫，加数滴异戊醇可除去。

(3) 如样品有色，应把样品上层液 20 mL 倒入锥形瓶中，加入 1 勺白陶土，振摇数次，使其充分脱色，静置后取上层液测定。同时，取一锥形瓶，加入 1% 草酸 20 mL，加入 1 勺白陶土，振摇数次，作为空白。

(4) 应选择脱色力强、不吸附抗坏血酸的白陶土，每批新的白陶土要测定回收率。

(5) 样品如不易过滤，可离心取上清液测定。

(6) 样品中可能有其他杂质也能还原 2,6 - 二氯酚靛酚，但还原染料的速度较抗坏血酸慢，所以滴定时以 15 秒粉红色不褪去为止。

Experiment 28　Determination of Methanol Content in Liquor

Ⅰ. Objectives

(1) Learn and master the principle and method of methanol content determination in liquor.
(2) To understand the harm of methanol in liquor to health.

Ⅱ. Principle

Methanol in liquor is oxidized to formaldehyde by potassium permanganate in phosphoric acid solution, excess potassium permanganate and manganese dioxide that produced in the reaction can be removed with oxalic acid sulfate solution, formaldehyde reacts with magenta sulfite to produce blue purple quinone pigment, then quantitated by comparison with standard series.

Ⅲ. Materials

1. Samples

Liquor, prepare samples A and B, and add a small amount of methanol to one of the samples.

2. Reagents

(1) Potassium permanganate-phosphoric acid solution: Weigh 3 g potassium permanganate, add it into the 85% phosphoric acid solution 15 mL and water 70 mL mixture, wait for potassium permanganate to dissolve, and then determine with water to the constant volume of 100 mL. This reagent should be stored in a brown bottle to prevent oxidation and the storage time shall not be too long.

(2) Oxalic acid-sulfuric acid solution: 5 g anhydrous oxalic acid or 7 g oxalic acid containing 2 crystal water are weighed and dissolved in 1 + 1 cold sulfuric acid, and determine with 1 + 1 cold sulfuric acid to the constant volume of 100 mL. Mix well and set aside in a brown bottle.

(3) Magenta bisulfite solution: Weigh 0.1 g finely grind alkaline magenta, add 6 mL water that at 80℃ several times, and grind to dissolve while adding water. After it is fully dissolved, filter it into a 10 mL volumetric flask, cool it, add 10 mL sodium sulfite solution (100 g/L), 1

Chapter Five Experiments and Cases of Nutrition and Food Hygiene
第五章 营养与食品卫生学实验及案例

mL hydrochloric acid, add water to the scale, mix it thoroughly, and leave it overnight. If the solution has color, add a small amount of activated carbon, stir and filter it, store it in a brown bottle in the dark. The solution should be discarded and reformulated when it turns red.

(4) Standard methanol solution: Accurately weigh 1.000 g methanol (equivalent to 1.27 mL), add it into a 100 mL volumetric flask with a small amount of distilled water, dilute with water to the scale, and mix well. This solution is equivalent to 10 mg of methanol per milliliter and should be stored at low temperature.

(5) Standard methanol application solution: Attract 10.0 mL standard methanol solution and add it into a 100 mL volumetric flask, dilute it with water to the scale, and mix well. This solution is equivalent to 1 mg methanol per milliliter.

(6) Methanol and formaldehyde-free ethanol: Take 0.3 mL ethanol and check it according to the experimental operation method. It should not be colored. If it is colored, it needs to be processed. Processing method: Take 300 mL ethanol (95%), add a little potassium permanganate, distillation, and collect the distillate. Add silver nitrate solution (1 g silver nitrate dissolved in a little water) and sodium hydroxide solution (1.5 g sodium hydroxide dissolved in a little water) in to the distillate, shake well, take the supernatant and distill, discard the initial 50 mL distillate and collect about 200 mL of the intermediate distillate, its concentration is measured with an alcohol hydrometer and then prepared the methanol-free ethanol with water (volume fraction approximately 60%).

(7) Sodium sulfite solution (10 g/L).

3. Instrument

Spectrophotometer.

Ⅳ. Experiment Procedures

1. Experimental procedure

(1) Appropriately sampling according to the amount of ethanol in the liquor sample (30% ethanol take 1.0 mL; 40% ethanol take 0.8 mL; 50% ethanol take 0.6 mL; 60% ethanol take 0.5 mL) and add it into a 25 mL colorimetric tube with plug.

(2) Precisely attract of 0 mL, 0.2 mL, 0.4 mL, 0.6 mL, 0.8 mL, 1.0 mL methanol standard application solution (equivalent to 0 mg, 0.2 mg, 0.4 mg, 0.6 mg, 0.8 mg, 1.0 mg methanol) and add it into 25 mL colorimetric tube with plug respectively, add 0.5 mL of methanol and formaldehyde-free ethanol into each tube (volume fraction is about 60%).

(3) Add water to 5 mL scale line in the sample tube and standard tube, mix well each tube and add 2 mL potassium permanganate – phosphoric acid solution, mix well, place it for 10 mins.

(4) Add 2 mL oxalic acid – sulfuric acid solution into each tube, mix well and let it stand until the solution fade.

(5) Add 5 mL magenta bisulfite solution into each tube, mix well, and stand still at above 20℃ for 0.5 h.

(6) Set zero with a zero tube, the absorbance was measured at the wavelength of 590 nm, compare with standard curve or visual comparison with standard series to quantify.

2. Calculation of results

$$X = \frac{m}{\frac{V}{10} \times 1000} \times 100$$

In the formula,

X—Content of methanol in the sample (g/100 mL);

m—The standard mass equivalent to the methanol contained in the measured sample (mg);

V—Sample volume (mL).

Calculate and retain two effective digits.

3. Notice

(1) When the magenta bisulfite solution is red, it should be reformulated. The newly prepared magenta bisulfite solution should be put in the refrigerator for 24 – 48 h before being used.

(2) Other aldehydes in liquor and aldehydes converted from alcohols by potassium permanganate oxidation (such as acetaldehyde, propionaldehyde, etc.), also react with magenta sulfite to coloration. However, in a certain concentration of sulfuric acid solution, except for formaldehyde which can form long-lasting purple, other aldehydes will fade in no time or show no color after a long time, so there is no interference, but the time conditions in the operation must be strictly controlled.

(3) The ethanol concentration in the sample and the standard solution has a certain influence on the colorimetric assay, so the ethanol content in the sample and the standard tube should be approximately equal.

实验二十八　白酒中甲醇含量的测定

一、实验目的

（1）学习和掌握白酒中甲醇含量测定的原理和方法。

（2）了解白酒中甲醇对机体健康的危害。

二、实验原理

白酒中甲醇在磷酸溶液中被高锰酸钾氧化成甲醛，过量的高锰酸钾及在反应中产生的二氧化锰被酸草酸溶液除去，甲醛与品红亚硫酸作用生成蓝紫色醌型色素，然后与标准系列进行比较定量。

三、实验材料

1. 样品

白酒，准备 A、B 样，其中一份添加少量甲醇。

2. 试剂

（1）高锰酸钾-磷酸溶液：称取 3 g 高锰酸钾，加入 15 mL 85%磷酸溶液及 70 mL 水的混合液中，待高锰酸钾溶解后用水定容至 100 mL。贮于棕色瓶中备用，防止氧化能力下降，储存时间不宜过长。

（2）草酸-硫酸溶液：称取 5 g 无水草酸或 7 g 含 2 个结晶水的草酸，溶于 1+1 冷硫酸中，并用 1+1 冷硫酸定容至 100 mL。混匀后，贮于棕色瓶中备用。

（3）品红亚硫酸溶液：称取 0.1 g 研细的碱性品红，分次加入 6 mL 80℃的水，边加水边研磨使其溶解，待其充分溶解后滤于 10 mL 容量瓶中，冷却后加 10 mL 亚硫酸钠溶液（100 g/L），1 mL 盐酸，再加水至刻度，充分混匀，放置过夜。如溶液有颜色，可加少量活性炭搅拌后过滤，贮于棕色瓶中，置暗处保存。溶液呈红色时应弃去重新配制。

（4）甲醇标准溶液：准确称取 1.000 g 甲醇（相当于 1.27 mL）置于预先装有少量蒸馏水的 100 mL 容量瓶中，加水稀释至刻度，混匀。此溶液每毫升相当于 10 mg 甲醇，置低温环境下保存。

（5）甲醇标准应用液：吸取 10.0 mL 甲醇标准溶液置于 100 mL 容量瓶中，加水稀释至刻度，混匀。此溶液每毫升相当于 1 mg 甲醇。

（6）无甲醇无甲醛的乙醇：取 0.3 mL 乙醇按实验操作方法检查，不应显色。如显色须进行处理。处理方法：取 300 ml 乙醇（95%），加高锰酸钾少许，蒸馏，收集馏出液。在馏出液中加入硝酸银溶液（取 1 g 硝酸银溶于少量水中）和氢氧化钠溶液（取 1.5 g 氢氧化钠溶于少量水中），摇匀，取上清液蒸馏，弃去最初 50 mL 馏出液，收集中间馏出液约 200 mL，用酒精比重计测其浓度，然后加水配制成无甲醇的乙醇（体积分数约为 60%）。

（7）亚硫酸钠溶液（10 g/L）。

3. 仪器

分光光度计。

四、方法和步骤

1. 实验步骤

（1）根据待测白酒中含乙醇多少适当取样（含乙醇 30%取 1.0 mL；40%取 0.8 mL；50%取 0.6 mL；60%取 0.5 mL）于 25 mL 具塞比色管中。

（2）精确吸取 0 mL、0.2 mL、0.4 mL、0.6 mL、0.8 mL、1.0 mL 甲醇标准应用液（相当于 0 mg、0.2 mg、0.4 mg、0.6 mg、0.8 mg、1.0 mg 甲醇）分别置于 25 mL 具塞比色管中，各加入 0.5 mL 无甲醇无甲醛的乙醇（体积分数约为 60%）。

（3）于样品管及标准管中各加水至 5 mL，混匀，各管依次加入 2 mL 高锰酸钾-磷酸溶液，混匀，放置 10 min。

（4）各管加 2 mL 草酸－硫酸溶液，混匀后静置，使溶液褪色。

（5）各管再加入 5 mL 品红亚硫酸溶液，混匀，于 20℃ 以上静置 0.5 h。

（6）以零管调零点，于 590 nm 波长处测吸光度，与标准曲线比较定量或与标准系列目测比较。

2. 结果计算

$$X = \frac{m}{\frac{V}{10} \times 1000} \times 100$$

式中，X：样品中甲醇的含量（g/100 mL）；

m：测定样品中所含的甲醇相当于标准的质量（mg）；

V：样品取样体积（mL）。

计算结果保留两位有效数字。

3. 注意事项

（1）亚硫酸品红溶液呈红色时应重新配制，新配制的亚硫酸品红溶液放冰箱中 24～48 小时后再用为好。

（2）白酒中其他醛类以及经高锰酸钾氧化后由醇类变成的醛类（如乙醛、丙醛等）与品红亚硫酸作用也显色。但在一定浓度的硫酸酸性溶液中，除甲醛可形成经久不褪的紫色外，其他醛类则历时不久即自行消退或不显色，故无干扰，但操作中的时间条件必须严格控制。

（3）白酒样品和标准溶液中的乙醇浓度对比色有一定的影响，故样品与标准管中乙醇含量要大致相等。

Experiment 29　Anthropometric Measuring

Ⅰ. Objective

Master the methods and the key to operation of anthropometry.

Ⅱ. Principle

Anthropometric index can comprehensively reflect the nutritional status of human body, which is one of the important contents of nutrition investigation. Anthropometry usually includes two aspects: One is measurement of growth and development, including measurement of head circumference, weight and height (length); The other one is measurement of body composition, such as skin fold thickness, upper arm circumference, waist circumference and hip circumference. Different age groups select different indicators.

Ⅲ. Materials

(1) Body weight scales (beam balance).

Chapter Five　Experiments and Cases of Nutrition and Food Hygiene

(2) Height bar.

(3) Measuring bed.

(4) Tape.

(5) Skin thickness gauge.

Ⅳ. Experiment Procedures

1. Measurement of body weight

(1) Equipment: beam balance.

(2) Measuring method: The accuracy and sensitivity of the instrument should be checked before using. The standard weights are used to ensure the accuracy error is less than 0.1%. The beam balance should be calibrated for each measurement. Place it on flat ground and adjust zero point to scale level. The subjects should stand in the center of the scale, wearing shorts and a vest. The reading is in kilograms (kg) to one decimal.

2. Measurement of height

(1) Equipment: height bar.

(2) Measuring method: The zero point should be checked before using, and the height of the red marks on the reference plane should be measured with a steel ruler to determine whether the mark is 10.0 cm. At the same time, check whether the column is vertical, whether the joint is tight, whether there is shaking, weather the zero point is loose and so on, and calibrated if it's necessary. The upper limbs of the subject should be naturally drooping, with their feet close together and their toes 60 degrees apart. The heel, sacrum and the middle of the two scapula are in contact with the column, keep the torso naturally straight. The surveyor stands to the right of the subject, slide the horizontal plate down the column gently and press it on the head of the subject. The tester's eyes should be as high as the plate surface when reading, and the reading should be accurate to one decimal place (0.1 cm). The measurement process should be strictly abided by the principle of "three points against the column" and "two points on the horizontal".

3. Measurement of body length (for children under 3 years of age)

(1) Equipment: measuring bed.

(2) Measuring method: Place the measuring bed on a flat floor or table, take off the shoes, hat, and thick clothes of the child, make the child lie on his back in the midline of the measuring plate, fix his head, keep his ears on the same horizontal line, and make him touch the head plate. The surveyor stands on the right side of the child, and the left hand holds on to the child's knee to make it fixed, then slide the board with the right hand to keep it close to the child's heel, and take the readings and accurate to one decimal place (0.1 cm).

4. Measurement of upper arm circumference

(1) Equipment: tape.

(2) Measuring method: The measurement position of the upper arm circumference is the arm

circumference from the acromion to the midpoint of the line of the olecranon of the left upper arm, including upper arm tension circumference and upper arm relaxation circumference. The difference between the two is indicative of muscle development, while the greater is the difference, the better is the muscle development. The upper arm circumference reflects the nutritional status, it is closely related to body weight.

Upper arm tension circumference measurement: The upper arm tension circumference is the circumference of the upper arm when the upper arm biceps maximum contract. The subject raises his upper arm at an oblique level about 45 degrees, clenches his fist upward and bends his elbow hard. The surveyor stands to the side or opposite, measure around the thickest part of the biceps of the upper arm by tape. The tested muscles need to fully contract during measurement, the tightness of the tape measure should be appropriate, and the measurement error is less than 0.5 cm.

Upper arm relaxation circumference measurement: After measuring the upper arm tension circumference, keep the tape in its original position, let the subject slowly straighten his upper arm, take a tape measure around the thickest part of his upper biceps. When measuring the relaxation circumference of the upper arm, the tape should not move during muscles' shifting from tension to relaxation, and the measurement error is less than 0.5 cm.

5. Measurement of skin fold thickness

(1) Equipment: skin thickness gauge.

(2) Measuring method: The subject stands naturally with the tested part fully exposed, the surveyor stands behind the subject and finds the acromion and the olecranon, mark the midpoint of the line from acromion to olecranon behind the left arm with a pen. Lift the skin and subcutaneous tissue with left thumb, index finger and middle finger, the thickness of skin fold is measured below the point. Loosen the caliper handle of the skin thickness gauge, so that the tips of the caliper fully hold the skin fold, immediately read the number when the pointer of skin thickness gauge quickly fall back. Continuous measure 3 times to get the average, with mm as a unit, precise to 0.1 mm.

The thickness of skin fold is a good index to measure individual nutrition status and obesity level. We generally measure the thickness of skin fold of upper arm triceps, subscapular angle, beside the umbilicus, trunk, waist, abdomen and other parts to estimate the subcutaneous fat accumulation.

6. Measurement of waist circumference

(1) Equipment: tape (made of non-scalable materials, scale of 0.1 cm).

(2) Measuring method: The subject stands naturally and looks straight ahead, the surveyor takes the midpoint of the line between the lowest level of the costal margin and the highest point of the anterior superior iliac ridge, place the tape horizontally around the waist and take a reading at the end of breath but before inhale of the subject.

实验二十九 人体测量

一、实验目的
掌握人体测量的方法和操作要点。

二、实验原理
人体测量指标可以综合地反映人体的营养状况,是营养调查的重要内容之一。人体测量通常包括两个方面:一是生长发育测量,包括头围、体重及身高(长)等的测量;二是机体组成测量,如皮褶厚度、上臂围、腰围及臀围等。不同年龄组选择的指标不同。

三、实验材料
(1)体重计(杠杆秤)。
(2)身高计。
(3)量床。
(4)卷尺。
(5)皮褶厚度计。

四、方法和步骤
1. 体重的测量
(1)使用器材:杠杆秤。
(2)测量方法:使用前应检查仪器的准确性和灵敏度。用标准砝码进行检验,使其准确度误差不超过0.1%。每次测量时,杠杆秤要进行校正。将其放在平坦的地面上,调整零点至刻度尺呈水平位。受试者身着短裤、背心,站立于秤中央。读数以千克(kg)为单位,精确到小数点后一位。

2. 身高的测量
(1)使用器材:身高坐高计。
(2)测量方法:使用前应校对零点,用钢尺测量基准板平面红色刻线的高度是否为10.0 cm。同时应检查立柱是否垂直,连接处是否紧密,有无晃动,零点有无松脱等情况并加以校正。被测者上肢自然下垂,足跟并拢,足尖分开呈60°,足跟、骶骨及两肩胛区与立柱接触,躯干自然挺直;测试者站在被测者右侧,将水平板轻轻沿立柱下滑,轻压于被测者头顶,测试者读数时两眼应与压板平面等高,读数精确到小数点后一位(0.1 cm)。测量过程要严格遵守"三点靠立柱""两点呈水平"的原则。

3. 身长的测量(3岁以下的儿童)
(1)使用器材:卧式量板或量床。
(2)测量方法:将量板放在平坦的地面或桌面上,脱去儿童的鞋帽和厚衣裤,使其仰卧于量板中线位置，固定小儿头部，两耳在同一水平线上，并使其接触头板。测量者位于小儿右侧，将左手置于小儿膝部，使其固定；用右手滑动滑板，使之紧贴小儿足跟，读数至小数点后一位（0.1 cm）。

4. 上臂围的测量

（1）使用器材：无伸缩性材料制成的卷尺，刻度为 0.1 cm。

（2）测量方法：上臂围测量位置为左上臂从肩峰至尺骨鹰嘴连线中点的部位臂围长，包括上臂紧张围和上臂松弛围。两者之差可反映肌肉发育状况，差值越大，肌肉发育状况越好。上臂围可反映营养状况，它与体重密切相关。

上臂紧张围测量：上臂紧张围是指上臂肱二头肌最大限度收缩时的围度。被测者上臂斜平举约 45°，手掌向上握拳并用力屈肘；测量者站于侧面或对面，将卷尺在上臂肱二头肌最粗处绕一周进行测量，测量时被测者的肌肉要充分收缩，卷尺的松紧度要适宜，测量误差小于 0.5 cm。

上臂松弛围测量：在测量上臂紧张围后，将卷尺保持原来位置不动，让被测者将上臂缓慢伸直，将卷尺在上臂肱二头肌最粗处绕一周进行测量，测量上臂松弛围时应注意肌肉由紧张变换到松弛时，勿使卷尺移位，测量误差小于 0.5 cm。

5. 皮褶厚度的测量

（1）使用器材：皮褶厚度计。

（2）测量方法：被测者自然站立，被测部位充分裸露，测试者站在被测者身后，找到肩峰、尺骨鹰嘴部位，用油笔标记出左臂后从肩到尺骨鹰嘴连线中点。用左手拇指和食指、中指将被测部位皮肤及皮下组织夹提起来，在其下方用皮褶厚度计测量厚度，松开皮褶厚度计的卡钳钳柄，使钳尖部充分夹住皮褶，皮褶厚度计指针快速回落后立即读数。连续测量 3 次，以 mm 为单位，精确到 0.1 mm。

皮褶厚度是衡量个体营养状况和肥胖程度的较好指标，主要测量皮下脂肪厚度，可以间接反映人体肥胖程度。一般测量上臂肱三头肌、肩胛下角、脐旁、躯干、腰腹等部位的皮下脂肪堆积情况。

6. 腰围的测量

（1）使用器材：无伸缩性材料制成的卷尺，刻度为 0.1 cm。

（2）测量方法：被测者自然站立，平视前方；测试人员先取肋下缘最底部和髂前上脊最高点之间连线的中点处，将卷尺水平围绕腰一周，并在被测者呼气末而吸气未开始时进行读数记录。

 Experiment 30　Dietary Survey

Ⅰ．Objectives

（1）Understand the purpose, significance, and implementation process of dietary survey, and master the methods of dietary calculation, evaluation, and improvement.

Chapter Five Experiments and Cases of Nutrition and Food Hygiene
第五章 营养与食品卫生学实验及案例

(2) To further understand the significance of proper nutrition and a balanced diet for body health.

Ⅱ. Principle

The dietary survey is the basis of nutrition investigation, through the investigation of individual or population's daily intake of various foods, the daily energy and intake of various nutrients, and the mutual proportional relationship between various nutrients are calculated, and the food sources of energy and nutrients are analyzed. The dietary survey can not only comprehensively understand the nutritional intake of a certain population or individual, evaluate the advantages and disadvantages of their dietary structure, but also find out the population with unbalanced nutrition, providing basic information for nutrition monitoring and nutrition policy formulation and modification. Besides, it can provide reference data for studying the correlation between certain diseases and nutrition.

The methods of the dietary survey are as follows:

(1) Weighing method: Weigh the daily food consumption of each meal of an organization or individual, and then calculate the daily nutrients intake of each person. Because this method can accurately reflect the food intake and food distribution of each meal, the weighing method is often used as the gold standard of the dietary survey to measure the accuracy of other methods.

(2) Bookkeeping method: This method is suitable for organizations that have established detailed accounts of foods. According to the consumption of all kinds of food and the number of diners during a certain period of time of the organization, the average daily food consumption per capita is roughly estimated and the energy and nutrients intake per capita of each day is calculated according to the food composition table. This method can also be applied to the family. This method is easy to operate, easy to be accepted by the dietary management personnel. However, this method is not very accurate, and it is difficult to analyze the individual dietary intake status.

(3) Chemical analysis method: Collect all main foods and non-staple foods ingested in each meal of the object, and the quantity and quality of energy and nutrients in foods are determined by the chemical analysis method in the laboratory. Due to the complexity and high cost of this method, it is generally only used for small-scale investigation, such as nutrient metabolism experiments, to understand the absorption and metabolism of nutrients in the body.

(4) Food frequency method: The food frequency method is able to obtain the dietary intake and dietary patterns of the participants over a period of time. The eating habits of participants are not affected. Therefore, this method is widely used in the epidemiological study of diet and chronic diseases. This survey method is simple and low cost, but cannot estimate the food consumption accurately.

(5) 24-hour dietary retrospection method: Participants are asked to review the type and amount of all foods consumed in the previous 24 hours. The surveyors should receive unified training, to guide and help the participants to review their previous diet, and they can use food models and measurement tools to conduct quantitative accounting of the food intake of the participants.

III. Materials

(1) Recording table.
(2) Food composition table.
(3) Calculator.

IV. Experiment Procedures

1. Calculation of food intake

Conduct a mutual investigation in pairs, and fill your partner's intakes of staple food, non-staple food, snacks and condiments within 24 hours in the following table.

Table 30 – 1 Food diary record

	Breakfast		Lunch		Dinner	
	Recipe	Food weight	Recipe	Food weight	Recipe	Food weight
Staple food	Red bean bun	Flour, 100 g red bean paste, 40 g	Rice	Rice, 100 g	Rice	Rice, 100 g
Non-staple food 1	Milk	Milk, 250 g	Bouilli	Pork, 75 g Sauce, 10 g Salt, 2 g Oil, 5 g	Scrambled eggs	Egg, 75 g Salt, 2 g Oil, 10 g
Non-staple food 2	Tuber mustard	Tuber mustard, 25 g	Sauteed cabbage	Cabbage, 200 g Salt, 3 g Oil, 5 g	Sauteed celery and bean curd	Celery, 200 g Bean curd, 50 g Oil, 5 g Salt, 3 g
Non-staple food 3					Apple	Apple, 150 g

2. Calculation of energy and nutrient intake

Refer to the food composition table to calculate the energy and nutrients of each food. Summarize the meal and daily calories and nutrient intakes and fill in the table below.

Table 30 – 2 Calculation of food composition

	Food name	Weight/ g	Proteins/ g	Fats/ g	Carbohydrates/ g	Energy/ kcal	Calcium/ mg	Iron / mg	VA/ mg	VD/ mg
Breakfast										
Lunch										
Dinner										
In total										

Note: If the rows and columns are not enough, they can be added.

3. Evaluation of dietary energy and nutrient intake

(1) According to the gender, age and labor intensity of the recipe user, find the appropriate recommended nutrient intake (RNI) or appropriate intake (AI) and fill in the table below to calculate the percentage of actual intake to RNI or AI.

Table 30-3 Diet evaluation

Nutrients	Proteins/g	Fats/g	Carbohydrates/g	Energy/kcal	Calcium/mg	Iron/mg	VA/mg	VD/mg
Recommended daily intake								
Average daily intake								
Intake/RNI or AI (×100%)								

(2) Calculate the source distribution of energy and protein.

Table 30-4 Sources of nutrient foods

	Energy	Protein
Animals/%		
Beans/%		
Others/%		

(3) Calculate the energy distribution of three meals.

Table 30-5 Energy distribution of three meals

	Breakfast	Lunch	Dinner
energy/%			

(4) Calculate the energy supply ratio of the three main energy productive nutrients.

Table 30-6 Energy supply ratio of the three main energy productive nutrients

	Intake/g	Energy/kcal	Energy/%
Protein			
Fats			
Carbohydrate			

4. Dietary assessment, and put forward suggestions for improvement

(1) Whether the intake of various nutrients and energy is insufficient or excessive?

(2) Whether the energy distribution of three meals in one day is reasonable?

(3) Whether the food sources distribution of energy and protein is reasonable?

(4) Whether the energy supply ratio of the three energy producing nutrients is reasonable?

(5) Finally, please put forward the improvement plan according to the actual situation.

实验三十　膳食调查

一、实验目的

(1) 了解膳食调查的目的、意义、实施过程，掌握膳食计算、评价和改进的方法。

(2) 进一步了解合理营养和平衡膳食对机体健康的意义。

二、实验原理

膳食调查是营养调查的基础，通过对个人或人群每天各种食物摄入量的调查，计算出每人每天能量和各种营养素的摄入量、各种营养素之间的相互比例关系，分析能量和营养素的食物来源等。膳食调查不仅可以全面了解某人群或个体的营养摄入情况，评价其膳食结构的优缺点，还能够发现营养不平衡人群，为营养监测和营养政策的制定和修改提供基础资料。另外，可以为研究某些疾病与营养的相关关系提供参考数据。

膳食调查的方法有以下几种：

(1) 称重法：对某一单位或个人一日各餐食物的消费量进行称重，然后计算每人每日的营养素摄入量。由于该方法能准确反映食物的摄入情况，以及各餐次食物的分配情况，故常将称重法作为膳食调查的金标准，用来衡量其他方法的准确性。

(2) 记账法：此法适用于有详细伙食账目的集体单位，根据该单位在一定时期内的各种食物消耗总量和就餐者的人数，粗略估算出平均每人每日的食物消耗量，再根据食物成分表计算每人每日的能量和营养素的摄入量，此法也可应用于家庭。该方法操作简便，易于被膳食管理人员所接受，不足之处是不太准确，而且很难对个体膳食的摄入状况进行分析。

(3) 化学分析法：此法是指对调查对象一日各餐膳食中要摄入的主、副食品进行收集，在实验室用化学分析的方法测定其所含的能量和营养素的数量和质量。由于此法分析过程较复杂，成本较高，一般只用于较小规模的调查，如营养代谢实验，了解营养素在体内的吸收及代谢状况等。

(4) 食物频率法：食物频率法能够得到被调查者在过去一段时间内的膳食摄入量及膳食模式。调查者的饮食习惯不受影响，因此在膳食与慢性病相关流行病学研究中应用广泛。该调查方法简单且费用低，但对食物摄入量的估计不准确。

(5) 24小时膳食回顾法：要求被调查者回顾调查时刻前24小时内摄入的所有食物的

种类和数量。调查者应经过统一培训，引导和帮助被调查者对既往的膳食情况进行回顾，可以借助实物模型和测量工具，对调查对象的食物摄入量进行定量核算。

三、实验材料

（1）记录表。
（2）食物成分表。
（3）计算器。

四、方法和步骤

1. 食物摄入量的计算

两人一组相互调查，将对方24小时内主食、副食、零食、调味品等的摄入情况填入下表。

表 30-1 食谱

	早餐		午餐		晚餐	
	食谱	食物重量	食谱	食物重量	食谱	食物重量
主食	豆沙包	面粉，100 g 红豆沙，40 g	大米饭	粳米，100 g	大米饭	粳米，100 g
副食1	牛奶	牛奶，250 g	红烧肉	猪肉，75 g 酱油，10 g 盐，2 g 油，5 g	炒鸡蛋	鸡蛋，75 g 盐，2 g 油，10 g
副食2	榨菜	榨菜，25 g	清炒小白菜	小白菜，200 g 盐，3 g 油，5 g	芹菜炒香干	芹菜，200 g 豆腐干，50 g 油，5 g 盐，3 g
副食3					苹果	苹果，150 g

2. 能量及营养素摄入量的计算

查阅食物成分表，计算出每种食物所供给的能量和各种营养素，并对各餐次、每日热能和各种营养素摄入量进行汇总，填入下表。

表 30-2 食物营养成分计算

	食物名称	重量/g	蛋白质/g	脂肪/g	糖类/g	能量/kcal	钙/mg	铁/mg	VA/mg	VD/mg
早餐										
午餐										
晚餐										
总计										

注：如行、列不够可以增加。

3. 膳食能量及营养素摄入量评价

（1）根据食谱使用者的性别、年龄、劳动强度等，查找相应的推荐摄入量（RNI）或适宜摄入量（AI）并填入下表，计算实际摄入量占 RNI 或 AI 的百分比。

表 30-3　膳食评价

各种营养素	蛋白质/g	脂肪/g	糖类/g	能量/kcal	钙/mg	铁/mg	VA/mg	VD/mg
推荐的每日摄入量								
平均每日摄入量								
摄入量/RNI 或 AI（×100%）								

（2）计算能量、蛋白质的来源分配。

表 30-4　营养素食物来源分配

	能量	蛋白质
动物食物/%		
豆类食物/%		
其他食物/%		

（3）计算三餐的能量分配情况。

表 30-5　三餐能量分配

	早餐	午餐	晚餐
能量百分比/%			

（4）计算三大产能营养素的供能比。

表 30-6　三大产能营养素供能比

	摄入量/g	供能量/kcal	占能量的百分比
蛋白质			
脂肪			
碳水化合物			

4. 进行膳食评价，提出改进建议

（1）各种营养素及能量的摄入量是否不足或过剩？

（2）一日三餐的能量分配是否合理？

（3）能量、蛋白质的食物来源分配是否合理？

（4）三大产能营养素的供能比是否合理？

（5）请结合实际提出改进方案。

Experiment 31　Case Analysis of Nutrition Intervention

Ⅰ. Background

×× county of ×× province in the south of China is a poverty-stricken county in our country. The residents have low economic and cultural level, and the awareness rate of the prevention and treatment of iron deficiency anemia is very low. In this region, 30% of school-age children aged 6 to 12 years old have iron deficiency anemia, and the awareness rate among patients is only 35%. Less than 30% of school routine physical examinations include hemoglobin measurement items.

Ⅱ. Procedures and methods of nutritional intervention for school-age children

（1）Formulation of intervention programs for iron deficiency anemia in school-age children.

（2）Evaluation of nutrition intervention projects.

Ⅲ. Case analysis of nutritional intervention for school-age children

1. What are the short-term and long-term goals of the project

（1）Short-term goals: Through nutrition education and iron supplement and other intervention measures, improve the target population's cognitive level of rational nutrition-related knowledge; Increase the intake of iron-rich animal foods; Increase the production and supply of iron-rich foods; Establish a monitoring system for iron deficiency anemia in school-age children; Increase the diagnosis rate of children with iron deficiency anemia.

（2）Long-term goal: Reduce the prevalence of iron deficiency anemia among school-age children in this poverty-stricken county.

2. How to formulate the overall plan

（1）Get the basic information: Before the implementation of the project, it is necessary to know the epidemiological information of iron deficiency anemia among the target population, as well as local main food resources, nutritional knowledge, dietary habits and other information of the local residents.

(2) Identify the main problems:

①Who are in the high-risk groups? (children aged 6 to 12);

②What is the main nutrition problem? (Iron deficiency anemia);

③How serious is it? (Prevalence rate is as high as 30% among children aged 6 to 12);

④What could be the reasons? (unreasonable dietary habits, lack of nutrition knowledge, lack of social attention)

(3) Formulate intervention measures and time limit: It is planned to adopt the intervention measures based on iron-fortified soy sauce, combined with nutrition knowledge publicity and education, with the intervention period of 1 year.

(4) Obtain social surroundings support: including the approval of the ethics committee of the implementation organization, the informed consent of the target group, the support of the local government, the cooperation of the participating organizations, and the publicity of the local media.

3. How to determine the target group

In order to promote the solution of iron deficiency problem, students, parents and teachers in the poverty-stricken county should also be listed as the priority objects of intervention, while other groups in the poverty-stricken county should be the general objects of intervention.

Two primary schools in the county were randomly selected as the target population, including children aged 6 to 12 and their parents and teachers. One intervention group and the other control group were randomly selected as the target population, and then stratified by age, and integrally sampling by class.

4. How to formulate the nutrition intervention plan

(1) Health education: According to the local actual situation, students, parents and teachers in the intervention group received the health education of unified form and content to improve the awareness of the iron deficiency anemia dangers and prevention skills. The main contents include: carrying out reasonable diet education for students, parents and teachers; promote the use of iron-rich foods at home in a planned way.

(2) Nutrition intervention: The intervention group adopted iron-fortified soy sauce for a period of 12 months. Soy sauce was distributed monthly for each family, designed at 15 mL per person per day (about 4.4 mg of iron), and the actual daily consumption of each person was recorded in detail. The control group was only reminded of regular healthy diet, not strengthened.

(3) Social support: Train canteen staff and encourage students to eat nutritious meals; Encourage home farming and cultivation, and also contact relevant enterprises to adjust the industrial structure and increase the supply of iron-rich food; Establish student health records and incorporate hemoglobin measurement into routine physical examination.

5. How to evaluate the effect of intervention

(1) Whether the expected goal is achieved? What changes have taken place in the nutritional knowledge, attitude and behavior of the object? The evaluation indicators should be

Chapter Five　Experiments and Cases of Nutrition and Food Hygiene
第五章　营养与食品卫生学实验及案例

corresponding, such as: the change of prevalence rate of iron deficiency anemia, the awareness rate of people on iron-rich foods and influencing factors of iron absorption, the intake of iron-rich foods, the market coverage rate of iron-fortified soy sauce and the household utilization rate, etc.

（2）Evaluation of the design, implementation and evaluation of the intervention plan, such as: Is the project for the prevention and treatment of iron deficiency anemia in the community proceeding as plan? Including time, coverage, cost, material sorting and data analysis, etc.

（3）Causal analysis of project implementation and behavior change.

（4）Analysis of supporting factors and obstacle factors for intervention.

（5）Whether it has been modified during the implementation of the plan and its natural character analysis.

（6）Summarize the lessons learned from the project.

6. Notes for nutrition intervention

（1）The goal of intervention should be clear and the plan of intervention should be specific.

（2）Interventions should be targeted and operable, and should base on safety and harmlessness.

（3）Interventions should consider the acceptability of the target population and be consistent with the selection preferences of the target population.

（4）The duration of observation and follow-up should be the minimum period for the occurrence of a measurable result.

（5）The evaluation index of intervention effect should be objective, specific, non-invasive and quantifiable.

（6）Ethical requirements should be met. Subjects should sign informed consent, and the whole experiment should conform to the ethical principles in the *Declaration of Helsinki*.

（7）The economy of interventions should be considered, and a relatively small input should be exchanged for a relatively large return as far as possible.

实验三十一　营养干预案例分析

一、背景资料

我国南方××省××县为我国贫困县，居民经济、文化水平较低，对缺铁性贫血防治知识的知晓率很低。该区域30%的6～12岁学龄儿童患有缺铁性贫血，患者中知晓率仅为35%，学校常规体检包含血红蛋白测定项目的不到30%。

二、学龄期儿童营养干预的程序与方法

（1）学龄期儿童缺铁性贫血干预方案的制订。

（2）营养干预项目的评价。

三、学龄期儿童营养干预案例分析

1. 项目的近期目标和远期目标

（1）近期目标：通过营养宣教和铁剂补充等干预措施，提高目标人群对合理营养相关知识的认知水平；提高含铁丰富的动物性食物的摄入量；提高含铁丰富的食物的生产和供给能力；建立学龄期儿童缺铁性贫血的监测系统；提高缺铁性贫血儿童的就诊率。

（2）远期目标：降低该贫困县学龄儿童缺铁性贫血的患病率。

2. 如何制定总体方案

（1）了解基本情况：在项目实施前须了解目标人群的缺铁性贫血流行病学资料，以及当地主要食物资源，当地居民的营养知识、饮食生活习惯等信息。

（2）确定主要问题：

①哪些人群是高危人群？（6～12岁学龄儿童）

②主要问题是哪种营养问题？（缺铁性贫血）

③严重程度如何？（6～12岁学龄儿童中患病率高达30%）

④原因可能是什么？（不合理的饮食生活习惯、营养知识缺乏、社会关注度不够）

（3）拟定干预措施和期限：拟采用以铁强化酱油为主的干预措施，配合营养知识宣教等方式，干预期为1年。

（4）获得环境支持：包括执行单位伦理委员会的批准、目标人群的知情同意、当地政府的支持、参与单位的配合、当地媒体的宣传。

3. 如何确定目标人群

为了促进铁缺乏问题的解决，该贫困县的学生、家长和教师应同时列为重点干预对象，该贫困县的其他人群为一般干预对象。

随机选择该县两所小学6～12岁学龄儿童及其家长和教师为目标人群，随机确定其中一所为干预组，另一所为对照组，进一步以年龄分层，以班级为整群抽样。

4. 如何制定营养干预方案

（1）健康教育：根据当地实际情况，干预组学生、家长和教师均采用统一形式和内容的健康教育，提高对缺铁性贫血危害的认识和预防技能。主要内容包括：对学生、家长及老师开展合理膳食教育；有计划地宣传家庭使用富铁食品。

（2）营养干预：干预组采用铁强化酱油进行为期12个月的干预，酱油以家庭为单位按月发放，按每人每天15 mL设计（约含4.4 mg铁），详细记录每人每日的实际食用量。对照组仅做常规健康膳食提醒，不予强化。

（3）社会支持：对食堂工作人员进行培训，鼓励组织学生食用营养餐；鼓励家庭养殖和种植，也可以与相关企业联系，调整产业结构，增加富铁食物供应；建立学生健康档案，把血红蛋白测定纳入常规体检中。

5. 如何评估干预效果

（1）是否达到预期目标？受干预对象的营养知识、态度和行为发生了哪些变化？评价指标应与之对应，如缺铁性贫血患病率的变化、人群对富含铁的食物及铁吸收影响因素的知晓率、含铁丰富的食物的摄入情况、铁强化酱油的市场覆盖率和家庭使用率等。

（2）干预计划的设计、实施以及评价等各阶段过程评价，如：社区缺铁性贫血防治项目是否按计划进行？包括时间、覆盖人群、经费、材料整理和数据分析等。

（3）项目实施与行为改变的因果分析；

（4）干预成功与否的支持因素和障碍因素分析；

（5）计划实施过程中是否被修正及其性质分析；

（6）总结该项目得到的经验教训。

6. 营养干预的注意事项

（1）干预的目标要明确，干预的方案要具体。

（2）干预措施要有针对性、可操作性，要以对人安全、无害为前提。

（3）干预措施要考虑目标人群的可接受性，与目标人群的选择偏好一致。

（4）观察随访的期限应以出现某种可测量的结果的最短期限为原则。

（5）干预效果的评价指标应具有客观性、特异性，且无损伤，最好可定量。

（6）应符合伦理学要求，实验对象签署知情同意书，整个试验要符合《赫尔辛基宣言》中的伦理原则。

（7）要考虑干预措施的经济性，尽可能以较小投入换取较大收益。

Experiment 32 Case Analysis of Food Poisoning Investigation and Treatment

Ⅰ. Background

Health supervision institute of a tropical coastal tourism city received a telephone report from ×× Hospital at 8:00 a.m. on October 3, 2019. It is reported that the hospital has admitted 34 suspected food poisoning patients, all of whom are individual tourists. After eating at a seafood restaurant at noon on October 2, they developed symptoms and went to ×× Hospital in the afternoon. The main symptoms were paroxysmal colic in the upper abdomen, diarrhea and vomiting, and some patients had slight fever.

Ⅱ. Procedures and methods for investigation and treatment of food poisoning

(1) The main purpose of on-site investigation and treatment of food poisoning.

(2) Registration of reports.

(3) Food poisoning investigation.

(4) Technical analysis of survey data.

(5) Control and treatment of food poisoning incidents.

Ⅲ. Case analysis of food poisoning investigation and treatment

1. What emergency measures should be taken

(1) Establish a food poisoning investigation and treatment team.

(2) Treatment of patients.

(3) Control of suspected food.

2. What preparations should be made before the survey

After receiving the report of food poisoning, in addition to the above emergency measures, preparations shall be made for on-site investigation and treatment of food poisoning.

(1) Personnel preparation: Generally, more than two food hygiene professionals should be assigned to the scene for investigation. When food poisoning that involving a wide range of problems, inspectors and other professionals should be assigned to assist the investigation.

(2) Material preparation: Essential items for food poisoning investigation, including sampling supplies.

(3) Legal documents: on-site health supervision records, investigation records, sampling records, opinions of hygiene supervision, etc.

(4) Forensic tools: recorder, camera, etc.

(5) Food poisoning rapid detection box.

(6) Vehicle preparation: Special vehicles for epidemic investigation should be prepared and ready at any time so as to get to the scene quickly.

3. How to conduct the on-site investigation, how to determine the cause of food poisoning

(1) To understand the situation of the disease: Investigators rushed to the scene to hear the introduction of the disease.

(2) Investigation of clinical manifestations and meal history of poisoning patients: Fill in each item according to the unified "Food poisoning clinical manifestations questionnaire", and ask the patients to sign for approval.

The clinical investigation results of this food poisoning incident are as follows: The main symptoms of the patients were gastrointestinal symptoms, 80% of the patients had an incubation period of 6 - 8 hours, the shortest wsa 4 hours, and the longest was 20 hours. The main clinical symptoms of the patient were upper abdominal paroxysmal colic, followed by diarrhea, which 4 - 6 times or more than 10 times a day. The stool was watery or mushy. About 15% of the patients had blood watery stools. A few had mucous or mucinous stools, but there was no tenesmus. Most of the patients had nausea and vomiting after diarrhea, and the body temperature was 37.5 - 39.5℃. There was obvious tenderness in the ileum, and the course of disease was 1 - 8 days, most of which were 2 - 4 days.

(3) The dining investigation shall be completed item by item according to the unified table of "Eating conditions for patients with food poisoning" about the eating conditions that 24 to 48 hours before the onset of the disease, so as to determine the suspicious food. The results of the food poisoning investigation are as follows: There were 34 people in total, all of whom were tourists from other places. They had lunch in a seafood restaurant at noon on October 2. The preliminary estimate is a bacterial food poisoning.

Chapter Five Experiments and Cases of Nutrition and Food Hygiene
第五章 营养与食品卫生学实验及案例

(4) Suspicious food survey: According to the analysis results of questionnaire on eating conditions of patients with food poisoning, investigators traced to a seafood stall and investigate the raw materials, quality, processing and cooking methods, heating temperature and time, cleanliness of utensils and containers and food storage conditions of the suspected poisoned food. Meanwhile, they collected the remaining suspected food and the sample of the links that may be contaminated.

After investigation and inquiry, the food poisoning patients are tourists, who have eaten seafood in a seafood stall. Further investigation showed that the majority of the patients were men, and fewer were women. The reason was that a dish called "minced garlic scallop" had only been cooked for a short time. Most of the female tourists thought it was too fishy and did not eat it, but the male tourists did not care and ate it. All the people who ate the dish fell ill, and none of whom didn't fell ill. A search of epidemic data proved that there was no recent epidemic of infectious diseases with similar clinical characteristics. Therefore, the onset of the day at noon is the toxic meal, "minced garlic scallop" is the suspected poisoning food.

4. How to obtain further evidence

The whole process of food poisoning investigation, in a sense, is a process of obtaining evidence, therefore, the investigators must pay attention to the objectivity, scientificalness, and the legal nature of evidence, and should make full use of tape recorders, cameras to record the conversation with the client and the sanitary condition of the survey site objectively. When inquiring the relevant personnel, the case investigation records must be made and signed by the respondent for approval. The cause of food poisoning can be determined based on field epidemiological investigations and laboratory tests.

In this food poisoning incident, investigators conducted an epidemiological investigation of the suspected poisoning food. According to the investigation, this restaurant purchased scallops from ×× seafood wholesaler in the afternoon of the previous day (Oct. 1). The batch of scallops with a total weight of 20 kg were fresh. The scallops were raised in seawater for dinner, midnight snack on Oct. 1 and lunch on Oct. 2. Due to the large number of people eating lunch on October 2, the cooking staff was busy and forgot the cooking time, and the scallops were brought to the table without being cooked thoroughly. The diners at this table were all tourists from inland cities. They thought the seafood would be fresh only if it was "half-cooked". They did not give feedback on the quality of the dishes.

5. How to conduct on-site sampling and inspection

(1) Vomitus collection: Vomitus collection should be done before the patient takes the medicine. For suspected bacterial food poisoning, 3 mL venous blood should be collected in the acute phase (within 3 days) and the convalescent phase (about 2 weeks), respectively.

(2) Food collection: Collect the leftover suspicious food, and if necessary, collect the semi-finished products or raw materials of the suspicious food as well.

In this case, investigators collected one portion of scallops from the seafood sales booth, one portion of remained scallops from the restaurant, one portion of scallops from the table, six portions of vomitus, 14 portions of the patient's blood and stools at the time of illness and the same person's blood and stools 2 days after the illness. After the sample was labeled, numbered, sealed tightly, and the sampling time, conditions, and the pathogen (*Vibrio parahaemolyticus*) were attached, the sample was signed and sent to the laboratory for inspection. According to the routine test of intestinal pathogenic bacteria, vibrio parahaemolyticus was detected in all scallops and vomitus and stools of the patients by adding bacteria, isolating bacteria, pure culture, biochemical test and serological identification. Serum lectin titers of 14 patients were significantly higher than that at the time of onset, increasing to 1∶40 – 1∶320.

6. How to deal with food poisoning

(1) Control measures: After confirmation of suspected food poisoning, investigators shall take administrative control measures according to law to prevent the scope of food poisoning from expanding.

(2) Scope of control: including sealing up suspicious food and its raw materials, contaminated food utensils, processing equipment and containers, and ordering them to be cleaned and disinfected.

(3) The administrative control: Seal the suspected food and its raw materials with paper strip seals sealed by the administrative department of public health, "Administrative control decision" should be assigned. In an emergency, the investigator may seal up and keep records on the spot and report them to the health authority for approval of "Administrative control decision". The administrative control time is 15 days, and the health administration department should complete the inspection or evaluation of the sealed objects within 15 days from the date of sealing, and make a decision of destroying or unsealing.

The food poisoning treatment is as follows: The health supervision department immediately ordered the restaurant, stop supplying scallop, sealed on the spot, find the scallop stall through the purchase channel, also sealed on the spot, all tools and utensils contacted with scallop should be disinfected.

(4) Recall and destroy the food that caused the poisoning: According to the results of on-site investigation and inspection, the confirmed poisoning food may be destroyed directly by food safety departments. It may also be destroyed by the unit that caused the incident on its own under the supervision of the public health administration department. Those who have sold the poisoned food shall be ordered to take back and destroy it.

(5) The disposal of the poisoning place: According to the different nature of food poisoning, appropriate measures shall be taken for the poisoning place. Tableware, utensils, containers and equipment that contact with bacterial food poisoning shall be sterilized by boiling 1% – 2% lye water or soaked in chlorine preparation solution with effective chlorine content of 150 – 200 mg/L, for similar items that contact with chemical food poisoning, wash them thoroughly with lye.

(6) The emergency treatment plan shall be corrected and supplemented as necessary.

7. How to carry out administrative punishment

After the on-site investigation, the investigators should sort out and analyze the epidemiological investigation data, make a final diagnosis based on the laboratory results, and write a complete investigation report.

The departments of public health supervision may, in general, take some punitive measures against the production and business operation entities. The punishment measures include warning, suspension of business for rectification, time limit for improvement, destruction of food, confiscation of illegal income, fine, revocation of hygiene permit, etc. The specific punishment measures shall be taken by the administrative departments of public health according to the illegal facts, evidence and the application of relevant laws, making law enforcement documents and carrying out administrative punishment according to the law enforcement procedures.

实验三十二 食物中毒调查处理案例分析

一、背景资料

某热带沿海旅游城市卫生监督所于2019年10月3日早8时接到××医院的电话报告。报告称该医院收治了34名疑似食物中毒病人，这些病人均为散客团游客，10月2日中午在某海鲜大排档就餐后，下午陆续出现症状而到××医院就诊，主要表现为上腹部阵发性绞痛、腹泻、呕吐等症状，部分患者轻微发热。

二、食物中毒调查处理程序与方法

（1）食物中毒现场调查处理的主要目的。
（2）报告登记。
（3）食物中毒的调查。
（4）调查资料的技术分析。
（5）食物中毒事件的控制和处理。

三、食物中毒调查处理案例分析

1. 要采取哪些应急措施

（1）成立食物中毒调查处理小组。
（2）对患者的救治。
（3）对可疑食物的控制。

2. 调查前要做哪些准备工作

接到食物中毒报告后，除做好以上应急措施，同时应进行食物中毒现场调查处理的各项准备工作。

（1）人员准备：一般要指派两名以上食品卫生专业人员赶赴现场调查，对涉及面广、疑难的食物中毒应配备检验人员和有关专业人员协助调查。

（2）物资准备：食物中毒调查必备物品，包括采样用品。

（3）法律文书：现场卫生监督记录、调查记录、采样记录、卫生监督意见书等。

（4）取证工具：录音机、照相机等。

（5）食物中毒快速检测箱。

（6）交通工具准备：应备有疫情调查专用车，随时待命，以便迅速赶赴现场。

3. 如何开展现场调查？如何确定食物中毒的致病原因

（1）了解发病情况：调查人员赶赴现场听取病情介绍。

（2）中毒患者临床表现和进餐史调查：按统一制定的"食物中毒临床表现调查表"逐项填写，并请患者签字认可。

本次食物中毒事故，临床调查结果如下：患者均以胃肠道症状为主，80%病人潜伏期为6~8小时，最短4小时，最长20小时。病人主要临床症状为上腹阵发性绞痛，继而腹泻，每日4~6次，多者达10次以上。粪便为水样或糊状，约有15%的患者出现洗肉水样血水便，少数有黏液或黏液血便，但没有里急后重症。多数患者在腹泻后出现恶心、呕吐，体温为37.5℃~39.5℃。回盲肠部有明显压痛，病程1~8天，大部分2~4天。

（3）进餐调查：按统一制定的"食物中毒患者进餐情况调查表"对患者发病前24~48小时进餐情况逐项询问填写，以便确定可疑食物。本次食物中毒调查结果为：本次中毒共34人，都是外地游客，10月2日中午在某海鲜大排档就餐，初步印象是一起细菌性食物中毒。

（4）可疑食物调查：根据"食物中毒患者进餐情况调查表"的分析结果，调查人员追踪至某海鲜大排档，对可疑中毒食物的原料与质量、加工烹饪方法、加热温度与时间、用具容器的清洁度和食品储备条件进行调查，同时采集剩余的可疑食物并对可能污染的环节进行采样。

经过调查询问，本次食物中毒病人都是外地游客，都在某海鲜大排档吃过海鲜。进一步调查发现，发病者绝大多数是男性，女性较少，原因是有一道蒜蓉粉丝扇贝烹饪时间过短，多数女性游客认为腥气太重而没吃这个菜，但男性游客则不以为然。所有吃过这道菜的人都发病，而未吃者无一发病。查询疫情资料证明，近期当地没有类似临床特征的传染病流行。由此认为，发病当天中午是中毒餐次，蒜蓉粉丝扇贝是可疑中毒食物。

4. 如何进一步取证

食物中毒调查的整个过程，从某种意义上讲是一个取证过程。因此，调查人员必须注意证据的客观性、科学性、法律性，要充分利用录音机、照相机等手段，客观地记录下与当事人的谈话和现场卫生状况，向有关人员询问时，必须做好个案调查记录，并经被调查者签字认可。根据现场流行病学调查和实验室检验可确定食物中毒的原因。

本次食物中毒事件，调查人员对中毒可疑食物进行了流行病学调查。经调查，该酒店是前一天（1日）下午从××海鲜批发商购买的扇贝，该批次共20 kg，均为鲜活。在海水中暂养，分别供应10月1日晚餐、夜宵和10月2日午餐，由于10月2日午餐就餐人数多，炊事人员忙中生乱忘了烹饪时间，扇贝没有蒸熟就端上了餐桌。而该桌就餐人员都是内陆城市游客，以为海鲜就要"半生不熟"才新鲜，并没有对菜品质量进行反馈。

5. 如何进行现场采样和检验

（1）患者呕吐物的采集：患者呕吐物采集应在患者服药前进行。对疑似细菌性食物中毒，应采集患者急性期（3天内）和恢复期（2周左右）静脉血3 mL。

（2）食物采集：采集剩余可疑食物，必要时也可采集可疑食物的半成品或原料。

本起食物中毒事件调查人员以无菌操作，采集了海鲜销售摊点、酒店剩下的扇贝及餐桌剩下的扇贝各一份，呕吐物6份，病人发病时血液及同一人2天后血液、粪便各14份。样品经加注标签，编号，严密封袋，并附加采样时间、条件、重点怀疑病原（副溶血性弧菌），签字后送至实验室检验。实验室按肠道致病菌检验常规，经增菌、分离、纯培养，生化检验、血清学鉴定，从所有扇贝及病人的吐、泻物中均检出了副溶血性弧菌。14份病人血清凝集效价均比发病当时显著升高，均增至1∶40～1∶320。

6. 对食物中毒如何处理

（1）控制措施：确认疑似食物中毒后，调查人员要依法采取行政控制措施，防止食物中毒范围扩大。

（2）控制范围：包括封存可疑食物及其原料，被污染的食品用具、加工设备、容器，并责令其清洗、消毒。

（3）行政控制：使用加盖卫生行政部门印章的封条封存可疑食物及其原料，下达"行政控制决定书"。在紧急情况下，调查人员可现场封存并做记录，然后报卫生行政部门批准，补送"行政控制决定书"。行政控制时间为15天，卫生行政部门应在封存之日起15天内完成对封存物的检验或做出评价，并做出销毁或解封决定。

本次食物中毒处理如下：卫生监督部门当即责令该酒店，停止供应扇贝，就地封存，并通过进货渠道，找到卖扇贝的摊点，也一并就地封存，凡接触过扇贝的工具、器皿一律消毒处理。

（4）追回、销毁导致中毒的食物：根据现场调查与检验结果，对确认的中毒食物卫生部门可直接予以销毁，也可在卫生行政部门的监督下，由肇事单位自行销毁，对已经售出的中毒食物要责令肇事者追回销毁。

（5）中毒场所处理：根据不同性质的食物中毒，对中毒场所采取相应措施。对接触细菌性食物中毒的餐具、用具、容器、设备等，用1%～2%碱水煮沸消毒或用有效氯含量为150～200 mg/L的氯制剂溶液浸泡消毒；对接触化学性食物中毒的类似物品，要用碱液进行彻底清洗。

（6）对急救治疗方案进行必要的纠正与补充。

7. 如何进行行政处罚

现场调查处理后，调查人员应对流行病学调查资料进行整理分析，结合实验室结果做出最后的诊断，写出完整的调查报告。

卫生监督部门对生产经营单位一般可采取一些处罚措施。处罚措施包括警告、停业整顿、限期改进、销毁食品、没收违法所得、罚款、吊销卫生许可证等。具体采取哪种处罚措施，卫生行政部门应按违法事实、证据、适用有关法律，制作执法文书，按执法程序进行行政处罚。

（李彦川）

Chapter Six | Cases and Practices of Health Education
第六章 | 健康教育案例与实践

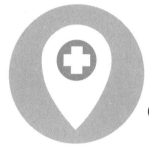

Chapter Six Cases and Practices of Health Education
第六章 健康教育案例与实践

Experiment 33 Design and Evaluation of Audience-centered Health Communication Materials

Ⅰ. Objectives

(1) To master the production process of audience-centered health communication materials.

(2) To familiarize with the principles of making audience-centered health communication materials.

(3) To understand the evaluation method of audience-centered health communication materials and the significance of pre-experimentation.

Ⅱ. Practice Contents

1. Health communication and health communication materials

Health communication is a kind of behavior to transform the research results in the medical field into popular health knowledge which is widely accepted by the public, and to reduce the morbidity and mortality of diseases in the population by changing the public's attitude and behavior towards health, so as to improve the quality of life and health of the public. Health communication is also a process of making, transmitting, communicating, and sharing health information for the purpose of maintaining and promoting human health, with the health of everyone as the starting point and using various media and methods.

Health communication materials are the carriers of health information in health education communication activities. Health communication materials can generally be divided into three types. Type Ⅰ: Text printing materials, including leaflets, folding pages, brochures, posters, picture albums, magazines, books, etc. Type Ⅱ: Audio-visual materials, including television, radio, movies, electronic slides, video, audio, mobile phone SMS, Internet, etc. Type Ⅲ: Physical materials. When developing health communication materials, consideration should first be given to selecting available materials from existing communication materials in order to save time and resources.

The design and manufacture of health communication materials should follow the following principles:

(1) The form and content of materials should be closely related to the theme of communication.

(2) Communication materials should be targeted.

(3) The production capacity, technical level, resource conditions and the difficulty of the materials to be produced should be considered to ensure the feasibility of the production plan.

(4) When making materials, it should be considered to being suitable for the selected medium.

(5) Health communication materials should conform to the psychosocial, ethical, and cultural characteristics of the target population.

(6) The communication materials should be unified and harmonious overall, with prominent emphasis.

The 20th century saw three leaps in the health communication media: radio, television, and the Internet. The Internet has formed a cross-country, cross-language and cross-culture space for the exchange of health information. With the rapid development of Internet and computer technology, new media emerged at the right moment, such as digital newspaper, digital magazine, microblog, WeChat, Tik Tok and so on. At present, the health education content on the Internet mainly involves general disease prevention knowledge, health preserving in four seasons, prevention and treatment of common diseases, mental health, prevention and control of infectious diseases (such as SARS, influenza, AIDS, dengue fever, Ebola, COVID-19, etc.).

New media has gradually integrated the communication characteristics of all traditional media and gradually became an omnimedia, bringing about the renewal of health communication methods and communication concepts. New media is built based on digital technology and network technology, taking multimedia as the presentation form of information. It is characterized by flexibility, diversity, large amount of information, rich content, storageable of information, continuity of dissemination, low cost, fast dissemination, fast update, convenient retrieval, and wide audience.

New media has significant advantages in the dissemination of health information. Firstly, traditional media is mainly one-way communication, and the feedback channels of the audience are not smooth. However, new media can realize the process of asking and answering, showing a good interactive advantage. Secondly, new media can quickly obtain the latest health information, and spread the latest and most timely content to the audience at the fastest speed, showing a good timeliness advantage. Thirdly, new media can provide "one-on-one" personalized information to the audience and meet the different needs of different groups of people for different information. Therefore, it has the advantage of clustering. Fourthly, the Internet allows communicators to publish multiple health information at the same time, and the audience can choose their own appropriate time to watch or receive health information, so it has the advantage of non-synchronicity. Finally, new media is also economical and efficient. However, in the continuous development of new media, its disadvantages are also appearing constantly. For example, the standardized management of information is weak and false information is rampant, information homogenization and dilution, uneven distribution of information resources, the professional quality of communicators is uneven, privacy breach and so on.

2. Production procedures for health communication materials

Effective health communication activities must aim at assisting target populations in changing unhealthy behavior and adopting healthy lifestyles. This requires health educators to strengthen the idea that the target population is the center, to strengthen the research on the target population in health communication activities, to formulate appropriate communication strategies, and to develop suitable communication materials.

(1) Analysis of needs and identification of communication topics.

Through literature review, audience survey and other methods, the characteristics and needs of the audience were investigated and analyzed in order to collect first-hand information to produce health communication materials. Preliminarily determine the information content of health communication materials.

(2) Plan for production of health communication materials.

Based on the demand analysis, according to its own production capacity, technology level and economic situation, determine the content and type of health communication, health materials plan is constructed. The plan should include determining the determination of the target population, the types of materials, usage scope, distribution channel, usage method, preliminary experiment, evaluation method and budget, etc.

(3) Completion of the first draft of health communication materials.

The design process of the first draft is the process of information research and formation. According to the determined information content and production requirements, design the first draft of materials. The complexity of information and the amount of information are determined according to the education level and acceptance ability of the target population.

(4) Preliminary experiment of health communication materials.

Pre-experiment refers to the process in which a small part of the target population is selected for experimental use of the health communication material before the final draft production, the target population's response to the material is systematically collected, and the communication material will be repeatedly modified according to the feedback of the target population. The number of preliminary experiments should be determined according to the quality of the first draft, the opinions of the experimental subjects, and the treatment of the revised draft. It takes 2 – 3 times in general.

(5) Design and manufacture of health communication materials.

After the preliminary experiment, the final draft of the health communication materials shall be determined according to the principles of timeliness, scientificity, artistry and economy.

(6) Production, distribution, and usage.

The final draft of the health communication materials shall be submitted to the responsible personnel for review and approval, and production shall be arranged according to the plan. Determine distribution channels of communication materials to ensure adequate distribution of communication materials to the target population. At the same time, provide the necessary training to the disseminators of communication materials so that they know how to use these communication materials effectively.

(7) Monitoring and evaluation.

Evaluate the production quality, distribution, usage status and communication effect of materials under actual conditions, so as to summarize the experience and find out deficiencies, and guide the production plan of new communication materials.

3. **Requirements and methods for making common health communication materials**

(1) Leaflets.

Production requirements:

①Define the theme.

②Pictures in the health communication materials should be novel. Through the publicity of pictures, people will have a deeper understanding of health knowledge and finally accept relevant health knowledge.

③Words should be concise. The text should have affinity with the audience, respect the audience, and make the audience easy to accept.

Manufacture method: A leaflet generally consists of three parts: title, body, and contact information.

①The title is the most important element of a leaflet. The title should be attractive enough to draw the audience's attention and guide the audience to read the text of the leaflet and watch the illustrations of the leaflet. The title should be in a larger font size and should be placed in the most prominent position on the leaflet.

②The text of the leaflet is the content of the leaflet, which is basically an extension of the title. The text of the leaflet is centered and usually arranged around or above the illustration.

③The illustration of the leaflet, the color version should be bright and gorgeous, black and white version should be layered.

④The contact information of the leaflet is the name, address and telephone number of the unit that distributing the leaflet. Contact information can be placed under the title or at the end of the article.

(2) Poster.

Production requirements: The general requirement is to be clear. A poster usually contains three elements: color, picture, and text. Among them color is more important. We first need to set a theme to collect materials around this topic, and then determine the main tone of the poster, the use of graphic fonts, etc.

Manufacture method:

①Full visual impact, can be achieved through the image and color. The color matching should make the audience feel comfortable without visual fatigue, and it should apply color based on the premise of people's perception of color.

②Keep it short and to the point.

③Picture is the main part, text as a supplement.

④Subject font should be bold, text left aligned is neat, clear, and orderly. Text right alignment is suitable for a small number of texts, and it will produce a specific visual effect. Text center alignment appears to be solemn, traditional, classic. Free typesetting is suitable for a small number of words or headings, it appears to be perceptual freedom, relaxed and lively.

⑤Important content should be placed at the height 2/3 of the poster.

4. Case analysis

The Fei-Long lake area is one of the endemic areas of schistosomiasis in China. Schistosomiasis control among fishermen in the region is a priority for local public health. To elevate the prevention awareness of fishermen, develop healthy behaviors and lifestyles, and reduce the risk of schistosomiasis infection, the local Center for Disease Control and Prevention (CDC) launched a "behavior-oriented" popularization activity for schistosomiasis control. The local health education institute in CDC plans to carry out health education on schistosomiasis and develop a set of health communication materials targeted at the local schistosomiasis.

Before to the material design, the team of health communication materials research and development personally conducted a field survey in the Fei-Long lake area. Yun-Long village is a village around Fei-Long lake with a total of 432 households and 1983 fishermen. The field survey found out that this village has the village committee, village clinic, kindergarten, primary school, fishing self-help team and other organizations and groups. According to the survey, there are 4 fixed propaganda columns, 1 activity room and 1 library, and 1 recreational team of fishermen square dancing in the village. In each year's fishing off season, the Mid-Autumn Festival, the Double Ninth Festival and the Spring Festival, there are folk performances and fishermen's spontaneous recreational activities in the Yun-Long village.

A sampling survey was conducted among 350 adult fishermen in Yun-Long village, 180 males and 170 females, aged from 21 to 70 years old, with an average age of 43 years old. The respondents generally have a low level of education, with illiteracy accounting for 9.5%, primary school and junior high school education accounting for 43% and 32% respectively, and senior high school education accounting for 6.8%. The survey also indicated that 17% (61/350) of the fishermen were unaware that schistosomiasis was harmful to the human body and 31.42% (110/350) of the fishermen were unaware of the risk of transmission of schistosomiasis by means of direct discharge of feces into the lake water. 90.57% (117/350) of the fishermen expressed their willingness to undergo schistosomiasis testing, and control. Exposure of fishermen to infected water: 84.86% (297/350) of fishermen spent more than 5 hours a day in contact of infected water due to fishing in the lake. When washing clothes and vegetables in the lake water, 92.57% (324/350) of the fishermen did not wear rubber clothes or gloves.

According to the results of the survey, 84.86% (297/350) of the respondents consider the posters about the protection against schistosomiasis with the fishermen companion as one of their preferred methods. In addition, 54.85 percent (192/350) of the respondents said that skits and popular songs about schistosomiasis may help them remember the dangers of schistosomiasis and how to control it.

Based on the above results of field survey, please analyze the following questions:

(1) Please set the educational goals for the local health communication materials for

schistosomiasis control.

(2) As the person in charge of the project, please determine the target audience and the purpose of health communication for schistosomiasis control.

(3) Based on the above survey results, please analyze the knowledge, attitude, and behavior of the local fishermen on schistosomiasis control.

(4) What health communication materials are suitable for the local fishermen and why?

(5) What do you learn from the practice of this case?

Ⅲ. Practice tasks

According to the content of this case, one poster in A3 paper size and one leaflet in A4 paper size will be made in the form of a team. Topics are optional.

Ⅳ. Exercises

(1) What are the production procedures for audience-centered health communication materials?

(2) What are the general categories of health communication materials?

(3) What are the advantages of new media in the dissemination of health information?

(4) What challenges do new media face in dissemination of health information?

实验三十三 以受众为中心的健康传播材料设计与评价

一、实习目的

(1) 掌握以受众为中心的健康传播材料的制作程序。

(2) 熟悉以受众为中心的健康传播材料的制作原则。

(3) 了解以受众为中心的健康传播材料的评价,预实验的意义。

二、实习内容

1. 健康传播与健康传播材料

健康传播(health communication)是一种将医学领域的研究成果转化为大众能够广泛接受的通俗易懂的健康知识,并通过改变大众对健康的态度和行为,降低疾病在群体中的患病率和死亡率,最终达到有效提高大众生活质量和健康水平的行为。健康传播也是以人人健康为出发点,运用各种传播媒介和方法,为维护和促进人类健康的目的而制作、传递、交流、分享健康信息的过程。

健康传播材料(health communication materials)是在健康教育传播活动中健康信息的载体。健康传播材料一般可分为三类:第一类是文字印刷材料,包括宣传单、折页、小册子、宣传画、海报、画册、杂志、书籍等。第二类是音像视听材料,包括电视、广播、电影、电子幻灯片、视频、音频、手机短信、网络等。第三类是各种实物材料。在制作健康传播材料时，首先应该考虑从现有的传播材料中选择可利用的材料，以便节约时间和资源。

健康传播材料设计制作应该遵循以下原则：

（1）材料的形式和内容应紧扣传播的主题。

（2）传播材料要具有针对性。

（3）要考虑制作机构的制作能力、技术水平、资源条件、拟制作材料的难易程度等以保证制作计划具有可行性。

（4）制作材料时应考虑要适合于所选择的媒介。

（5）健康传播材料应符合目标人群的社会心理、伦理和文化特点。

（6）传播材料应从总体上保持统一与和谐，重点突出。

健康传播媒体在20世纪经历了三次飞跃：广播、电视和网络。互联网形成了跨国家、跨语言和跨文化的健康信息交流空间。目前互联网的健康教育内容主要涉及一般疾病预防知识、四季养生、常见病防治、心理健康、传染病防控［如严重急性呼吸综合征（SARS）、流感、艾滋病、登革热、埃博拉、新冠肺炎等］。伴随着互联网和计算机技术的迅猛发展，新媒体应运而生，例如数字报纸、数字杂志、微博、微信、抖音等。新媒体逐渐整合了所有传统媒体的传播特征，逐渐变成了一种全媒体，带来了健康传播方式和传播理念的更新。新媒体是建立在数字技术和网络技术的基础上，以多媒体作为信息的呈现形式。新媒体具有灵活多样、信息量大、内容丰富，信息可储存、传播的再延续性，成本低、传播快、更新快、检索方便、受众广等特点。

新媒体传播健康信息具有显著优势。第一，传统媒体主要是单向性传播，受众反馈渠道不通畅，然而新媒体可以实现一问一答的过程，展现出很好的互动性优势。第二，新媒体能迅速获取最新健康信息，并以最快的速度将最新、最及时的内容传播给受众，展现出良好的时效性优势。第三，新媒体能向受众提供"一对一"的个性化信息，满足不同人群对不同信息的不同需求，具有分群性优势。第四，互联网使传播者可以同时发布多条健康信息，而受众可以随意选择自己合适的时间观看或接受健康信息，具有非同步性优势。最后，新媒体也具有经济性和高效性。然而，在新媒体的不断发展中，其弊端也在不断显现，如信息的规范化管理薄弱，虚假信息泛滥；信息同质化、飞沫化；信息资源分配不均；传播者专业素质参差不齐；隐私泄露等诸多问题。

2. 健康传播材料的制作程序

有效的健康传播活动必须致力于协助目标人群改变不良的行为习惯，采纳健康的生活方式。这就要求健康教育工作者强化以目标人群为中心的思想，在健康传播活动中加强对目标人群的研究，制定适宜的传播策略，研制适用的传播材料。

（1）分析需求和确定传播主题。

通过查阅文献、受众调查等方法对受众的特征及其需求进行调查分析，为制作健康传播材料收集第一手资料。初步确定健康传播材料的信息内容。

（2）制订健康传播材料的计划。

在需求分析的基础之上，根据自身的制作能力、技术水平、经济状况，确定健康传播的内容和种类，制订健康材料制作计划，计划应包括确定目标人群、材料的种类、材料的内容、使用范围、发放渠道、使用方法、预实验、评价方法和经费预算等。

（3）形成初稿。

初稿的设计过程是信息的研究与形成过程。根据确定的信息内容和制作要求，设计出材料初稿。根据目标人群的文化程度和接受能力决定信息复杂程度和信息量的大小。

（4）预实验。

预实验是指传播材料在最终定稿和投入生产之前，选取少部分目标人群进行试验性使用，系统收集目标人群对该信息的反映，并根据反馈意见对传播材料进行反复修改的过程。预实验的次数需要根据初稿的质量、预实验对象的意见、修改稿的治疗等情况来确定。一般来说需要 2～3 次。

（5）设计制作。

预实验后，根据时效性、科学性、艺术性、经济性的原则，确定健康传播材料的终稿。

（6）生产、发放与使用。

确定健康传播材料终稿后，应交付有关负责人员审阅批准，按照计划安排生产。确定和落实传播材料的发放渠道，以保证足够的传播材料发放到目标人群。同时对传播材料的发放人员进行必要的培训，使他们懂得如何有效地使用这些传播材料。

（7）监测与评价。

在实际条件下对材料的制作质量、发放、使用状况、传播效果做出评价，以便总结经验、发现不足，用以指导新的传播材料的制作计划。

3. **常见健康传播材料的制作要求与方法**

（1）宣传单。

制作要求：①明确主题。②图片要新颖。通过图片的宣传，使人们对健康知识有更深入的了解，最终接受相关健康知识。③文字要精简。文字对受众要有亲和力，尊重受众，使受众容易接受。

制作方法：宣传单一般由标题、正文和联系信息三部分组成。①标题是宣传单制作的最重要元素。标题应具有吸引力，能使受众注目，引导受众阅读宣传单正文、观看宣传单插图。标题要用较大号字体，要安排在宣传单画面最醒目的位置。②宣传单正文是说明宣传单内容的文字，基本上是标题的扩展。宣传单正文文字居中，一般都安排在插画的左右或上下方。③宣传单的插画，彩色版要鲜艳绚丽，黑白版要层次分明。④宣传单的联系方式即传单派发单位的名称、地址和电话。联系方式可以放在标题下面，也可以放在文末。

（2）海报。

制作要求：海报制作的总要求是使人一目了然。海报一般包含三个元素——色彩、图像和文字，其中色彩较为重要。制作时，首先需要设定一个主题，围绕着这个主题收集素材，然后确定好海报的主色调、图形字体的运用等。

制作方法：①充分的视觉冲击力，可以通过图像和色彩来实现。配色应使受众视觉感到舒适而不会产生视觉疲劳，以人们对色彩的感受为前提来应用色彩。②内容精练，抓住要点。③以图为主，以文案为辅。④主题字体醒目，文字左对齐，整齐划一，清晰有序；

文字右对齐适合少量文字，会产生特定的视觉效果；文字中心对齐显得庄严、传统、经典；文字自由排版适合少量文字或标题，显得感性自由，轻松活泼。⑤重要内容放置在海报的 2/3 高度处。

4. 案例分析

飞龙湖地区是我国血吸虫病流行区之一，该地区渔民的血吸虫病防治是当地公共卫生的重点工作。为了提高渔民自我防范意识并养成健康的行为生活方式，降低血吸虫病的感染风险，当地疾病预防控制中心开展了一项"行为导向"的血吸虫病防治的科普活动。当地健康教育所准备开展血吸虫病的健康教育并研发一套针对当地的血吸虫病健康传播材料。

在开展材料设计之前，健康传播材料研发团队亲自到飞龙湖地区开展了实地调查。云龙村是环绕飞龙湖的一个村庄，共有 432 户人家，有渔民 1983 人。该村有村委会、村卫生室、幼儿园、小学、渔业自助小队等组织和团体。调查发现，村里用于宣传的资源有固定宣传栏 4 块，村活动室和图书馆各 1 间，渔民广场舞文娱团队 1 支。在每年的禁渔期、中秋节、重阳节和春节都有民俗表演活动及渔民自发的文娱活动。

采用抽样调查的方式调查了云龙村 350 名成年渔民。其中，男性 180 人，女性 170 人，年龄为 21～70 岁，平均年龄为 43 岁。被调查者受教育程度普遍偏低，文盲者占比 9.5%，小学和初中文化分别占比 43% 和 32%，高中文化占比 6.8%。调查还发现有 17%（61/350）的渔民不知道血吸虫病对人体会造成伤害，31.42%（110/350）的渔民不知道粪便直接排入水中的方式具有传播血吸虫病的风险。90.57%（117/350）的渔民表示愿意接受血吸虫病检查和防治。渔民接触疫水情况：渔民因在湖里捕鱼，每天接触时间在 5 个小时以上，占 84.86%（297/350）。在用湖水洗衣洗菜时，有 92.57%（324/350）的渔民不穿橡胶衣裤或戴橡胶手套。

调查结果显示，有 84.86%（297/350）的调查对象认为张贴有渔民同伴的血吸虫病防护方法的海报是他们乐于接受的方式之一。此外，有 54.85%（192/350）的被调查者认为有关血吸虫病的小品和相关脍炙人口的歌曲可能有助于他们记住血吸虫病的危害和防治方法。

根据以上实地调查结果，请分析以下问题：
（1）请为当地的血吸虫病防治健康传播材料设定教育目标。
（2）作为该项目的负责人，请你为本次血吸虫病防治拟定受众对象和健康传播目的。
（3）结合上述调查结果，请分析当地渔民的血吸虫病防治知识、态度和行为情况。
（4）针对当地渔民，适合他们的健康传播材料有哪些，为什么？
（5）通过本案例的实践，你从中获得哪些启示？

三、练习任务

根据本次案例内容，主题自选或以上面的案例内容为主题，以小组为单位分别制作 A3 纸大小的海报 1 份、A4 纸大小的宣传单 1 份。

四、练习

（1）以受众为中心的健康传播材料制作程序有哪些？

（2）健康传播材料一般可分为几类？

（3）新媒体传播健康信息的优势有哪些？

（4）新媒体传播健康信息面临的挑战有哪些？

Experiment 34　Assessment of Community Health Education

Ⅰ. Objectives

(1) To master the concepts and procedures of community assessment, and the design principles and procedures of health education intervention plans.

(2) To familiarize with the purpose of community assessment.

(3) To understand the content of community assessment.

Ⅱ. Practice Contents

1. Community assessment and the Green model

The first task of health education and health promotion practice is how to design, implement and evaluate the health education and health promotion project in combination with the theories of health education and health promotion, so as to ensure the pertinence and effectiveness of behavioral intervention for a certain target behavior. Behavior occurs in a certain environment and situation. How to analyze the environmental factors that influence behavior is also an important aspect of health education and health promotion practice.

Community assessment means that community health service workers use sociology, epidemiology, anthropology, and other research methods to comprehensively investigate the resources of target communities, find problems, and collect data through qualitative and quantitative investigation and research methods. Through scientific and objective analysis, the main public health problems in this community are determined and the main health problems and influencing factors that need to be solved urgently in this community are found out, so as to provide scientific basis for the establishment of community health service plan. Making a good community assessment is the basis and key to make the intervention plan of community health education and health promotion.

In community assessment, the guiding theory that frequently used is the Green model, which provides an effective and simple method for community assessment. According to the Green model, the following five assessment steps are performed in sequence before an intervention or

Chapter Six Cases and Practices of Health Education
第六章　健康教育案例与实践

education plan is developed.

Firstly, sociological assessment is made to identify various problems related to healthy life in specific communities, starting from the current situation and social problems of the community. These problems are then prioritized according to different indicators such as degree of need, importance, and impact. At this stage, the social problems currently facing of the community should be identified, and the quality of life and health service needs of the community residents should be evaluated.

Secondly, epidemiological assessment should be carried out based on social assessment. Prioritize the health issues and understand the surveillance data for target populations. These data include life expectancy, birth rate, morbidity rate, mortality rate, etc. And then select the most urgent health issues that are likely to be addressed, based on considering the resources currently available to the community and its problem-solving capacity.

Thirdly, from the perspective of behavior and environment assessment, identify the factors that are most likely to affect health problems and most likely to change, and then set the goals of health intervention based on this. In the assessment of behavior and environment at this time, we should first start from the individual behavior or lifestyle, then evaluate from influential people around the individual, and finally from the influential factors in his life environment.

Fourthly, educational and ecological assessment explores the factors that affect the health behaviors of the target population, and finds out the motivation for behavioral change and the factors that make the new behaviors sustainable. The Green model classifies the factors that affect human health behavior into three categories: predisposing, enabling, and reinforcing factor. Predisposing factor, which is also called antecedent factor, refers to the existing influencing factors before an individual engages in a certain behavior, namely the reason for the occurrence of a certain behavior, including the individual's knowledge, attitude, belief, and values, as well as demographic characteristics such as age, gender, race, family income and occupation. Enabling factor refers to the factors contributing to behavioral change, that is, the factors enabling an individual to carry out a certain behavior. Enabling factor can influence behavior directly or indirectly through the environment, including the resources and skills needed to achieve a certain behavior. Reinforcing factor refers to the factors that affect the persistence or repetition of behaviors, such as the reward after the formation of good behaviors, family support, and behavior demonstration by important figures.

Fifthly, administrative and policy assessment should be carried out. Identify appropriate strategies based on the impact factors established in the previous phases, and consider the resources, equipment, and policies needed to implement and sustain the plan, as well as the obstacles that may be encountered.

2. **Procedures for community health education assessment**

(1) Preparation for community assessment.

In the case of community assessment, community mobilization should be initiated in order to obtain the cooperation of all sectors and to mobilize the active participation of families and individuals in the community. Secondly, the methods of diagnosis, sampling, information (data) collection, statistical analysis of data, standards of quality control and budget should be determined.

(2) Information collection.

Data collection is an important part and a key link of community assessment. The work of data collection mainly includes collection of the existing data and data from specific surveys in community.

①Demographic information of the community, including the information of the registered population and the information of the temporary residents, which can be obtained from police stations of street.

②Information on the community environment, including physical environment, cultural facilities, community economy, community institutions, floating population, and community services, which can be obtained from sub-district offices and neighborhood committees.

③Information on poverty and disability in the community which can be obtained from the civil affairs office and the disabled persons' federation.

④Information on community health resources, including health institution resources and health human resources, which can be obtained from the health administration.

⑤Statistics on the incidence and death of infectious diseases in the community which can be obtained from local disease prevention and control agencies.

⑥ Information on the prevalence of diseases among community residents which can be obtained from on-the-spot investigations of residents.

⑦Information on the main behavioral risk factors and bad living habits of community residents which can be consulted on the health records of community residents or the special investigation of community residents.

(3) Information sorting, statistical description, and analysis of data.

After being examined, the collected data will be put into the database, the appropriate indicators for statistical description and analysis will be selected. It is suggested that the data should be collated and analyzed according to Green assessment model.

① Demographic assessment: analyze the features of the community, the demographic characteristics of the community, the payment of the medical expenses of residents, and the environmental resources of the community.

② Epidemiological assessment: death statistical analysis, analysis on the incidence of infectious diseases, analysis on the incidence of chronic diseases, etc.

③Behavioral and environmental assessment: risk factor analysis of behavioral and lifestyle, analysis of the basic health knowledge of the population, analysis of enabling and reinforcing factor.

④ Management and policy assessment: analysis of data from community health service centers, the implementation of community health education, the supply of basic medical services

Chapter Six Cases and Practices of Health Education

in the community.

(4) Determination of the major health issues in the community.

A comprehensive analysis is carried out to identify the major health problems in the community based on the prevalence and severity of disease in the community. At this step, the community health issues should be listed. The following principles should be followed in determining the list of major issues.

①A disease that causes many deaths or those in the first order of death.

②The main causes of potential life loss and disease.

③Morbidity and mortality rates in the community are higher than the national average.

④The main risk factors including behavioral and non-behavioral risk factors, which are associated with death from these diseases.

(5) Selection of target behavior for intervention.

After identifying the target disease in the community, all factors that influence the development of the disease including behavioral and non-behavioral factors, should be found. According to the importance and variability principles of determining priority intervention factors, the target behaviors of intervention will be selected based on the information of all behavior risk factors related to the occurrence and development of the disease obtained through the community survey.

3. Case on community health education assessment

Sunshine community is in the south of an urban area, 30 kilometers away from the downtown area, and covers an area of about 80 square kilometers, among which there are more than 10 provincial and municipal enterprises and institutions, more than 50 private enterprises and individual commercial outlets. These enterprises are mainly engaged in chemical industry, smelting, papermaking, building materials, food and so on. This community is a mixed community for residents, mainly for trade, industry, agriculture, and travel. In recent years, with the development of the community economy, the continuous improvement of people's living conditions, and the acceleration of the aging process of the population, the prevalence of cerebrovascular diseases among the community residents has been rising significantly. Stroke mortality and paralysis rates among people over 60 years old are higher than this city's average.

There are four neighborhood committees in the community. The total number of households is 9723. The permanent population is 22015 and the floating population is 2323. There are 11212 males and 10803 females in this community. There are 3753 women of childbearing age and 92 low-income households. The number of persons with disabilities is 401, including 111 persons with mental disabilities. The number of annual deaths in the community is 131, with a mortality rate of 5.95‰. The number of people born in the community is 112, with the birth rate of 5.05‰. The number of natural population growth is −19, with the natural growth rate of −0.85‰. The natural population growth is declining in Sunshine community. Most of the residents are Han Chinese, accounting for 99.7%.

This survey uses random cluster sampling method to randomly select 200 households in each neighborhood committee, a total of 800 households, 2373 people as the survey objects, among which 1183 are males and 1190 are females. People over 60 years old is for accounted 25.46% Most of the occupation are workers, accounting for 30.21%, followed by domestic workers, accounting for 20.34%. Other population distribution characteristics are shown in Table 34 – 1 and Table 34 – 2.

Table 34 – 1   Age composition of residents in Sunshine community

Ages/year	Numbers	Proportion/%
0 –	229	
10 –	243	
20 –	273	
30 –	454	
40 –	327	
50 –	243	
60 –	489	
70 –	115	
Total	2373	

Note: Proportion (%) = (the number of people at a certain age ÷ the total number of people in this survey) ×100%.

Table 34 – 2   The composition of the educational level of some community residents

Degrees of education	Numbers	Proportion/%
Primary schools and below	243	
Junior high school	281	
Senior high school	1004	
University and above	845	
Total	2373	

Note: Proportion (%) = (the number of people with some degree of education ÷ the total number of people) ×100%.

According to the survey, the medical payments of the residents in this community are urban basic health insurance programs for urban staff and workers, accounting for 45.73%, followed by the medical insurance for urban residents and self-pay, accounting for 23.02% and 16.66% respectively. Rural cooperative health insurance is accounted for 8.47% and commercial insurance is accounted for 6.11%. There are 6 kindergartens, 3 primary schools, 2 junior high schools and 1 senior high school in the community. According to the investigation, 131 residents died in this

Chapter Six Cases and Practices of Health Education

community in the past year, and the top five causes of death are shown in Table 34-3.

The investigation found out that the occurrence of infectious diseases was mainly dominated by tuberculosis in the community. The incidence of tuberculosis in 2019 was on the rise from 0.34‰ to 1.02‰ compared with that in 2018. The incidence of chronic diseases in this community is shown in Table 34-4. The number of pregnant women in this community was 218: 208 were registered for early pregnancy, 204 were managed during pregnancy, 86 were in high-risk pregnancy. There were 82 cases of common diseases in pregnant women, including 1 case of gestational hypertension, 1 case of gestational diabetes, 5 cases of gestational anemia, and 75 cases of other diseases.

Table 34-3 The causes of death and the sequence of causes of death throughout the year

Diseases	Numbers of deaths	Proportion of death/%	Mortality rate/ (1/100000)	Rank of death cause
Cadiocerebrovascular diseases	46			
Tumors	37			
Respiratory diseases	26			
Digestive system diseases	9			
Urinary system disease	6			
Other diseases	6			
Total	131			

Note: Mortality rate = (the number of deaths from diseases ÷ the registered population of the street) × 100000 (1/100000). Rate of death cause = (the number of deaths from a disease ÷ total number of deaths from a disease) × 100%.

Table 34-4 The prevalence of chronic diseases in Sunshine Community

Name of disease	Number	Proportion/%	Prevalence/%
Hypertension	345		
Coronary heart disease	106		
Diabetes	34		
Tumor	15		
Chronic gastritis	56		
Other	25		
Total	581		

Note: Prevalence = the number of new and old cases of a disease in a population in a specific period ÷ the number of observed population in the same period, Proportion (%) = the number of people with certain disease ÷ the total number of people.

The main risk factors affecting chronic diseases of the community residents are shown in Table 34-5. The survey found out that 547 (28.77%) of the community surveyed population aged 20 or above had attended the health knowledge lecture in the institutions of community health service, and 71.23% of the community residents have not attended any lectures. The total awareness rate of hypertension prevention knowledge, diagnostic criteria and risk factors were 67.69%, 48.23% and 56.52% respectively. Those who believed that reducing salt intake could prevent high blood pressure accounted for 36.34%. Among those with salty taste, only 16.75% were willing to reduce salt intake. And only 18.2% of the smokers were willing to quit.

Only 12.03% of the respondents used salt spoons to control their salt intake. Only 15.65% of the smokers were willing to quit and knew how to control withdrawal symptoms during the quitting process. There is no free place to measure blood pressure in the community. Residents can only measure their blood pressure when they register for medical treatment at the community health service center. The percentage of respondents with an electronic blood pressure meter was 13.37%. When asked whether they supported the use of a low-salt diet for people with high blood pressure at home (If they did), 21.78% of families supported it. 66.32% of hypertensive patients (If any) were encouraged to take the prescribed medication at home.

Table 34-5 Prevalence of major risk factors for chronic diseases

Risk factors	Number	Prevalence/%
Lack of physical exercise	872	
Overweight, obesity	719	
Eat salted food often	653	
Intake of fruits and vegetables is less than half jin /day	592	
Smoking	539	
High intake of salt	267	
Drink	392	

The survey found out that the total value of fixed assets of the community health service center was 2607300 yuan, among which 25 professional equipment that above 10000 yuan were worth 923600 yuan. There are 85 staff members in the community health service center, including 32 males and 53 females. There are 70 registered health technicians, including 25 medical practitioners, 4 assistant medical practitioners, 16 registered nurses, 13 pharmaceutical personnel, 2 inspectors and 8 others. There are 4 registered technical personnel of other profession. According to the professional and technical titles, there are 13 people of undetermined level, 26 people of primary level, 27 people of intermediate level and 4 people of deputy high level.

This community health service center has a total of 97327 person-times of outpatient and emergency, 41457 person-times of general practice, 13729 person-times of medical insurance, 191 person-times of family ward and 62 person-times of family diagnosis and treatment. The main diseases in the outpatient department are cold, tracheitis, hypertension, arthritis, etc. The main diseases of family ward are cerebral apoplexy sequelae, hypertension, and lumbar fracture.

The community has four bulletin boards, which are replaced every two months. More than 20 kinds of health education prescriptions were issued, a total of 32700 copies. Regularly carry out health education in the community, a total of 7 lectures, 32 times of health education guidance in key places. Social publicity activities on various health awareness days were held six times.

Ⅲ. Practice Tasks

According to the above cases and combined with the methods of community assessment, please complete the following practice contents:

(1) How do you identify the current major health problems in the community?

(2) What needs to be prepared at the beginning of community assessment?

(3) What information should be collected for community assessment? How do you get it?

(4) Please calculate and fill in the blanks in Table 34-1 to Table 34-5.

(5) Based on the information in this case, what do you think are the major health problems in the community? What are the prior health issue to solve?

(6) What are the risk factors of major health problems in the community? What can be interfered with? What can not be interfered with?

Ⅳ. Exercises

(1) What are the definitions of predisposing factor, enabling factor and reinforcing factor?

(2) What are the idea of community assessment in health education?

(3) What are the procedures of health education assessment in community?

实验三十四　社区健康教育诊断

一、实习目的

（1）掌握社区诊断的概念、步骤，健康教育干预计划的设计原则和步骤。

（2）熟悉社区诊断的目的。

（3）了解社区诊断的内容。

二、实习内容

1. 社区诊断与格林模式

健康教育与健康促进实践的第一要务是如何利用健康教育与健康促进相关理论进行健康教育与健康促进项目的设计、实施与评价，从而保证对靶行为的干预有针对性和有效性。行为是在一定环境和情境下发生的，如何分析影响行为的环境因素也是健康教育与健康促进实践的重要方面。

社区诊断（Community assessment）是指社区卫生服务工作者运用社会学、流行病学及人类学等研究方法对目标社区的资源进行综合考察，发现问题，通过定性、定量的调查研究方法和手段收集资料。通过科学、客观的分析，确定该社区的主要公共卫生问题并找出该社区急需解决的主要健康问题及影响因素，为社区卫生服务计划的制订提供科学依据。做好社区诊断是制订社区健康教育与健康促进干预计划的依据和关键。

在社区诊断中，使用较多的指导理论是格林模式（Green model），该理论为社区诊断提供了行之有效且简便易行的诊断思路。格林模式认为，在制订一项干预计划或教育计划之前，要依次进行以下五个诊断步骤：

第一，进行社会学诊断（sociological assessment），即针对特定社区，从社区现况和社会问题入手，找出与健康生活有关的各种问题，然后根据需求程度、重要性和影响程度等不同指标，将这些问题按优先次序排列出来。在此阶段要提出社区面临的社会问题，评价社区居民的生活质量和卫生服务需求。

第二，在社会诊断的基础上开展流行病学诊断（epidemiological assessment），即确立健康问题的优先顺序，了解目标人群的监测资料，包括期望寿命、出生率、患病率、死亡率等，然后参考社区目前拥有的资源及解决问题的能力，选出最迫切需要又有可能解决的健康问题。

第三，从行为和环境的角度（行为与环境诊断，behavior and environment assessment）出发，找出最可能影响健康问题且最可能改变的因素，并据此制订健康干预的目标。在此时的行为与环境诊断中，首先，应该从个人行为或生活方式入手；其次，从个人周围有影响力的人那里进行评估；最后，从他生活的大环境中的影响因素进行评估。

第四，教育与生态学诊断（educational and ecological assessment），探讨影响目标人群健康行为的因素，找出引发行为改变的动机，以及使新行为得以持续的因素。格林模式将影响人类健康行为的因素总结为三类，即倾向因素、促成因素和强化因素。倾向因素（predisposing factor）又称为前置因素，是指个人从事某项行为之前，已经存在的影响因素，即某种行为发生的理由，包括个人的知识、态度、信念、价值观念，以及年龄、性别、种族、家庭收入、职业等人口学特征。促成因素（enabling factor），是指有助于实现行为改变的因素，即促使个人某种行为得以实现的因素。促成因素可以直接影响行为，或间接地通过环境影响行为，包括实现某种行为所需要的资源及技能。强化因素（reinforcing factor），是指影响行为持续或重复的因素，如良好行为形成后的奖励、家庭支持、重要人物的行为示范等。

第五，进行管理与政策诊断（administrative and policy assessment），根据前几个阶段确立的影响因素，分别找出合适的策略，并考虑执行和持续计划时所需要的资源、设备和政策，以及可能遇到的阻碍。

2. 社区健康教育诊断操作步骤

（1）社区诊断的前期准备工作。

在社区诊断时，首先应进行社区动员，以取得各部门的配合并动员家庭和个人积极参与；其次要确定诊断的方法、样本抽样方法、资料收集方法、数据统计分析方法、质量控制标准和经费预算等。

（2）资料收集。

资料收集是开展社区诊断的重要内容和关键环节。社区资料收集主要包括现有资料的收集和社区专项调查。

①社区人口学资料，包括户籍人口情况和暂住人口情况资料，可以从街道派出所获取。

②社区环境资料，包括自然地理环境、文化设施、社区经济、社区机构、流动人口及社区服务等资料，可以从街道办事处、居委会获取。

③社区贫困与残疾人资料，可以从民政与残联部门获取。

④社区卫生资源相关资料，包括卫生机构资源和卫生人力资源，可以从卫生行政部门获取。

⑤社区传染病发病和死亡统计资料，可以从当地疾病预防控制机构获得。

⑥社区居民患病情况资料，可以通过对居民进行现场调查获得。

⑦社区居民主要行为危险因素和生活不良习惯资料，可以查阅社区居民健康档案或对社区居民的专项调查。

（3）资料整理、数据统计描述与分析。

对收集到的社区资料核查以后录入数据库，然后选择合适的指标进行统计描述和统计分析。建议按照格林诊断模式进行资料的整理分析：

①人口学诊断：分析社区特点，社区人口学特征，社区居民医疗费用支付情况，以及社区环境资源情况。

②流行病学诊断：死亡统计分析、传染病发病情况分析、慢性病发病情况分析等。

③行为与环境诊断：行为和生活方式危险因素分析、居民基本卫生知识知晓情况分析、促成因素分析和强化因素分析。

④管理与政策诊断：社区卫生服务中心资源情况、社区健康教育开展情况、社区基本医疗服务供给情况。

（4）确定社区的主要健康问题。

结合疾病发生的普遍性和严重性进行综合分析，确定社区的主要健康问题。此时，应该列出社区主要卫生问题清单。主要问题清单的确定应遵循以下原则：

①引起大量死亡的疾病或死亡顺位中的前几位疾病。

②潜在寿命损失的主要原因和疾病。

③本社区发病、死亡情况严重于全国平均水平的疾病。

④与这些疾病死亡相关的主要危险因素，包括行为和非行为危险因素。

（5）选择靶标行为。

确定该社区的目标疾病后查找资料，找出影响该疾病发生、发展的所有因素，包括行为和非行为因素。结合本社区调查获得有关该疾病发生、发展的所有危险行为因素情况，同时根据确定优先干预因素的重要性和可变性原则，选择本次干预的靶标行为。

3. 案例分析

阳光社区地处某市区南部，距市中心30km，占地面积约80km^2，其中有10余家省、市企事业单位，50余户私人企业及个体商业网点。这些企业主要经营的产业有化工、冶炼、造纸、建材、食品等。该社区为居民混合型社区，以商贸、工业、农业、旅游为主。近年来，随着该社区经济的发展，人民生活条件不断改善；随着人口老龄化进程的加快，社区居民中心脑血管疾病患病率呈明显的上升趋势。60岁以上人群的中风死亡率和瘫痪的比例高出该市的平均水平。

社区内拥有4个居民委员会；有9723户人家；常住人口22015人，流动人口2323人；男性有11212人，女性有10803人，育龄妇女有3753人；低保特困户92户；残疾人数为401人，其中有精神残疾111人。本社区全年死亡人数为131人，死亡率为5.95‰；社区出生人口数为112人，出生率为5.05‰；人口自然增长数为-19人，自然增长率为-0.85‰，人口自然增长呈下降趋势。社区居民多为汉族，约占99.7%。

本次调查采用随机整群抽样方法，在各居委会随机抽取200户，共800户居民，2373人作为调查对象，其中男性1183人，女性1190人；60岁以上老年人比例达25.46%。职业中以工人居多，占30.21%；其次为家政人员，占20.34%。其他人群分布特征见表34-1和表34-2。

表34-1 阳光社区居民年龄构成

年龄/岁	人口数	构成比/%
0～	229	
10～	243	
20～	273	
30～	454	
40～	327	
50～	243	
60～	489	
70～	115	
合计	2373	

注：构成比=（某年龄段人口数÷本次调查总人数）×100%。

表34-2 阳光社区居民文化程度构成

文化程度	人数	构成比/%
小学及以下	243	
初中	281	
高中	1004	
大学及以上	845	
合计	2373	

注：构成比=（某种文化程度人数÷总人数）×100%。

调查发现该社区居民医疗费用支付方式主要以职工基本医疗保险为主，占45.73%；

其次为城镇居民医疗保险和自费,分别为23.02%和16.66%;农村合作医疗占8.47%;商业保险占6.11%。社区有幼儿园6所、小学3所、初级中学2所、高级中学1所。经调查发现,该社区近一年居民死亡人数为131人,死因顺位前五位见表34-3。

表34-3 阳光社区居民全年死亡原因及死因顺位

疾病	死亡人数	死因构成比/%	死亡率/(1/10万)	死因顺位
心脑血管疾病	46	36.8		
肿瘤	36	28.8		
呼吸系统疾病	25	20.00		
消化系统疾病	8	6.4		
泌尿系统疾病	5	4.00		
其他疾病	5	4.00		
合计	125	100.00		

注:死亡率=(疾病致死人数÷本街道户籍人口数)×10万(1/10万);死因构成比=(某疾病死亡人数÷疾病死亡总人数)×100%。

调查发现,该社区传染病的发生主要以肺结核为主。2019年肺结核发病率与2018年相比,呈上升趋势,由0.34‰上升为1.02‰。该社区慢性病患病的发生情况见表34-4。该社区妊娠妇女218人,早孕建卡数为208人,孕期管理数204人,高危妊娠人数86人。孕妇常见病检出人数82人,其中妊娠高血压1人,妊娠糖尿病1人,妊娠贫血5人,其他疾病75人。

表34-4 阳光社区慢性病患病情况

病名	患病人数	构成比/%	患病率/%
高血压	345		
冠心病	106		
糖尿病	34		
肿瘤	15		
慢性胃炎	56		
其他	25		
合计	581		

注:患病率=特定时期某人群中某病新旧病例数÷同期观察总人口数;某病构成比=(某病人数÷患病总人数)×100%。

影响该社区居民慢性病的主要危险因素见表34-5。调查发现20岁及以上的社区调查人群中参加过社区卫生服务机构卫生知识讲座的有547人,占28.77%;71.23%的社区居民没有听过任何讲座。高血压防病知识的总知晓率为67.69%,高血压的诊断标准知晓率为48.23%，高血压的危险因素知晓率为56.52%。认为通过减少盐摄入量可以预防高血压的人占比36.34%，在口味偏咸者中愿意减少盐摄入量的仅为16.75%，吸烟者愿意戒烟的仅为18.2%。

表34-5 阳光某社区居民慢性病主要危险因素流行情况

危险因素	人数	流行/%
不经常参加体育锻炼	872	
超重、肥胖	719	
常吃腌制品	653	
水果蔬菜摄入少于半斤/天	592	
吸烟	539	
口味偏咸	267	
饮酒	392	

调查人群中家庭平时使用盐勺控制盐摄入量的仅占12.03%。吸烟者中愿意戒烟者且知道戒烟过程控制戒断症状方法的仅为15.65%。社区中没有提供免费测量血压的场所，居民只能在社区卫生服务中心挂号看病时测量血压。被调查的家庭中有电子测血压仪的比例为13.37%。当被问及是否支持家中高血压病人（如果有的话）使用低盐饮食，表示支持的家庭比例为21.78%。鼓励家中高血压病人（如果有的话）按医嘱服药的比例为66.32%。

调查发现，该社区卫生服务中心固定资产总值为260.73万元，其中10000元以上专业设备有25台，总值92.36万元。社区卫生服务中心人员共85人，其中男性32人，女性53人；在册卫生技术人员70人，包括执业医师25人、执业助理医师4人、注册护士16人、药剂人员13人、检验人员2人、其他8人；在册其他技术人员4人。按专业技术职称分：未定级13人，初级26人，中级27人，副高4人。

该社区卫生服务中心一年门急诊量合计97327人次，全科41457人次，医保13729人次，家庭病床191人次，家庭诊疗62人次。门诊主要就诊病种前几位分别是：感冒、气管炎、高血压病、关节炎等。家庭病床病种排在前几位的分别是：脑中风后遗症、高血压病、腰椎骨折等。

该社区共设立4个宣传栏，每两月定期更换一次。印发健康教育处方20余种，共32700份。定期在社区内开展健康教育，共举办讲座7次，重点场所健康教育指导32次。举办各种卫生宣传日社会宣传活动6次。

三、实习任务

根据以上案例，结合社区诊断方法，请完成以下实习内容：
（1）如何确定目前该社区的主要卫生问题？
（2）社区诊断开始时需要从哪些方面进行准备？

(3) 进行社区诊断时需要收集哪些资料？这些资料如何获取？

(4) 请完成表 34-1 至表 34-5 中空格部分的计算。

(5) 根据本案例资料，你认为该社区的主要卫生问题有哪些？应优先解决的健康问题是什么？

(6) 影响本社区主要健康问题的危险因素有哪些？哪些是可以干预的？哪些是不可以干预的？

四、练习

(1) 倾向因素、促成因素和强化因素的定义是什么？

(2) 健康教育社区诊断的思路是什么？

(3) 社区健康教育诊断的操作步骤有哪些？

Answers for Exercises

Chapter One

Experiment 1
(1) A   (2) C   (3) A   (4) B   (5) C
Experiment 2
(1) B   (2) D   (3) B   (4) C   (5) C
Experiment 3
(1) C   (2) D   (3) B   (4) A   (5) D
Experiment 4
(1) A   (2) C   (3) C   (4) B   (5) B
Experiment 5
(1) A   (2) D   (3) C   (4) B   (5) C
Experiment 6
(1) A   (2) A   (3) D   (4) B   (5) A

Chapter Two

Experiment 7
(1) D   (2) C   (3) B   (4) C   (5) D
Experiment 8
(1) B   (2) D   (3) A   (4) C   (5) A
Experiment 9
(1) D   (2) C   (3) D   (4) C   (5) C
Experiment 10
(1) C   (2) D   (3) D   (4) A   (5) D
Experiment 11
(1) D   (2) C   (3) C   (4) B   (5) C
Experiment 12
(1) A   (2) C   (3) B   (4) D   (5) C
Experiment 13
(1) C   (2) A   (3) A   (4) A   (5) A

Chapter six

Experiment 33

(1) ① Analysis of needs and identification of communication topics. ②Plan for production of health communication materials. ③ Completion of the first draft of health communication materials. ④ Preliminary experiment of health communication materials. ⑤ Design and manufacture of health communication materials. ⑥ Production, distribution and usage. ⑦ Monitoring and evaluation.

(2) Health communication materials can generally be divided into three types: Type Ⅰ, text printing materials, including leaflets, folding pages, brochures, posters, picture albums, magazines, books, etc. Type Ⅱ, Audio-visual materials, including television, radio, movies, electronic slides, video, audio, mobile phone SMS, Internet, etc. Type Ⅲ, physical materials.

(3) ① interaction; ②timeliness; ③clustering; ④ non-synchronicity; ⑤ The economical and efficient character.

(4) The standardized management of information is weak and false information is rampant; Information homogenization and dilution; Uneven distribution of information resources; The professional quality of communicators is uneven; Privacy breach.

Experiment 34

(1) ① Predisposing factor, which is also called antecedent factor, refers to the existing influencing factors before an individual engages in a certain behavior, namely the reason for the occurrence of a certain behavior, including the individual's knowledge, attitude, belief and values, as well as demographic characteristics such as age, gender, race, family income and occupation. ②Enabling factor refers to the factors contributing to behavioral change, that is, the factors enabling an individual to carry out a certain behavior. Enabling factor can influence behavior directly or indirectly through the environment, including the resources and skills needed to achieve a certain behavior. ③Reinforcing factor refers to the factors that affect the persistence or repetition of behaviors, such as the reward after the formation of good behaviors, family support, and behavior demonstration by important figures.

(2) ① Sociological assessment; ② Epidemiological assessment; ③ Behavior and environment assessment; ④ Educational and ecological assessment; ⑤ Administrative and policy assessment.

(3) ① Preparation for community assessment; ②Information collection; ③Information sorting, statistical description, and analysis of data; ④ Determination of the major health issues in the community; ⑤ Selection of target behavior for intervention.

习题参考答案

第一章

实验一
(1) A (2) C (3) A (4) B (5) C

实验二
(1) B (2) D (3) B (4) C (5) C

实验三
(1) C (2) D (3) B (4) A (5) D

实验四
(1) A (2) C (3) C (4) B (5) B

实验五
(1) A (2) D (3) C (4) B (5) C

实验六
(1) A (2) A (3) D (4) B (5) A

第二章

实验七
(1) D (2) C (3) B (4) C (5) D

实验八
(1) B (2) D (3) A (4) C (5) A

实验九
(1) D (2) C (3) D (4) C (5) C

实验十
(1) C (2) D (3) D (4) A (5) D

实验十一
(1) D (2) C (3) C (4) B (5) C

实验十二
(1) A (2) C (3) B (4) D (5) C

实验十三
(1) C (2) A (3) A (4) A (5) A

第六章

实验三十三

（1）①分析需求和确定传播主题；②制订计划；③形成初稿；④预实验；⑤设计制作；⑥生产、发放与使用；⑦监测与评价。

（2）健康传播材料一般可分为三类：第一类是文字印刷材料，包括宣传单、折页、小册子、宣传画、海报、画册、杂志、书籍等。第二类是音像视听材料，包括电视、广播、电影、电子幻灯片、视频、音频、手机短信、网络等。第三类是各种实物材料。

（3）优势：互动性、时效性、非同步性、分群性、经济性和高效性。

（4）信息的规范化管理薄弱，虚假信息泛滥；信息同质化、飞沫化；信息资源分配不均；传播者专业素质参差不齐；隐私泄露等。

实验三十四

（1）①倾向因素又称为前置因素，是指个人从事某项行为之前，已经存在的影响因素，即某种行为发生的理由，包括个人的知识、态度、信念、价值观念，以及年龄、性别、种族、家庭收入、职业等人口学特征。②促成因素，是指有助于实现行为改变的因素，即促使个人某种行为得以实现的因素。促成因素可以直接影响行为，或间接地通过环境影响行为，包括实现某种行为所需要的资源及技能。③强化因素是指影响行为持续或重复的因素，如良好行为形成后的奖励、家庭支持、重要人物的行为示范等。

（2）①社会学诊断；②流行病学诊断；③行为与环境诊断；④教育与生态学诊断；⑤管理与政策诊断。

（3）①社区诊断的前期准备工作；②资料收集；③资料整理、数据统计描述与分析；④确定社区的主要健康问题；⑤选择靶标行为。

参考文献

[1] 陈冰冰,李慧泉,潘欣婷,等.鸡蛋摄入与非酒精性脂肪肝病患病风险的病例对照研究[J].中华疾病控制杂志,2020,24(7):767-772.

[2] 陈兴才,孔存青,玉洪荣,等.广西少数民族中老年人骨质疏松性少肌性肥胖的现况调查[J].现代预防医学,2020,47(12):2117-2120.

[3] 陈禹存,杨世宏,安庆玉,等.2020年7—8月辽宁省大连市新型冠状病毒肺炎暴发疫情流行病学调查分析[J].疾病监测,2021,36(2):127-130.

[4] 傅华.健康教育学[M].3版.北京:人民卫生出版社,2017.

[5] 龚瑞,李涛,孙伟,等.宁夏新冠肺炎流行病学特征分析[J].现代预防医学,2020,47(20):3688-3691.

[6] 李海龙,夏彬彬,李倩,等.云南省边境地区人群弓形虫感染血清流行病学调查[J].中国血吸虫病防治杂志,2019,31(2):216-217,221.

[7] 李晓阳,周德华.健康教育与健康促进[M].北京:北京大学医学出版社,2011.

[8] 李载红,洪燕,覃伶伶,等.海口地区正常单胎胎儿妊娠早期NT厚度参考值的建立[J].东南大学学报(医学版),2016,35(2):202-204.

[9] 马骁.健康教育学[M].2版.北京:人民卫生出版社,2012.

[10] 史静琤,莫显昆,孙振球.量表编制中内容效度指数的应用[J].中南大学学报(医学版),2012,37(2):49-52.

[11] 孙可欣,郑荣寿,张思维,等.2015年中国分地区恶性肿瘤发病和死亡分析[J].中国肿瘤,2019,28(1):1-11.

[12] 王静雷,马吉祥,杨一兵,等.全民健康生活方式行动工作现况分析[J].中国慢性病预防与控制,2019,27(10):724-727,731.

[13] 吴蕊,常明泉,陈芳,等.妇安消疹洗液治疗手部汗疱疹的临床研究[J].中医药导报,2019,25(13):69-70,73.

[14] 杨克敌.环境卫生学[M].8版.北京:人民卫生出版社,2017.

[15] 杨土保,胡国清.医学科学研究与设计[M].3版.北京:人民卫生出版社,2020.

[16] 于帅,黄用文,吴月青,等.海南地区悬浮红细胞实际容量调查[J].海南医学,2014,25(15):2247-2249.

[17] HE M, XIANG F, ZENG Y, et al. Effect of time spent outdoors at school on the development of myopia among children in China[J]. JAMA, 2015, 314(11):1142.

[18] RATTRAY J, JONES M C. Essential elements of questionnaire design and development [J]. Journal of clinical nursing, 2010, 16 (2): 234-243.

[19] SIDHU J K, SINGH S, KATHURIA P. How to design and validate a questionnaire [J]. A guide. Current clinical pharmacology, 2018, (13): 210-215.